Biomedical Application
of Nanoparticles

OXIDATIVE STRESS AND DISEASE

Series Editors

LESTER PACKER, PhD
ENRIQUE CADENAS, MD, PhD

UNIVERSITY OF SOUTHERN CALIFORNIA SCHOOL OF PHARMACY
LOS ANGELES, CALIFORNIA

Biomedical Application of Nanoparticles

Edited by
Bertrand Henri Rihn
Université de Lorraine

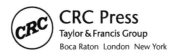

CRC Press
Taylor & Francis Group
Boca Raton London New York

CRC Press is an imprint of the
Taylor & Francis Group, an **informa** business

CRC Press
Taylor & Francis Group
6000 Broken Sound Parkway NW, Suite 300
Boca Raton, FL 33487-2742

First issued in paperback 2020

ISBN-13: 978-1-4987-5001-1 (hbk)
ISBN-13: 978-0-367-73581-4 (pbk)

Library of Congress Cataloging-in-Publication Data

Library of Congress Cataloging-in-Publication Data
Names: Rihn, Bertrand, 1955- editor.
Title: Biomedical application of nanoparticles / editor, Bertrand Rihn.
Description: Boca Raton : Taylor & Francis, 2017. | Includes bibliographical references.
Identifiers: LCCN 2017010537 | ISBN 9781498750011 (hardback : alk. paper)
Subjects: | MESH: Nanoparticles | Nanotechnology--methods | Biocompatible Materials | Biomedical Technology--methods
Classification: LCC R857.M3 | NLM QT 36.5 | DDC 610.28--dc23
LC record available at https://lccn.loc.gov/2017010537

Visit the Taylor & Francis Web site at
http://www.taylorandfrancis.com

and the CRC Press Web site at
http://www.crcpress.com

Contents

SECTION I   Nanoparticle Characterization

SECTION II   Interaction with Biological Systems

SECTION III Safety Assessment for Human Use

SECTION IV Medical Use

Foreword

Nanotechnology is a field of research and development that focuses on structures, devices, and processes based on the atomic, molecular, or supramolecular modeling of matter at scales typically of the order of one to one hundred nanometers (1–100 nm).

The constituents—sometimes referred to as elementary bricks—are nanomaterials that are produced only in small quantities. Nanomaterials include nanoparticles, nanostructured coatings, dense bulk materials, and nanocomposites (with an organic, inorganic, or metal matrix). These materials are expected to show novel types of behavior due to the relative importance of quantum phenomena at this scale. Many potential industrial and medical applications are emerging, and some nanomaterials are already in use. The European Commission estimated that the nanotechnology world market amounted to slightly over €40 billion in 2001. By 2008, the global market for nanotechnology products is expected to top €700 billion. Between 2010 and 2015, the economic stakes via the advent of nanotechnology worldwide are set to rise to €1,000 billion per year across all sectors (according to the National Science Foundation) of which nanomaterials specifically account for almost €340 billion (Hitachi Research Institute). BCC Research (https://www.bccresearch.com /market-research/nanotechnology/nanocomposites-global-markets-nan021e.html) estimated that in 2016, the nanocomposite market reached 333,043 metric tons and $2.4 billion with an annual growth rate around 20% in both unit and value terms. Over the same period, the nanotechnology industry is estimated to employ two to three million people worldwide.

On the basis of such figures, many see the advent of nanosciences—nanotechnologies and nanomaterials—as a major turning point in twentieth and twenty-first century industrial development. However, as in other industries, questions must be asked about the introduction of these new products; notably, how to measure their impact on health, the environment, and society. This is essential to guarantee the responsible, safe, and controlled development of nanoscience applications.

The world nanoparticle market for biomedical, pharmaceutical, and cosmetic applications was estimated at €85 million in 2000 (*Rapport de la Direction Générale de l'Industrie, des Technologies de l'Information et des Postes*, 2004) and reached €126 million in 2005 (i.e., an average yearly growth rate of 8.3%). This market concerns inorganic particles used in the production of antimicrobial agents, biological markets for research and diagnosis, biomagnetic separation, drug carriers, MRI contrast medium, and in orthopedic devices and sunscreens. As reported by the European Technology Platform (ETP) on Nanomedicine, nanomedicine has the potential to enable early detection and prevention and to drastically improve diagnosis, treatment, and follow-up of many diseases, including cancer. Overall, the ETP on Nanomedicine has identified more than 70 products under clinical trial that cover all major diseases, including cardiovascular, neurodegenerative, musculoskeletal, and inflammatory, as well as enable technologies in all healthcare areas. Nanomedicine has been reported to account for 77 marketed products, ranging from nanodelivery (44) and pharmaceutical (18) to imaging, diagnostics, and biomaterial (15).

Taking into account such developments of nanomaterials, nanoparticles, and nanodevices in the fields of medical application, and including nanomedicine as an offshoot of nanotechnology, *Biomedical Applications of Nanoparticles* was written to report on the exploration of nanoparticles. It includes reporting on their chemical and physical properties, with a focus on description of the various types of nanoparticles, how they can be synthesized, and their interaction in biological systems with proteins, immune system, and targeted cells. Risk assessment of nanoparticles for humans is also described, including cellular paradigms, transcriptomics, and toxicogenomics, and provides guidance on safe use of nanoparticles. Finally, the application of nanoparticles in medicine and antioxidant regenerative therapeutics are presented in several chapters, with emphasis on how nanoparticles enhance transport of drugs across biological membrane barriers and therefore may enhance drug bioavailability.

The book explores the following aspects in respect to the elements previously discussed:

- In Section I, titled Nanoparticle Characterization, the following points will be discussed. Nanoparticle world: a history and introduction to the diversity, dispersion, and characterization of nanoparticles. Manufacturing nanoparticles: A pharmacist's approach, green synthesis, and characterization of semiconductor and metal nanoparticles.
- In Section II, titled Interaction with Biologicial Systems, nanoparticle interaction with proteins and the corona formation will be described as well as the question of the nanoparticle and virus as mitophagy inducers in immune cells.
- In Section III, titled Safety Assessment for Human Use, attention will be paid to rodent inhalation in nanoparticle risk assessments, *in vivo* hepatoxicity nephrotoxicity of polymeric nanoparticles, and *in vitro* exposure systems of nanoparticles.
- In Section IV, medical use is detailed in relation to some particular behaviors of nanoparticules, that is, the transbarrier trafficking of nanoparticles in perspectives for cancer therapeutics, the involvement of nanoparticles as a vehicle of antioxidants in diseases, the application of nanoparticles in photodynamic therapy, and the use of nanoparticles as nitroso-glutathion vehicles.

As emphasized by the ETP and described in the various sections of this book, nanomedicine is a key enabling instrument for personalized, targeted, and regenerative medicine by delivering the next level of drugs, treatments, and implantable devices to clinicians and patients for real breakthroughs in healthcare. Beyond that, nanomedicine provides important new tools to deal with the grand challenge of an aging population and is thought to be instrumental for improved and cost-effective healthcare—a crucial factor for making medicine and treatment available and affordable to all.

Dr. Eric Gaffet
Institut Jean Lamour
UMR 7198 Centre National de Recherche Scientifique—Université de Lorraine

Series Preface: Oxidative Stress in Health and Disease

Oxidative stress is an underlying factor in health and disease. In this series of books, the importance of oxidative stress and disease associated with cell and organ systems of the body is highlighted by exploring the scientific evidence and the clinical applications of this knowledge. This series is intended for researchers in the biomedical sciences, clinicians, and all persons with an interest in the health sciences. The potential of such knowledge for healthy development, healthy aging, and disease prevention warrants further knowledge about how oxidants and antioxidants modulate cell and tissue function.

Bertrand Rihn is to be congratulated for producing this very excellent and timely book, *Biomedical Application of Nanoparticles*, in the ever-growing field of importance of the application of nanoparticle technology as a vehicle to deliver nutrients and pharmaceuticals for human health.

Lester Packer
Enrique Cadenas
Oxidative Stress and Disease Series Editors

Editor

Bertrand Henri Rihn, MD, DSc, professor of biochemistry and molecular biology at Lorraine University, France, is a leading expert in the field of particulate toxicology, with research topics including safety toxicology, immunotoxicology, and investigating the transcriptomic changes in macrophages following nanoparticle exposure. In addition to his research, Professor Rihn has also worked as a clinical toxicologist, and was awarded the Baratz Award (2004) and the E. Taub Award (2011) from the National Academy of Medicine (France). He also served as the president of the French Society of Toxicology from 2007 to 2009, and was a EUROTOX Registered Toxicologist.

Contributors

Khaled G. Abdel-Wahhab
Medical Physiology Department
National Research Center
Cairo, Egypt

Mosaad A. Abdel-Wahhab
Food Toxicology and Contaminants
    Department
National Research Center
Cairo, Egypt

Jean-Claude André
CNRS
Nancy, France

Sneha Bhagyaraj
Centre for Nanomaterials Science
    Research
University of Johannesburg
Doornfontein, South Africa

Nadia Canilho
SRSMC UMR 7565
Université de Lorraine–Centre National
    de Recherche Scientifique
Vandœuvre-lès-Nancy, France

Flemming R. Cassee
National Institute for Public Health and
    the Environment
Bilthoven, the Netherlands

and

Institute for Risk Assessment Studies
Utrecht, the Netherlands

Alain Celzard
Institut Jean Lamour
UMR 7198–Centre National de
    Recherche Scientifique—Université
    de Lorraine
Épinal, France

Yahya E. Choonara
Wits Advanced Drug Delivery Platform
    Research Unit
Department of Pharmacy and
    Pharmacology
School of Therapeutic Sciences
Faculty of Health Sciences
University of the Witwatersrand
Johannesburg, South Africa

Frédéric Cosnier
Institut National de Recherche et de
    Sécurité
Département Toxicologie et
    Biométrologie
Vandœuvre-lès-Nancy, France

Roudayna Diab
SRSMC UMR 7565
Université de Lorraine–Centre National
    de Recherche Scientifique
Vandœuvre-lès-Nancy, France

Silvia Diabaté
Karlsruhe Institute of Technology
    (KIT)
Institute of Toxicology and Genetics
Eggenstein-Leopoldshafen, Germany

Marco Dilger
Karlsruhe Institute of Technology (KIT)
Institute of Toxicology and Genetics
Eggenstein-Leopoldshafen, Germany

Ghislain Djiokeng-Paka
Institut Armand Frappier
Institut National de la Recherche
    Scientifique
Laval, Quebec, Canada

Zahra Doumandji
CITHEFOR
Faculté de Pharmacie
Université de Lorraine
Nancy, France

Lisa C. du Toit
Wits Advanced Drug Delivery Platform
    Research Unit
Department of Pharmacy and
    Pharmacology
School of Therapeutic Sciences
Faculty of Health Sciences
University of the Witwatersrand
Johannesburg, South Africa

Housam Eidi
Department of Ophthalmology and
    Visual Sciences
University of British Columbia
Vancouver, British Columbia, Canada

Ahmed A. El-Kady
Food Toxicology and Contaminants
    Department
National Research Center
Cairo, Egypt

Aziza A. El-Nekeety
Food Toxicology and Contaminants
    Department
National Research Center
Cairo, Egypt

Olayemi J. Fakayode
Department of Applied Chemistry
University of Johannesburg
and
Centre for Nanomaterials Science
    Research
Doornfontein, South Africa

Luc Ferrari
CITHEFOR
Faculté de Pharmacie
Université de Lorraine
Nancy, France

Solenne Fleutot
Institut Jean Lamour
Université de Lorraine
Vandœuvre-lès-Nancy, France

Eric Gaffet
Institut Jean Lamour
UMR CNRS 7198
Université de Lorraine
Nancy, France

Laurent Gaté
Institut National de Recherche et de
    Sécurité (INRS)
Department Toxicologie et
    Biométrologie
Vandœuvre-lès-Nancy, France

Fernanda Bianca Haffner
SRSMC UMR 7565
Université de Lorraine–Centre National
    de Recherche Scientifique
Vandœuvre-lès-Nancy, France

Nabila S. Hassan
Pathology Department
National Research Center
Cairo, Egypt

Olivier Joubert
Institut Jean Lamour
UMR CNRS 7198
Université de Lorraine
and
CITHEFOR
Faculté de Pharmacie
Université de Lorraine
Nancy, France

Sanghoon Kim
SRSMC UMR 7565
Université de Lorraine–Centre National
    de Recherche Scientifique
Vandœuvre-lès-Nancy, France

Tobias Krebs
VITROCELL Systems, GmbH
Waldkirch, Germany

Pradeep Kumar
Wits Advanced Drug Delivery Platform
    Research Unit
Department of Pharmacy and
    Pharmacology
School of Therapeutic Sciences,
Faculty of Health Sciences
University of the Witwatersrand
Johannesburg, South Africa

Emmanuel Lamouroux
SRSMC UMR 7565
Université de Lorraine–Centre National
    de Recherche Scientifique
Vandœuvre-lès-Nancy, France

Sijin Li
SRSMC UMR 7565
Université de Lorraine–Centre National
    de Recherche Scientifique
Vandœuvre-lès-Nancy, France

Fathia A. Mannaa
Medical Physiology Department
National Research Center
Cairo, Egypt

Thashree Marimuthu
Wits Advanced Drug Delivery Platform
    Research Unit
Department of Pharmacy and
    Pharmacology
School of Therapeutic Sciences
Faculty of Health Sciences
University of the Witwatersrand
Johannesburg, South Africa

Sonja Mülhopt
Karlsruhe Institute of Technology (KIT)
Institute for Technical Chemistry
Eggenstein-Leopoldshafen, Germany

Christophe Nemos
Neurotoxicologie Alimentaire et
    Bioactivité
Université de Lorraine
Metz, France

Van Son Nguyen
Institut Jean Lamour
Université de Lorraine
Vandœuvre-lès-Nancy, France

Oluwatobi Samuel Oluwafemi
Department of Applied Chemistry
University of Johannesburg
and
Centre for Nanomaterials Science
    Research
Doorfontein, South Africa

Andreea Pasc
SRSMC UMR 7565
Université de Lorraine–Centre National
    de Recherche Scientifique
Vandœuvre-lès-Nancy, France

Hanns-Rudolf Paur
Karlsruhe Institute of Technology (KIT)
Institute for Technical Chemistry
Eggenstein-Leopoldshafen, Germany

Ileana-Alexandra Pavel
SRSMC UMR 7565
Université de Lorraine–Centre National
    de Recherche Scientifique
Vandœuvre-lès-Nancy, France

Viness Pillay
Wits Advanced Drug Delivery Platform
    Research Unit
Department of Pharmacy and
    Pharmacology
School of Therapeutic Sciences
Faculty of Health Sciences
University of the Witwatersrand
Johannesburg, South Africa

Priyamvada Pradeep
Wits Advanced Drug Delivery Platform
    Research Unit
Department of Pharmacy and
    Pharmacology
School of Therapeutic Sciences
Faculty of Health Sciences
University of the Witwatersrand
Johannesburg, South Africa

Chloe Puisney
CITHEFOR Faculté de Pharmacie
Université de Lorraine
Nancy, France

Jean-Michel Rabanel
Institut Armand Frappier
Institut National de la Recherche
    Scientifique
Laval, Quebec, Canada

Charles Ramassamy
INRS-Institut Armand-Frappier
Laval, Quebec, Canada

Bertrand Henri Rihn
Institut Jean Lamour
UMR CNRS 7198
Université de Lorraine
and
CITHEFOR
Faculté de Pharmacie
Université de Lorraine
Nancy, France

Phèdre Rihn
University of California, Berkeley
Department of Integrative Biology
Berkeley, California

Carole Ronzani
CITHEFOR
Faculté de Pharmacie
Université de Lorraine
Nancy, France

Didier Rouxel
Institut Jean Lamour
Université de Lorraine
Vandœuvre-lès-Nancy, France

Ramia Safar
CITHEFOR
Faculté de Pharmacie
Université de Lorraine
Nancy, France

Annette B. Santamaria
Toxicology and Food Safety Practice
Rimkus Consulting Group
Houston, Texas

Jonathan Simon
Archives Poincaré
UMR 7117
Université de Lorraine
Nancy, France

Christoph Schlager
Karlsruhe Institute of Technology (KIT)
Institute for Technical Chemistry
Eggenstein-Leopoldshafen, Germany

Sandile P. Songca
Department of Chemistry
University of Zululand
Kwadlangezwa, South Africa

Lucija Tomljenovic
Department of Ophthalmology and
    Visual Sciences
University of British Columbia
Vancouver, British Columbia, Canada

Ncediwe Tsolekile
Department of Applied Chemistry
University of Johannesburg
and
Centre for Nanomaterials Science
    Research
University of Johannesburg
Doorfontein, South Africa

Mihayl Varbanov
SRSMC UMR 7565
Université de Lorraine–Centre National
    de Recherche Scientifique
Vandœuvre-lès-Nancy, France

Section I

Nanoparticle Characterization

1 Nanoparticle World
History and Introduction to Their Diversity in Medicine

Annette B. Santamaria

CONTENTS

1.1 INTRODUCTION

Nanotechnology is a means to develop and use chemical substances, materials, devices, structures, and systems that have novel properties and functions due to their small size. Nanoparticles have at least one dimension on the nanoscale (1–100 nanometers, nm) and exhibit novel properties compared to the non-nanoscale form of a material of the same composition. The dimension of 1–100 nm may be considered an intermediate state between atomic or molecular/bulk state, where materials exhibit some unexpected and unusual new properties that cannot be defined by classical laws of physics. Unique physical properties (e.g., magnetic, optical, mechanical, and electrical) and quantum mechanics (e.g., electron configuration and confinement) can vary continuously or abruptly with changes in the size of some materials produced at the nanoscale. Nanomaterials are used because they have desirable properties, including enhanced pharmacokinetic and targeting properties, optical properties, catalytic properties, porosity properties, electromagnetic properties, mechanical properties, and material and structural surface properties (e.g., stiffness; elasticity; strength; weight reduction; increased stability; or improved functionality, such as "easy to clean," "antifog," "anti-fingerprint," or "scratch resistance"). The unique physicochemical properties of nanomaterials are being exploited for use in several fields of research, including science and medicine.

There was a significant increase in the popularity of nanotechnology and the development of diverse nanomaterials in the 1990s and the 2000s, with the incorporation of nanomaterials into a wide variety of consumer products. Nanoparticles are not new, as they have been around in the atmosphere since the dawn of the universe. In the field of medicine, historical evidence suggests that gold nanoparticles were used as drug products by the Chinese as early as 2500 BC, and that red colloidal gold is still in use under the name of Swarna Bhasma and Makaradhwaja in Ayurveda, the traditional medicine system of India, which dates back to the first millennium BC (Bhattacharya and Mukherjee 2008). More recently, scientists have been studying nanoscience phenomena for many decades in several fields of science and medicine. For example, Watson and Crick's discovery of the structure of DNA in 1953 can be considered nanoscience, just as can the identification of and research on carbon fullerenes in the 1980s. The first observations and size measurements of nanoparticles was made early in the twentieth century by Richard Adolf Zsigmondy, who used the term *nanometer* to characterize a particle size of 1/1,000,000 of a millimeter. He developed the first system of classification based on particle size in the nanometer range (Zsigmondy 1914). In 1912, Zsigmondy applied for a patent for the immersion ultramicroscope, which permitted investigation of the behavior of colloidal solutions. The first time the idea of nanotechnology was introduced was in 1959, when Richard Feynman, a physicist and Nobel prizewinner from Caltech, gave a talk entitled "There's Plenty of Room at the Bottom" (Feynman 1960). Feynman's talk has been viewed as the first academic talk that dealt with a main tenet of nanotechnology, the direct manipulation of individual atoms or molecular manufacturing. Although he did not use the term *nanotechnology*, he suggested that it would be eventually possible to manipulate atoms and molecules to create "nanoscale" machines, through a cascade of billions of factories (Fanfair et al. 2007). Feynman proposed that these tiny "machine shops" would then eventually be able to create billions of tinier factories, and that as the scale got smaller and smaller, gravity would become more negligible, while both van der Waals attraction and surface tension would become more significant. Following Feynman's talk, two directions of thought arose describing the various possibilities for producing nanostructures, including the "top-down approach," corresponding to Feynman's comments on stepwise reduction in the size of already existing machines and instruments; and the "bottom-up approach," involving the construction of nanostructures atom for atom by physical and chemical methods and by using controlled manipulation of the self-organizing forces of atoms and molecules.

The term *nanotechnology* was first used in a publication in 1974 by a student named Norio Taniguchi from the Tokyo Science University who stated, "Nanotechnology mainly consists of the processing of, separation, consolidation, and deformation of materials by one atom or one molecule" (Taniguchi 1974). In 1979, Eric Drexler, a scientist at the Massachusetts Institute of Technology, expanded upon Feynman's vision of molecular manufacturing with contemporary developments in understanding protein function. Many believe that this is when the field of nanotechnology was created, and, in 1981, Drexler published his first article on the subject, entitled "Molecular Engineering: An Approach to the Development of General Capabilities for Molecular Manipulation" in the journal *Proceedings of the National Academy of Sciences* (Drexler 1981). In this article, Drexler discussed the possibility of molecular manufacturing as a process of fabricating objects with specific atomic specifications using designed protein molecules. Drexler took these concepts and expanded their potential in a book titled *Engines of Creation: The Coming Era of Nanotechnology* (Drexler 1986). While nanotechnology came into existence through Feynman's and then Drexler's visions of molecular manufacturing, the field has evolved to include research in chemistry, materials science, medicine, toxicology, ecotoxicology, and industrial hygiene. The goal for nanotechnology research is not to create billions of assemblers that will revolutionize our world, but rather to explore both the manufacturing and nonmanufacturing aspects of nanotechnology through a combination of chemistry, materials science, molecular biology, and molecular engineering.

As with any new technology, identification of potential health risks is a prerequisite for a proper assessment of the usefulness and safety of the new chemicals, materials, and products that may be developed. Although impressive from a physicochemical viewpoint, the novel properties of nanomaterials raise concerns about potential adverse effects on biological systems. Beginning in the early 2000s, concerns about the potential human and environmental health effects of nanomaterials were being expressed by many scientists, regulators, and nongovernmental agencies because particles and materials in the nanosize range may pose toxicological hazards due to their enhanced reactivity (e.g., chemical, electrical, magnetic) and potential for systemic availability and environmental occurrence (Santamaria 2012). Because of the physicochemical properties of nanomaterials, they may modify cellular uptake, protein binding, translocation from portal of entry to the target site, and may even have the potential to cause tissue injury. There has also been an increasing amount of research to evaluate the toxicokinetics and toxicodynamics of nanomaterials. The inhalation and dermal routes of exposure have been the primary focus for health effects research of nanomaterials; however, research on the ingestion of nanomaterials from food, or the intravenous exposure from the use of nanomaterials in medical devices, diagnostics, and therapeutics also increased significantly during the 2000s (Santamaria 2012). During this time, multidisciplinary research programs were initiated in the United States by the National Center for Environmental Research of the U.S. Environmental Protection Agency (USEPA), National Toxicology Program (NTP), National Institute of Environmental Health (NIEH), and National Institutes of Health (NIH) to address the impact of nanoparticles on human health and the environment. There were also multidisciplinary nanotechnology research programs implemented by groups in Europe, such as the European Commission (EC), the World Health Organization (WHO), U.K. Royal Society and Royal Academy of Engineering, Germany's Federal Institute for Risk Assessment (BfR), and the Organization for Economic Co-operation and Development (OECD). During the early 2000s, several groups recommended frameworks or screening strategies for developing nanomaterials that may be used safely, including the International Life Sciences Institute (ILSI), the European Centre for Ecotoxicology and Toxicology of Chemicals (ECETOC), and the collaborative partnership between DuPont Corporation and the non-governmental organization Environmental Defense. The intent of these frameworks or screening strategies was to define a systematic process for identifying, managing, and reducing potential environmental, health, and safety risks of engineered nanomaterials from production through manufacture, use, disposal, and ultimate fate. The screening strategies are targeted toward companies and public and private research institutions that are actively working with nanomaterials and developing associated products and applications.

Interest in engineered nanoparticles and their potential uses in medicine has increased significantly over the past several decades. Developments in the field of nanotechnology and nanomedicine have been driven by the development of instrumentation and the availability of tools that allow scientists to see things that they were not able to see in the past. In 1931, the transmission electron microscope (TEM) was developed by Max Knoll and Ernst Ruska. It allowed for significantly better resolution than the light microscope. Insight into the atomic range, however, first became possible with the field electron microscope developed by Erwin Müller in 1936 and its further development to the field ion microscope (FIM) in 1951, which allowed physicists to see individual atoms and their arrangement on a surface. The scanning tunneling microscope (STM) was invented by Gerd Binnig and Heinrich Rohrer in 1981 and, with this technology, individual atoms could be clearly identified for the first time, a breakthrough essential to the development of the field of nanotechnology because what had previously been concepts now could be viewed and tested (Fanfair et al. 2007). Some of the limitations in STM were eliminated through the development of the Atomic Force Microscope (AFM) in 1986, a microscope that could image non-conducting materials such as organic molecules and could be used to study biological macromolecules and living organisms. AFM was integral to the study of carbon fullerenes (also known as buckyballs), which fall within the angstrom (Å) range (10 Å = 1 nm) and were first identified and produced in Richard Smalley's laboratory at Rice University in Texas in 1985 (Kroto et al. 1985). The fullerene was named after Richard Buckminster Fuller because of its resemblance to the late architect's geodesic domes. The structure is approximately 1 nm in diameter and consists of a 60 carbon atom cage that forms the shape of a soccer ball. Research with fullerenes marked the beginning of the current era of nanoscale science and technology and its unprecedented impacts across broad sectors of society (Santamaria 2012). The idea that one could actually in some sense "touch" atoms and molecules also came about in the 1980s, when scientists attempted to further study Drexler's proposed theory regarding the ability to manipulate atoms and molecules. Using the various methods of scanning probe microscopy, it became possible not only to demonstrate nanoscale structures precisely, but also to position and manipulate them in a controlled way (Krukemeyer et al. 2015).

In 2001, the National Nanotechnology Initiative (NNI) was approved in the United States. The program had the following goal:

> National Nanotechnology Initiative defines the strategy of interaction between federal departments of the USA for the purpose of prioritizing nanotechnology development, which should become a basis for the economy and national security of the USA in the first half of the 21st century.

Extensive governmental financial support greatly stimulated the launch of interdisciplinary research and the launch of the NNI supported and coordinated the design, study, and exploration of nanomaterials, which has had a significant impact on nanomedicine-related research and development and the incorporation of nano-materials into consumer products.

The major types of nanomaterials in consumer products include (1) nanometals (e.g., titanium dioxide, silver, iron oxide, nickel, cobalt, zinc, aluminum, silica, copper, gold, and molybdenum), (2) ceramic or polymer nanoparticles, (3) quantum dots, (4) nanoencapsules, (5) nanoclay particles, (6) nanofibers, (7) carbon nanotubes (CNTs), and (8) fullerenes (Sayes and Santamaria 2014). Nanomaterials such as nano-titanium dioxide, nano-zinc oxide, and nanosilver are used in personal care products such as sunscreen, toothpaste, facial creams, hair products, and makeup. Carbon nanotubes are being used to reinforce a variety of sporting goods, such as bicycle frames, tennis rackets, baseball bats, and hockey sticks, because they offer greater strength and reduced weight while increasing stiffness. Carbon nanotubes are also used in a variety of other products, including automobile and airplane parts; in several biomedical applications, diagnostics, drug delivery systems; and in electrical and computer components. The continued miniaturization of electrical components using nanotechnology has facilitated enhancements to a number of consumer electronics, including cell phones, personal computers, and televisions. Nanomaterials may be incorporated into a variety of building materials to increase energy efficiency, reduce aging due to sunlight, make steel stronger, make concrete more durable and more easily placed, and for antimicrobial purposes. Functional textiles are being manufactured with nanomaterials that react to light to create power-generating clothing, and nanosilver is being used in clothing and in antimicrobial wound dressings. Nanomaterials are also being used in coatings to make fabric and clothing stain- and water-resistant and to provide nano-enabled surfaces that can remove scratches, stains, and scuff marks. Nanomaterials can be embedded on the surface of fabric fibers, creating a cushion of air around them. The fabric then allows perspiration to pass out while also causing surface water to bead up and roll off. Silver nanoparticles have been incorporated into washing machines, clothing, personal care products, and food contact products (e.g., utensils, cutting boards) as antimicrobial agents. Many of the world's largest food and food packaging companies are reported to be actively exploring the potential of nanotechnology for use in food, dietary supplements, or food packaging. There are four major types of applications of nanotechnology in the food industry: (1) agriculture, (2) food processing, (3) food packaging, and (4) dietary supplements (Santamaria 2012). Applications include the development of improved tastes, color, flavor, texture, and consistency of foodstuffs; increased absorption and bioavailability of nutrients and health supplements; new food packaging materials with improved mechanical, barrier, and antimicrobial properties; and nanosensors for traceability and monitoring the condition of food during transport and storage. Nanomaterials are being developed to more efficiently and safely administer pesticides, herbicides, and fertilizers by controlling more precisely when and where they are released. Extensive research efforts are also underway to produce nanoscale drug delivery systems, diagnostics, and therapeutics (Sandhiya et al. 2009). There are many benefits to formulating a pharmaceutical to be placed within a nanoparticulate, including increased bioavailability, faster onset of action, dose uniformity, reduction in fasted and fed variability, decreased toxicity, smaller dosage form, and stable dosage forms of drugs that could not previously be formulated conventionally.

The research, development, and production of nanomaterials are greatly outpacing the speed by which toxicological information is being acquired on engineered nanomaterials. An understanding of the mammalian and ecotoxicological profiles of nanomaterials will be necessary to ensure that nanomaterials are safe for use and to establish appropriate safety procedures for handling nanomaterials that may pose potential health hazards if there is sufficient exposure in the workplace, environment, or to consumers. For newly developed nanomaterials, it may be necessary to conduct a broad range of *in vitro* and *in vivo* studies to evaluate potential toxicological effects following oral, dermal, or inhalation exposure. The lessons we have learned from the chemical and biotechnology industries pave the way for the successful and safe incorporation of materials developed from technologies such as nanotechnology into products that can improve the quality of life. It is important that nanomaterials are developed responsibly with optimization of benefits, minimization of risks, and international cooperation to identify and resolve gaps in knowledge.

1.2   NANOMEDICINE

Nanobiotechnology and nanomedicine are concerned with molecular intra- and intercellular processes and are concentrated on research into the possibilities of controlling and manipulating cell processes, for example, by targeted transport of active substances (Krukemeyer et al. 2015).

Examples of applications of nanotechnology in biomedical sciences include drug delivery, nutraceuticals, production of biocompatible materials such as bone or tissue substitutes, implants, biosensors, tissue engineering, various diagnostic materials, and cosmetics (e.g., anti-aging formulations). Multifunctional nanoparticles for medical applications have been devised with (1) stealth-like features to evade the immune system and prevent opsonization; (2) protective layers to prevent the degradation of biologic cargo (e.g., proteins, DNA); (3) targeting moieties to improve specificity and tumor accumulation; (4) membrane-permeation moieties to improve cell uptake; (5) imaging agents to assess delivery and dosing; (6) endosome escape mechanisms, target-dependent assembly or disassembly to control drug release; (7) microenvironment sensors (pH, proteases, phospholipases) to trigger drug release and cell uptake; and (8) intracellular targeting moieties to direct drugs to specific intracellular compartments (Krukemeyer et al. 2015). There are several types of nanomedical applications of nanoparticles, including imaging and diagnostics, genetic screening, tests for viral or bacterial infection and the first signs of diseases before symptoms are manifested, the development of medicines and vaccines, drug delivery, treatments for diseases such as diabetes, cancer, heart disease, neurological diseases such as Alzheimer's and Parkinson's, organ implants, and targeted therapies. Nanoparticles and nanodevices under investigation for diagnostic or medicinal purposes are quantum dots, nanoshells, nanospheres, gold nanoparticles, paramagnetic nanoparticles, and carbon nanotubes. For pharmaceutical purposes, nanoparticles have been defined as solid colloidal particles ranging in size from 10 nm to 400 nm and consisting of macromolecular materials in which the active agent (drug or biologically active material) is dissolved, entrapped, or encapsulated, or to which the active agent is adsorbed or attached (Muthu and Singh 2009).

The use of nanotechnology for cancer and other disease diagnostics and therapeutics has been a rapidly advancing and evolving field (Samadian et al. 2016; Tatar et al. 2016; Pérez-Herrero and Fernández-Medarde 2015). Different cytotoxic drug carriers, such as liposomes, carbon nanotubes, dendrimers, polymeric micelles, polymeric conjugates, and polymeric nanoparticles are being developed and used in passive and active targeted cancer therapy. With respect to neurological diseases, the physicochemical features of the engineered nanomaterials confer to them different features, including the ability to cross the blood–brain barrier. Data from animal models for Parkinson's disease have shown an improvement of pharmacological properties, more stable drug concentrations, and longer half-life and attenuation of pharmacological adverse effects (Hawthorne et al. 2016).

The four main areas of nanomedicine include (1) diagnostics/imaging, (2) drug delivery, (3) therapeutics, and (4) tissue engineering (Hawthorne et al. 2016). Nanoparticles are smaller than human cells but similar in size to biological macromolecules such as enzymes and receptors, and they can be used as probes by conjugating them to peptides, antibodies, and nucleic acids to detect cellular movements and molecular changes associated with pathological states (Rawat et al. 2006). Such probes provide high levels of sensitivity, stability, and absorption coefficients across a wide spectral range, which allow them to be used for imaging and diagnostic purposes (Cuenca et al. 2006). Nanoparticles coated with antibodies, collagen, and other molecules are being used for early detection and diagnosis of diseases like cancer. Biologic robots designed with genes to synthesize vitamins, hormones, and enzymes may be used to treat congenital or acquired diseases (Freitas 2005). Nanodevices can be customized to carry large doses of anticancer drugs or genes into malignant and diseased cells while sparing normal healthy cells, which will help in achieving maximum beneficial effects with fewer side effects. In addition, nanocarriers can be engineered in such a way to be activated by stimuli like chemicals, magnetic field, heat, and pH to selectively kill cancer cells. For example, in 2002, Ishiyama and colleagues developed tiny magnetically driven spinning screws intended to swim along veins and carry drugs to infected tissues or even to burrow into tumors and kill them with heat (Ishiyama et al. 2002). These are just a few examples of the various uses of nanoparticles in nanomedicine. This review presents a brief overview of the application of nanotechnology in various aspects of medicine, including how nanoparticles are being used for diagnostics/imaging, therapeutics, drug delivery, and tissue regeneration.

1.3 DIAGNOSTICS/IMAGING WITH NANOMATERIALS

The use of nanomaterials as contrast media in diagnostic *in vivo* procedures, such as magnetic resonance imaging (MRI), enables imaging with an improved three-dimensional view by means of which types of tissue can be differentiated more easily. By virtue of a high payload of magnetic moieties, enhanced accumulation at disease sites and a large surface area for additional modification with targeting ligands, nanoparticle-based contrast agents offer promising new platforms to further enhance the high resolution and sensitivity of MRI for various biomedical applications (Mao et al. 2016). MRI is used as a powerful diagnostic tool for acquiring three-dimensional tomographical images of tissues and whole organs at high spatial and temporal resolution. To overcome difficulties in differentiating normal from diseased cells due to small native relaxation time differences, MRI contrast agents that have gadolinium and iron, two elements possessing a high number of unpaired electrons, are used for the enhancement of imaging sensitivities (Bobo et al. 2016). A significant drawback of gadolinium chelates is their rapid renal clearance, limiting the time window for an MRI. Therefore, efforts have been undertaken to incorporate gadolinium into or onto nanoparticles such as dendrimers, dextran, polymers, liposomes, and a variety of inorganic nanoparticles (Zhu et al. 2013). Noble metal nanostructures attract much interest in the field of imaging because of their unique properties, including large optical field enhancements resulting in the strong scattering and absorption of light.

Various studies have been performed on the development of micelles, polymeric nanoparticles, and dendrimers as imaging agents (Chan et al. 2016). However, the larger size of these macromolecular structures prevents their rapid clearance from the body through the renal system. The size and surface properties of nanoparticles can be modified to optimize their pharmacokinetics for imaging a specific disease, and increased imaging specificity would significantly improve accuracy in diagnosis, allowing better disease management planning and an improved prognosis (Chan et al. 2016). Agents such as superparamagnetic iron oxide (SPIO), manganese oxide, gold nanoparticles/nanorods, and quantum dots (QDs) possess specific properties like paramagnetism, superparamagnetism, surface plasmon resonance, and photoluminescence properties, which make them useful for single/multi-modal and single/multi-functional molecular imaging (Padmanabhan et al. 2016). Nanoparticles generally have nanomolar or micromolar sensitivity range and can be detected via imaging instrumentation. The distinctive characteristics of certain nanoparticles make them suitable for imaging, therapy, and delivery of drugs. There are many potential advantages of nanomaterial-based MRI contrast agents over low-molecular-weight complexes:

1. The possible variety of chemical composition, shapes, and sizes allows for the design of different degrees of biocompatibility and imaging properties.
2. Different degrees of biostability can be achieved via specific surface modifications.
3. Active targeting of nanoparticles is possible via attaching ligands to the particle surface.
4. Multimodal imaging can be achieved using a combination of optical and magnetic properties of nanomaterials (Zhu et al. 2013).

By imaging methods optimized by nanotechnology, the presence, position, and size of tumors can be determined more accurately than with conventional methods (Jain 2012). Due to stability and brightness, nanomaterial photoprobes display luminosity that is 1,000 times greater than that of conventional contrast media. Nanosized contrast agents have greater magnetic susceptibility than traditional MRI contrast agents (Mitra et al. 2006). Superparamagnetic nanoparticles are used to characterize hepatic tumors since they are rapidly taken up by the liver following intravenous administration (Wang et al. 2011). Nanoparticles from iron oxide have gained the attention of researchers because of their extraordinary magnetic and optical properties and have been used as a contrast agent for MRI. The ability of iron nanoparticles to be used as MRI contrast agents, together with their potential for selective targeting, has resulted in a wide range of studies for potential applications in MRI-based imaging and diagnostics. The unique advantage of iron oxide nanoparticles over low-molecular-weight gadolinium chelates as MRI contrast agents lies in their avoidance of renal clearance and their swift uptake by the reticuloendothelial system (Bourrinet et al. 2006). Superparamagnetic iron oxide nanoparticle (5–10 nm) contrast agents are taken up by lymph nodes and bone marrow. It has been well established that iron oxide nanoparticles are rapidly taken up by phagocytic cells like Kupffer cells, circulating monocytes/macrophages, mononuclear T cells, reactive astrocytes, microglia, and dendritic cells (Weinstein et al. 2010). They are used clinically to characterize lymph node status in patients with carcinoma of the breast, lung, prostate, endometrium, and cervix (Sandhiya et al. 2009). Furthermore, micro metastases that are less than 2 micrometers (mm) in diameter in lymph nodes, well below the limit of detection by positron emission tomography (PET), can be identified using iron oxide contrast agents (Torchilin 2007; Harisinghani et al. 2003). Several antibodies and other ligands has been conjugated to iron nanoparticles and tested for MRI imaging of tumors (Laurent et al. 2008). In addition, simultaneous MRI imaging and destruction of breast cancer cells has been demonstrated using targeted delivery of iron nanoparticles, entrapped into PLGA (Poly-D, L-lactide-co-glycolide) nanoparticles containing the anticancer drug Doxurubicin and antibody Herceptin1 (Dinarvard et al. 2011). Gold or silver nanoparticles have also been used for imaging purposes and have the advantage of being less susceptible to photobleaching, with absorption and emission orders of magnitude greater than those of small fluorescent dyes, making them better suited for imaging (Chan et al. 2016). Because these nanoparticles can generate heat by absorbing near-infrared light, they can also provide photothermal treatment and be formulated as theranostic agents (Chan et al. 2016). The term *theranostics* refers to the development of compounds that exhibit the characteristics of diagnostics and therapeutics in a single entity (Kang et al. 2015). The application of theranostic nanoparticles has probably been most successfully implemented in cancer research.

Quantum dots (QD) are small nanocrystals of semiconductor compounds (e.g., CdSe, CdTe, CdS, ZnSe, InP, and InS) that have been used for imaging because of their excellent fluorescence properties. QDs are novel nanocrystals composed of an inorganic elemental core like cadmium or mercury and a surrounding metal shell. The outer shell protects the QDs from photochemical damage and increases their water solubility. The unique optical properties of QDs make them excellent candidates for multiplex assays, enabling simultaneous probing of different molecules or cells labeled QDs with different colors, using a single excitation source. Genes, nucleic acids, proteins, molecules, and cell processes can be visualized in real time with the aid of QD, which can be diversely modified electronically and optically (Kosaka et al. 2010). QDs can be conjugated with antibodies or nucleic acids to target specific tissues or organs and can be used as fluorescent probes. Depending on their size and composition they have an intrinsic fluorescence emission spectra wavelength of 400–2000 nm. The potential use of QDs in humans may be limited because of their heavy metal composition and there have been reports of cytotoxicity attributed to the release of cadmium following exposure to ultraviolet radiation. This adverse effect can be limited by coating QDs with polyethylene glycol (PEG) or encapsulating them with micelles. Because of their unique features, QDs are considered next-generation fluorescence markers with the potential of revolutionizing the fields of diagnostics and imaging.

Hydrogel nanoparticles have been used for imaging because they have high hydrophilicity, biocompatibility, high colloidal stability, and tunable size in the nanometer range, which make them ideal for imaging. These nanogels (10 to 200 nm) can circumvent uptake by the reticuloendothelial system, allowing longer circulation times than small molecules and their size/surface properties can be further tailored to optimize their pharmacokinetics for imaging of a particular disease (Chan et al. 2016). Because of the availability of numerous formulation methods and building materials, nanogels can be utilized as imaging agents in many imaging modalities, making them very versatile (Chan et al. 2016). Specifically, due to flexibility in their constituents, biocompatible and less immunogenic materials, such as natural polymers (chitosan, dextran, and pullulan), can be used, which gives nanogels great potential as a platform for clinical contrast agents (Chan et al. 2016).

Carbon nanotubes (CNT) have been studied intensively for multiple imaging modalities, including fluorescence, photoacoustic, and Raman imaging (Bhattacharya et al. 2016). For example, De La Zerda et al. (2008) demonstrated that single-walled CNTs conjugated with cyclic Arg-Gly-Asp peptides can be used as a contrast agent for photoacoustic imaging of malignant glioma tumors in mice. Intravenous administration of these targeted nanotubes to mice bearing tumors showed eight times greater photoacoustic signal in the tumor than mice injected with non-targeted nanotubes (Bhattacharya et al. 2016). Single-walled CNTs were also used to visualize deep, disseminated tumors *in vivo*, which could facilitate surgical excision of model ovarian cancers with submillimeter precision (Bhattacharya et al. 2016). Delogu et al. (2012) demonstrated that the ultrasound signal of functionalized multi-walled CNTs was higher than graphine oxide, pristine MWCNTs, and functionalized SWCNTs. Similarly, graphene and its derivatives have also been investigated as optical or nonoptical imaging agents (Yoo et al. 2015).

1.4 NANOPHARMACEUTICALS

The merger of nanoscience and nanotechnology with pharmaceutical research and development opens new horizons for the creation of novel drugs, which will utilize the unique characteristics of nanosized materials (Weissig et al. 2004). Nanopharmaceuticals have been defined as "pharmaceuticals engineered on the nanoscale, i.e., pharmaceuticals where the nanomaterial plays the pivotal therapeutic role or adds additional functionality to the previous compound" (Rivera et al. 2010). To be classified as a nanopharmaceutical, Weissig et al. (2014) suggested that the drug product must meet two major criteria: (1) nanoengineering has to play a major role in the manufacturing process, and (2) the nanomaterial used has to be either essential for the therapeutic activity or has to confer additional and unique properties to the active drug entity. Others have defined nanomedicines as therapeutic or imaging agents which comprise a nanoparticle in order to control the biodistribution, enhance the efficacy, or otherwise reduce toxicity of a drug or biologic (Bobo et al. 2016).

When evaluating what types of pharmaceuticals qualify as nanopharmaceuticals, it is important to determine what a nanomaterial is, because in limiting the applicability of this term solely to the size range of 1–100 nm, all physiological macromolecules, derivatives, or self-assembled structures would qualify as nanomaterials. Interactions of nanomedicines with their biological surroundings (at the level of molecules, cells, organs, etc.) are dependent on a complex interplay between the controllable properties of the particles and the largely uncontrollable properties of the surrounding media (Bobo et al. 2016). When nanoparticles are exposed to the biological milieu, the process of non-specific protein adsorption results in the formation of a protein corona around the material (Bobo et al. 2016). It appears practically impossible to completely avoid the formation of this protein layer; however, its composition can be altered through the addition of polymer coatings on the particle surface (e.g., polyethylene glycol [PEG]; Bobo et al. 2016). Particle size, shape, and surface chemistry are key factors that determine performance criteria, including the degree of protein adsorption, cellular uptake, biodistribution patterns, and clearance mechanisms of nanoparticles (Santamaria and Sayes 2010). Particle size plays a key role in clearance of these materials from the body, with small particles (<10 nm) being cleared via the kidneys, and larger particles (>10 nm) being cleared through the liver and the mononuclear-phagocyte system (Bobo et al. 2016). The desired clearance mechanism can be a factor in the design of the nanomedicine, e.g., selecting small, actively targeted particles that are rapidly cleared if they are not taken up into the target organ after first-pass distribution.

The majority of the applications of nanotherapeutics have been related to treating cancer by killing cancerous cells using nanopharmaceuticals, heat, and gene transfections. Multifunctional nanoparticles have also been developed for the diagnosis and treatment of chronic neurodegenerative disorders such as Alzheimer's disease, Parkinson's disease, and strokes. For instance, multifunctional nanoparticles can be used for the amelioration of brain disorders that are associated with iron overload (Kang et al. 2015). Oxidative stress caused by metals like iron, which accumulate in the brain in excess, is considered one of the major causes of many neurodegenerative diseases, including Alzheimer's (Todorich et al. 2004). Iron chelators have been extensively used with the aim of removing the excess iron from the brain to improve these disease conditions.

In a recent review article, Bobo et al. (2016) identified 51 U.S. Food and Drug Administration (USFDA)–approved nanomedicines that correspond to their definition of a nanopharmaceutical and 77 products in clinical trials, with approximately 40 percent of clinical trials started in 2014 or 2015. Weissig et al. (2014) discussed 43 currently approved drug formulations that they identified as nanopharmaceuticals. While FDA-approved materials are heavily weighted to polymeric, liposomal, and nanocrystal formulations, there is a trend toward the development of more complex materials comprising micelles, protein-based nanoparticles, and also the emergence of a variety of inorganic and metallic nanoparticles in clinical trials (Bobo et al. 2016; Weissig and Guzman-Villanueva 2015; Weissig et al. 2014). Nanopharmaceuticals have unique physicochemical properties of the nanosized material made via nano-engineering, including nanotubes, nanoshells, nanoparticles, nanorods, and others, many of which are made from non-physiological inorganic atomic/molecular substances produced through nanoengineering. Nanoparticles have been used in cancer treatment wherein nanoparticles that have accumulated in the tumor tissue are heated by hyperthermia or thermoablation methods to weaken and destroy tumor tissue and increase the toxicity of chemotherapeutics (Krukemeyer et al. 2015). Clinical studies have shown that this method can be used safely on humans and that promising results can be achieved in combination with radiotherapy (Krukemeyer et al. 2015).

Nanocrystals constitute a unique group of pharmaceuticals, as they are composed of 100 percent water-insoluble drugs without any added excipient or any associated nanocarrier system (Weissig et al. 2014). Micronization is widely used as a common formulation method for sparingly soluble compounds, and the saturation solubility is a constant and depends on the chemical nature of the solid material, the dissolution medium, and the temperature (Weissig et al. 2014). However, below a critical size, the saturation solubility also becomes a function of the particle size, and below 1,000 nm it increases with decreasing particle size (Weissig et al. 2014). As a result, drug nanocrystals possess increased saturation solubility, which in turn increases the concentration gradient between gut lumen and blood, and thereby increases the absorption by passive diffusion (Junghanns and Miller 2008).

Gold nanoparticles are probably the most extensively studied nanoparticles that have been investigated for applications in nanomedicine. Among noble metal particles, gold nanoparticles have attracted intensive interest because they are easily prepared, have low toxicity, and can be readily attached to biological molecules. They have been used for a variety of applications in the fields of diagnostics, surgery, and medicine (Giasuddin et al. 2013). The use of gold has a long history in the field of medicine. For example, in China, gold was used in the treatment of ailments such as smallpox, skin ulcers, and measles; in Japan, thin gold foils placed in tea, sake, and food were seen as beneficial to one's health; in Bangladesh–Pakistan–India, traditional Ayurvedic medicines are still used widely with gold taken as a "rejuvenator" by millions of people each year with a typical daily dose consisting of 1–2 mg of gold incorporated into a mixture of herbs (Giasuddin et al. 2013). As medical science and medicine have advanced, so too have the biomedical uses and applications of gold. Gold has wide uses and applications in the fields of diagnostics, surgery, and medicine, particularly for labeling, delivering, heating, and sensing, primarily because of the inertness of gold as a material and resistance to bacterial infection (Giasuddin et al. 2013). A variety of methods are available for conjugation of ligands and biomolecules with gold nanoparticles for different biological applications. A common technique for a diagnostic test consists of an antibody attached to a fluorescent molecule—when the antibody attaches to a protein associated with the disease, the fluorescent molecule lights up under ultraviolet light. Instead of a fluorescent molecule, a gold nanoparticle can be attached to the antibody, and other molecules such as DNA can be added to the nanoparticle to produce bar codes (Jain 2012). Because many copies of the antibodies and DNA can be attached to a single nanoparticle, this approach is much more sensitive and accurate than the fluorescent molecule tests used currently (Jain 2012). In addition, gold nanoparticles are naturally taken up by many cell types and do not cause any detectable cytotoxicity, so they have been used to deliver DNA inside cells. Gold nanoparticles may also be excited with a suitable light source heat, producing localized heating resulting in cell death (e.g., cancer cells) or tissue environment manipulation. Gold nanoparticles have been used to collect specifically in a cancerous tumor by passing through the inherently leaky blood vessels attached to a tumor (Giasuddin et al. 2012).

Nanoparticles have also been used for gene therapy, which is the replacement of a faulty gene in the cell with a proficient gene or by overexpression or silencing of a gene by introducing a foreign DNA and modifying the cellular signaling. Nanoparticles have the capability to replace viral vectors because they are smaller in size and therefore can communicate with many biological moieties, like cytokines and proteins (Kang et al. 2015). Although nanoparticles have some drawbacks, such as inefficient transfecting efficiency, these can be overcome by chemical modification of the functional groups (Kang et al. 2015).

1.5 NANOPARTICLE-BASED DRUG DELIVERY

By combining both therapeutic and diagnostic functions in one delivery formulation, nanoparticle carrier agents may enable disease diagnosis, therapy, and real-time monitoring of treatment progress and efficacy, all with one pharmaceutical agent. There has been intensive research into the possible syntheses and uses of various carrier systems and physicochemical functionalization of their surface structure. In these areas of research, synthetic organic chemistry has played an important role in the creation of tailor-made molecules. The fact that nanoparticles exist in the same size domain as proteins makes nanomaterials suitable for biotagging or labeling with antibodies or drugs. In the early 1990s, nanoparticles were modified for the first time for transport of DNA fragments and genes and were directed into cells with the aid of antibodies (Kreuter 2007). The idea that pharmaceutical agents can be delivered specifically to diseased cells holds the promise of a variety of benefits. If, in addition, the pharmaceutical agent were to be adapted to the cell's genome, these benefits would be grouped under the heading *personalized medicine*. The use of nanoparticles for drug delivery involves at least two components, one to deliver the drug (transport device) and the other the active drug component. Nanospheres have been widely accepted as a useful tool for controlled or targeted drug delivery due to their inherently small size and corresponding large specific surface area, a high drug loading efficiency, a high reactivity towards surrounding tissues *in vivo*, and an ease of diffusion of drug-loaded particles (Walmsley et al. 2015). Drugs, growth factors, or genetic material may be delivered to cells and tissues by the encapsulation in either degradable or non-degradable nanospheres. Examples of non-degradable nanoparticles include hydroxyapatite, gold, dendrimer, and silica, while degradable nanoparticles include polymers such as poly(L-lactide) (PLA) or poly(L-lactide-co-glycolic) (PLGA). These polymers are known for both their biocompatibility and resorbability through natural pathways, and encapsulation of material in a shell comprised of a phospholipid bilayer can enhance tissue specific targeting, protection from degradation, and delivery of a large quantity of the drug. Encapsulating a drug within a polymer controls its pharmacokinetic profile by releasing it at a constant flow. The selection of the base biomaterial for nanosphere construction depends on the desired end application criteria (Walmsley et al. 2015). The selection of the nanosphere depends on factors such as size of the desired nanoparticles; properties of the drug (aqueous solubility, stability, etc.) to be encapsulated in the polymer; surface characteristics and functionality; degree of biodegradability and biocompatibility; and drug release profile of the final product (Mahapatro and Singh 2011). The small size of nanospheres allows them to quickly respond to stimuli from the surrounding environment (for example, pH, magnetic fields, ultrasounds, and irradiation) and thus these spheres can serve as stimulus-driven delivery for biologically or chemically active agents, and subsequently, establish triggered release by responding to external stimulation (Walmsley et al. 2015). Nanosize drug delivery systems generally focus on formulating bioactive molecules in biocompatible nanosystems, such as nanocrystals, solid lipid nanoparticles, nanostructure lipid carriers, lipid drug conjugates, nanoliposomes, dendrimers, nanoshells, emulsions, nanotubes, quantum dots, etc. Extensively versatile molecules, from synthetic chemicals to naturally occurring complex macromolecules such as nucleic acids and proteins, could be dispensed in such formulations, maintaining their stability and efficacy (Mukherjee 2013).

A drug may either be adsorbed or covalently attached to the nanocarrier's surface or encapsulated into it. Covalent linking has the advantage over other ways of attaching as it is able to control the number of drug molecules connected to the nanocarrier, i.e., a precise control of the amount of therapeutic compound delivered (Wilczewska et al. 2012). Cell-specific targeting with nanocarriers may be accomplished by using active or passive mechanisms. Active mechanisms rely on the attraction of a drug—the nanocarriers conjugate to the affected site by using recognition ligands, of conjugate antibodies or other substances and the active mechanism can be achieved through a manipulation of physical stimuli (e.g., temperature, pH, magnetism). Passive targeting is a result of enhanced vascular permeability and retention, which is characteristic of leaky tissues of tumors (Wilczewska et al. 2012). Once the drug–nanocarrier conjugates reach the diseased tissues, the therapeutic agents are released. A controlled release of drugs from nanocarriers can be achieved through changes in physiological environment (e.g., temperature, pH, osmolality) or via an enzymatic activity.

The achievements obtained so far in the field of nanocarriers for drug delivery include anticancer chemotherapeutics (doxorubicin, methotrexate, taxanes, platinum analogues, camptothecin, and gemcitabine), immunotherapeutics, and nucleic acids (Tripathi et al. 2015). The encapsulation of paclitaxel in biodegradable and nontoxic nano-delivery systems has been shown to protect the drug from degradation during circulation, and, in turn, protect the body from the toxic side effects of the drug, thereby lowering its toxicity, increasing its circulation half-life, exhibiting improved pharmacokinetic profiles, and demonstrating better patient compliance (Ma and Mumper 2013). Nanoparticle-based delivery systems can take advantage of the enhanced permeability and retention effect for passive tumor targeting. Thus, they are promising carriers to improve the therapeutic index and decrease the side effects of drugs such as paclitaxel (Ma and Mumper 2013). Paclitaxel albumin-bound nanoparticles (Abraxane®) have been approved by the USFDA for the treatment of metastatic breast cancer and non-small cell lung cancer, and there are a number of novel paclitaxel nanoparticle formulations currently in clinical trials (Ma and Mumper 2013). Drug nanocarriers not only transport the chemotherapeutic agents to tumors, avoiding normal tissues and reducing toxicity in the rest of the body, but they also protect cytotoxic drugs from degradation and increase the half-life, payload, and solubility of cytotoxic agents and reduce renal clearance. The magnetic property of iron nanoparticles has also been used for applications in drug and gene delivery, and application of strong magnetic pulses has been shown to promote transfection levels (Dobson 2006). Iron or gold nanoparticles can also be targeted to tumors for destruction by heating. Magnetic iron nanoparticles conjugated with the anticancer drug Methotrexate, which can target cancer cells that overexpress folate receptors on their surface, have been used for MRI imaging and to kill cultured breast and cervical cancer cells (Kohler et al. 2005). Nanoparticles, by being drug vectors, can also carry radio-sensitizer therapeutics to cancer cells. The ability of gold and iron nanoparticles to be targeted to tumors, used in MRI contrast agent, deliver anticancer drugs into tumor cells, and their role in hyperthermia makes them ideal candidates for cancer management.

Silica materials used in controlled drug delivery systems are classified as xerogels and mesoporous silica nanoparticles (MSNs), and they exhibit several advantages as carrier systems, including biocompatibility, highly porous framework, and an ease in terms of functionalization (Wilczewska et al. 2012). Among inorganic nanoparticles, silica materials are the carriers which most often are chosen for biological purposes (Wilczewska et al. 2012). Carbon nanomateials have provided an excellent technology platform in the field of drug delivery; specifically, carbon nanomaterials such as fullerenes, carbon nanotubes, and graphenes have exhibited wide applicability in drug delivery, owing to their small size and biological activity (Tripathi et al. 2015). Many achievements have been evidenced in delivering drugs using carbon nanomaterials for anticancer, neurodegenerative disorders, anti-mycobacterials, anti-inflammatory, topical agents, biomolecules, etc. Fullerenes, which are molecules of 60 carbon atoms that form a hollow sphere one nanometer in diameter, are entirely insoluble in water but suitable functionalization makes the molecules soluble. Initial studies on water-soluble fullerene derivatives led to the discovery of the interaction of organic fullerenes with DNA, proteins, and living cells (Jain 2012). Nanomolecular carbon cages like fullerenes are used for the delivery of drugs and imaging agents in several functional modes (Tripathi et al. 2015). These are also useful drug vectors or drug delivery scaffolds with non-covalent or covalent linkages between the fullerene and a bioactive moiety. Fullerenes have numerous points of attachments, which allow accurate grafting of active chemical groups in three-dimensional orientations (Tripathi et al. 2015). This attribute is the hallmark of rational drug design, which allows positional control in matching these carbon nanocompounds to biological targets (Tripathi et al. 2015). However, there are several limitations associated with the design and characterization of these nanomaterials, including cellular toxicity, the ability to achieve optimal drug loading on the carbon nanoparticles to control drug release and delivery, and uncertainties about pharmacokinetic profiles (Tripathi et al. 2015).

Several types of nanoparticles have been developed as nanocarriers, including polymeric nanoparticles, polymeric micelles, liposomal nanoparticles, protein nanoparticles, and inorganic nanoparticles. While the majority of FDA-approved nanomedicine nanocarriers rely on passive targeting via enhanced permeability and retention, there is a clear trend in emerging studies towards active targeting to further increase drug accumulation and ultimately efficacy at the disease site, while reducing toxicity in other organs (Bobo et al. 2016).

1.6   TISSUE ENGINEERING WITH NANOMATERIALS

Tissue engineering is the application of biomaterials, biomolecules, and cells to guide the construction, self-organization, or growth of renewed living material to replace tissues and functions in the body that have been lost or impaired. Nanobiotechnology opens up new possibilities above all in the field of regenerative medicine because, by stimulation and targeted control of cell growth, damaged or absent tissue—from hair, cartilage and bone, via muscles and organs, through to nerve cells—could be regenerated or produced artificially with the aid of nanomaterials (tissue engineering) (Krukemeyer et al. 2015). Nanoporous carrier materials are already used in wound healing and plastic surgery as matrices along which controlled cell growth takes place. If targeted growth of nerve cells were also to be successful, new possible treatments for neurological diseases such as Alzheimer's, Parkinson's, epilepsy, and multiple sclerosis could be developed. If targeted manipulation of adult stem cells can be accomplished, endogenous tissue which causes no rejection reactions could be cultured, and the use of embryonic stem cells could be abandoned (Krukemeyer et al. 2015). Nanostructured surfaces can serve as scaffolding for controlled tissue-growth and scaffolds possessing nanometer-scaled features are attracting increased attention for their application in tissue engineering. Creating nano-sized features on the surface of a hip or knee prosthesis could reduce the chances of rejection as well as to stimulate the production of osteoblasts. Although nanoparticle-based therapy is becoming more common in the treatment of cancer, integrating a nanosystem into the constructs of tissue engineering has proved challenging and has not been clinically validated. Tissue engineering involves seeding of cells on bio-mimicked scaffolds providing adhesive surfaces and has been successfully used for replacement of skin, bone, cartilage, and nerve tissue. Researchers face a range of problems in generating tissue that can be circumvented by employing nanotechnology because it provides substrates for cell adhesion and proliferation and agents for cell growth, and can be used to create nanostructures and nanoparticles to aid the engineering of different types of tissue.

1.7   TOXICOLOGY OF NANOPARTICLES
USED FOR MEDICAL PURPOSES

The development of nanoparticles has advanced the field of drug delivery and nanomedicine; however, it is relatively new to other forms of pharmaceutical formulations, and the mechanisms by which nanosystems can lead to toxicity have not been fully characterized. The potential adverse human health effects of nanopharmaceuticals and nanocarriers have raised concern for their use in the healthcare and consumer sectors (Yang et al. 2012; Love et al. 2012). The lack of availability of detailed toxicology data on nanocarrier systems makes it difficult to evaluate their potential toxicity, and currently there are no regulations available to assure the safety aspects of nanocarriers of drugs in healthcare and their impact on the environment (Mukherjee et al. 2016). The toxicity of nanoparticles depends on various conditions, including not only physicochemical properties of nanoparticles (e.g., size, shape, surface charge, chemical composition), but also physiological status (e.g., genetics, disease conditions; Kang et al. 2015). Although small size and large surface area are two of the unique properties making nanoparticles popular, these properties may also significantly affect toxicity. For example, because nanoparticles are smaller in size than cells and cell organelles, and they possess the potential to penetrate into these cellular structures in several organs by circulatory, nervous, and lymphatic systems, they can disrupt physiological functions and promote tissue inflammation, abnormal cell functioning, or even cell death (Wei 2012). Metallic nanoparticles (e.g., silver, gold) can enter the cells either by endocytosis or diffusion due to their relative small size. Upon their entry into the cell, they reach mitochondria and can impair the mitochondrial function by disturbing the electron transport chain, resulting in causing oxidative stress (Kang et al. 2015). In addition, metallic nanoparticles can generate reactive oxygen species, which enter the nucleus and cause oxidative stress, leading to DNA damage by cross-linking or formation of DNA adducts. The reactive oxygen species can also cause protein oxidation and lipid peroxidation, which may ultimately affect cell growth. Silica nanoparticles reduce levels of antioxidant glutathione as well as causing oxidative stress via ROS production, resulting in DNA damage (Kang et al. 2015). QDs can cause toxicity by disruption of mitochondrial function, which leads to DNA damage (Nguyen et al. 2015). Cationic carbon nanotubes may be more toxic than the neutral or negatively charged CNTs because they can cause platelet aggregation (Alkilany et al. 2010).

1.8 CONCLUSION

The scope of nanomedicine overlaps with several traditional medical and research fields. As our understanding of biology, pathology, tissue repair/regeneration, cancer, and other diseases develop, the use of nanomedical approaches will also continue to develop and provide new solutions and products to solve healthcare challenges in the future. The nanotherapy vision of the future is the treatment of patients with individually tailor-made medicines (personalized medicine) at the molecular level as soon as the disease is in the development stage. The preparation of nanodrugs and the various methods of targeted transport of active substances (drug delivery) will play a prominent role in the future (Krukemeyer et al. 2015). Nanotechnology may be yielding more medical benefits in the coming years, especially in the fields of imaging and drug delivery.

Many different types of nanoparticles have been successfully implicated in targeting and therapy of various diseases because of unique size-dependent optical or magnetic properties, multifunctionality, strong enhanced vascular permeability and retention effect, and long-term blood circulation. However, nanoparticles may lack important properties for clinical translation, such as high physiological stability, efficient clearance, minimum accumulation in non-targeted tissues and organs, and rapid distribution to various organs and tissues (Yu and Zheng 2015). The success of nanotechnology in medicine will depend on the rational design and use of nanoparticles and proper characterization of their toxicity. Nanomedicine has the potential to significantly improve the quality of life of patients; however, the new possibilities also involve risks and raise sociological and ethical questions which must be carefully studied and evaluated.

REFERENCES

Alkilany, A. M., and Murphy, C. J. 2010. Toxicity and cellular uptake of gold nanoparticles: What we have learned so far? *J Nanopart Res* 12:2313–2333.
Bhattacharya, K., Mukherjee, S. P., Gallud, A., Burket, S. C., Bistarelli, S., Belluci, S. et al. 2016. Biological interactions of carbon-based nanomaterials: From coronation to degradation. *Nanomedicine: NBM* 12:333–351.
Bobo, D., Robinson, K., Islam, J., Thurecht, K. J., and Corrie, S. R. 2016. Nanoparticle-based medicines: A review of FDA-approved materials and clinical trials to date. *Pharm Res* 33(10):2373–2387.
Bourrinet, P., Bengele, H. H., Bonnemain, B. et al. 2006. Preclinical safety and pharmacokinetic profile of ferumoxtran-10, an ultrasmall superparamagnetic iron oxide magnetic resonance contrast agent. *Invest Radiol* 41(3):313–324.
Chan, M., and Almutairi, A. 2016. Nanogels as imaging agents for modalities spanning the electromagnetic spectrum. *Mater Horiz* 3(1):21–40.
De la Zerda, A., Zavaleta, C., Keren, S., Vaithilingam, S., Bodapati, S., Liu, Z. et al. 2008. Carbon nanotubes as photoacoustic molecular imaging agents in living mice. *Nat Nanotechnol* 3:557–562.
Delogu, L. G. 2012. Functionalized multiwalled carbon nanotubes as ultrasound contrast agents. *Proc Natl Acad Sci* 109(41):16612–16617.
Dinarvand, R., Sepehri, N., Manoochehri, S., Rouhani, H., and Atyabi, F. 2011. Polylactide-co-glycolide nanoparticles for controlled delivery of anticancer agents. *Int J Nanomedicine* 6:877–95.
Drexler, K. E. 1981. Molecular engineering: An approach to the development of general capabilities for molecular manipulation. *Proc Natl Acad Sci* 78(9):5275–5278.
Drexler, K. E. 1986. *Engines of Creation: The Coming Era of Nanotechnology.* New York: Random House.
Fanfair, D., Desai, S., and Kelty, C. 2007. *The Early History of Nanotechnology.* Rice University, The Connexions Project, Module m14504.
Feynman, R. P. 1960. There's plenty of room at the bottom. *Eng Sci* 23(5):22–36.
Freitas, R. A. 2005. Nanotechnology, nanomedicine and nanosurgery. *Int J Surgery* 3(4):243–246.
Giasuddin, A. S. M., Jhuma, K. A., and Mujibul Haq, A. M. 2012. Use of gold nanoparticles in diagnostics, surgery, and medicine: A review. *Bangladesh J Med Biochem* 5(2):56–60.
Harisinghani, M. G., Barentsz, J., Hahn, P. F., Deserno, W. M., Tabatabaei, S., van de kaa, C. H. et al. 2003. Noninvasive detection of clinically occult lymph-node metastases in prostate cancer. *N Engl J Med* 348:2491–2499.

Hawthorne, G. H., Bernuci M. P., Bortolanza, M., Tumas, V., Issy, A. C., and Del-Bel, E. 2016. Nanomedicine to overcome current Parkinson's treatment liabilities: A systematic review. *Neurotox Res* 30(4):715–729.

Ishiyama, K., Sendoh, M., and Arai, K. I. 2002. Magnetic micromachines for medical applications. *J Magn Magn Mater* 242–245:1163–1165.

Jain, K. K. 2012. *The Handbook of Nanomedicine.* New York: Springer.

Junghanns, J. U., and Muller, R. H. 2008. Nanocrystal technology, drug delivery and clinical applications. *Int J Nanomedicine* 3(3):295–309.

Kang, H., Mintri, S., Menon, A. V., Lee, H. Y., Choi, H. S., and Kim, J. 2015. Pharmacokinetics, pharmacodynamics, and toxicology of theranostic nanoparticles. *Nanoscale* 7(45): 8848–18862.

Kohler, N., Sun, C., Wang, J., and Zhang, M. 2005. Methotrexate-modified superparamagnetic nanoparticles and their intracellular uptake into human cancer cells. *Langmuir* 13;21(19):8858–8864.

Kosaka, N., McCann, T. E., Mitsunaga, M., Choyke, P. L., Kobayashi, H. 2010. Realtime optical imaging using quantum dot and related nanocrystals. *Nanomedicine* 5:765–776.

Kroto, H., Health, J. R., O'Brian, S. C., Curl, R. F., and Smalley, R. E. C. 1985. C60: Buckminsterfullerene. *Nature* 318:162–163.

Krukemeyer, M. G., Krenn, V., Huebner, F., Wagner, W., and Resch, R. 2015. History and possible uses of nanomedicine based on nanoparticles and nanotechnological progress. *J Nanomed Nanotechnol* 6:6.

Love, S. A., Maurer-Jones, M. A., Thompson, J. W., Lin, Y. S., and Haynes, C. L. 2012. Assessing nanoparticle toxicity. *Annu Rev Anal Chem* 5:181–205.

Ma, P., and Mumper, R. J. Paclitaxel nano-delivery systems: A comprehensive review. 2013. *J Nanomed Nanotechnol* 4(2):1000164.

Mahapatro, A., and Singh, D. K. 2011. Biodegradable nanoparticles are excellent vehicle for site directed in-vivo delivery of drugs and vaccines. *J Nanobiotechnol* 9:55.

Mao, X., Xu, J., and Cui, H. 2016. Functional nanoparticles for magnetic resonance imaging. *Wiley Interdiscip Rev Nanomed Nanobiotechnol* 8(6):814–841.

Mitra, A., Nan, A., Line, B. R., and Ghandehari H. 2006. Nanocarriers for nuclear imaging and radiotherapy of cancer. *Curr Pharm Des* 12:4729–4749.

Mukherjee, B. 2013. Nanosize drug delivery system. *Curr Pharm Biotechnol* 14(15):1221.

Muthu, M. S., and Singh, S. 2009. Targeted nanomedicines: Effective treatment modalities for cancer, AIDS and brain disorders. *Nanomedicine* 4(1):105–118.

Nguyen, K. C., Rippstein, P., Tayabali, A. F., and Willmore, W. G. 2015. Pharmacokinetics, pharmacodynamics and toxicology of theranostic nanoparticles. *Tox Sci* 146:31–42.

Padmanabhan, P., Kumar, A., Kumar, S., Chaudhary, R. K., and Gulyás, B. 2016. Nanoparticles in practice for molecular-imaging applications: An overview. *Acta Biomater* 1(41):1–16.

Patra, C. R., Bhattacharya, R., Mukhopadhyay, D., and Mukherjee, P. 2010. Fabrication of gold nanoparticles for targeted therapy in pancreatic cancer. *Adv Drug Deliv Rev* 8;62(3):346–361.

Pérez-Herrero, E., and Fernández-Medarde, A. 2015. Advanced targeted therapies in cancer: Drug nanocarriers, the future of chemotherapy. *Eur J Pharm Biopharm* 93:52–79.

Rawat, M., Singh, D., Saraf, S., and Saraf, S. 2006. Nanocarriers: Promising vehicle for bioactive drugs. *Biol Pharm Bull* 29:1790–1798.

Rivera, G. P., Hühn, D., del Mercato, L. L., Sasse, D., and Parak, W. J. 2010. Nanopharmacy: Inorganic nanoscale devices as vectors and active compounds. *Pharmacol Res* 62(2):115–125.

Samadian, H., Hosseini-Nami, S., Kamrava, S. K., Ghaznavi, H., and Shakeri-Zadeh, A. 2016. Folate-conjugated gold nanoparticle as a new nanoplatform for targeted cancer therapy. *J Cancer Res Clin Oncol* 142(11):2217–2229.

Sandhiya, S., Dkhar, S. A., and Surendiran, A. 2009. Emerging trends of nanomedicine: An overview. *Fundam Clin Pharmacol* 23(3):263–269.

Santamaria, A. B. 2012. Historical overview of nanotechnology and nanotoxicology, in *Methods in Molecular Biology*, vol. 926, ed. J. Reineke. New York: Humana Press, Springer Publishing Group.

Santamaria, A. B., and Sayes, C. M. 2010. Toxicological studies with nanoscale materials, in *Nanotechnology Environmental Health and Safety*, eds. M. Hull and D. Bowman. Boston: Elsevier.

Sayes, C. M., and Santamaria, A. B. 2014. Toxicological issues to consider when evaluating the safety of consumer products containing nanomaterials, in *Nanotechnology Environmental Health and Safety: Risks, Regulation and Management*, eds. M. Hull and D. Bowman. Boston: Elsevier.

Taniguchi, N. 1974. On the basic concept of nano-technology. *Proceedings of the International Conference of Production Engineering*. Tokyo: Japan Society of Precision Engineering.

Tatar, A. S., Nagy-Simon, T., Tomuleasa, C., Boca, S., and Astilean, S. 2016. Nanomedicine approaches in acute lymphoblastic leukemia. *J Controlled Release* 28(238):123–138.

Todorich, B. M., and Connor, J. R. 2004. Redox metals in Alzheimer's disease. *Ann NY Acad Sci* 1012:171–178.

Torchilin, V. P. 2007. Targeted pharmaceutical nanocarriers for cancer therapy and imaging. *AAPS J* 9:E128–E147.

Tripathi, A. C., Saraf, S. A., and Saraf, S. K. 2015. Carbon nanotropes: A contemporary paradigm in drug delivery. *Materials* 8:3068–3100.

Walmsley, G. G. 2015. Nanotechnology in bone tissue engineering. *Nanomedicine* 11(5):1253–1263.

Wang, Y. X. 2011. Superparamagnetic iron oxide based MRI contrast agents: Current status of clinical application. *Quant Imaging Med Surg* 1(1):35–40.

Wang, Y. X., Hussain, S. M., and Krestin, G. P. 2006. Superparamagnetic iron oxide contrast agents: Physicochemical characteristics and applications in MR imaging. *Eur Radiol* 11:2319–2331.

Wei, A., Mehtala, J. G., and Patri, A. K. 2012. Challenges and opportunities in the advancement of nanomedicines. *J Controlled Release* 164:236–246.

Weinstein, J. S., Varallyay, C. G., Dosa, E., Gahramanov, S., Hamilton, B., Rooney, W. D. et al. 2010. Superparamagnetic iron oxide nanoparticles: Diagnostic magnetic resonance imaging and potential therapeutic applications in neurooncology and central nervous system inflammatory pathologies, a review. *J Cereb Blood Flow Metab* 30(1):15–35.

Weissig, V., and Guzman-Villanueva, D. 2015. Nanopharmaceuticals (part 2): Products in the pipeline. *Int J Nanomedicine* Feb 11(10):1245–1257.

Weissig, V., Pettinger, T. K., and Murdock, N. 2014. Nanopharmaceuticals (part 1): Products on the market. *Int J Nanomedicine* 15(9):4357–4373.

Yang, Z., Liu, Z. W., Allaker, R. P., Reip, P., Oxford, J., Ahmad, Z. et al. 2012. A review of nanoparticle functionality and toxicity on the central nervous system. *J R Soc Interface* 7(Suppl 4):S411–S422.

Yoo, J. M., Kang, J. H., Hong, B. H. 2015. Graphene-based nanomaterials for versatile imaging studies. *Chem Soc Rev* 44:4835–4852.

Yu, M., and Zheng, J. 2015. Clearance pathways and tumor targeting of imaging nanoparticles. *ACS Nano* 9:6655–6674.

Zhu, D., Liu, F., Ma, L., Liu, D., and Wang, Z. 2013. Nanoparticle-based systems for t1-weighted magnetic resonance imaging contrast agents. *Int J Mol Sci* 14(5):10591–10607.

Zsigmondy, R. 1914. *Colloids and the Ultramicroscope*. New York: Wiley.

2 Dispersion and Characterization of Nanoparticles

Didier Rouxel, Solenne Fleutot, and Van Son Nguyen

CONTENTS

2.1 INTRODUCTION

During the past few decades, nanoparticles (NPs) have emerged as a powerful tool for biomedical applications. For instance, as far as drug delivery is concerned, NPs can bring different precious potentials, like increased bioavailability; dose proportionality; increased surface area, which results in a faster dissolution of the active agent in an aqueous environment (such as the human body); smaller drug doses with less toxicity; and reduction in fed/fasted variability (Pal et al., 2011). Of course, this assumes that nanoparticles can be perfectly dispersed in a biosolution injectable in the human body and remain dispersed in order not to risk, for example, clogging capillaries or being unable to reach their target.

More generally, nanoparticles can be used not only as nanocarriers for transport of therapeutic agents to their target, but also as nanotracers for medical imaging, as nano-spyware inside the cells and even with magnetic nanoparticles as nano-burning agents for malignant cells, i.e., a variety of new diagnostic therapeutic and restorative solutions. They are also found in regenerative medicine for tissue engineering, prosthetics, and even cell therapy. For instance, while current prostheses for hips and knees are generally metal and polyethylene with an average lifetime of

10 years, the replacement of metal by ceramics reinforced with nanoparticles can increase this lifetime to 30 years. Coated with nanoparticles, prostheses also show better biocompatibility, stronger attachment to bone tissue, and better comfort for the patient. Additionally, surgery steel screws coated with a micrometer layer of diamond nanoparticles show ultra-resistance and a very low probability of rejection.

Along with the great hope for progress in medicine, electronics, and materials, some potential health risks have also appeared: Studies have shown toxicity in certain nanoparticles under certain conditions. This dilemma illustrates the modern paradox of perception in science: Hope and requirement on one hand; mistrust and suspicion on the other. Indeed, beyond medicine in everyday life, today more than 1000 products that use or include nanoparticles are on the market (mostly in the United States) and some "nano" products have been used for more than ten years, involving major societal as well as economic challenges. Because their number is expected to grow rapidly, a societal demand to control their potential risks for health throughout the life cycle has surfaced. And the major conclusion of nanotoxicological studies is that the toxicity may change dramatically, depending of physicochemical parameters of the nanoparticle.

Therefore, for biomedical applications of the nanoparticles, it is necessary

- First, to know most of their physicochemical and structural features, particularly to evaluate their possible toxicity.
- Second, to have perfectly dispersed nanoparticles solutions that permit their use *in vitro* or *in vivo* conditions.

It has been scientifically demonstrated that many physicochemical factors may strongly influence the toxicological properties of nanomaterials (Anses, 2015). The recent ISO/TR 13014 (August 2012) on "Guidance on Physico-Chemical Characterization of Engineered Nanoscale Materials for Toxicologic Assessment" identifies 57 physicochemical parameters characterizing a NP, of which eight are relevant physicochemical properties necessary for a risk assessment of nano-objects:

- Particle size/particle size distribution
- State of aggregation/agglomeration
- Shape
- Surface area or surface porosity
- Chemical composition, purity with impurity level
- Surface chemistry
- The surface charge
- Solubility and dispersibility

In practice, if we consider the literature on the subject and studies published in recent years, parameters generally used by authors to characterize NPs are the size (in nm), the size distribution (in % per class), size range (min-max size), the area of the surface of NPs, the number of particles per ml used in *in vitro* or *in vivo* solutions (in g/ml) and, when the NPs can be dissolved from metal ion, the concentration of these ions in the solution. Some articles also retain other parameters, such as the zeta potential of the nanoparticles. For nano-Ag, for example, various studies have suggested that dissolved ions play an essential role in the toxicity of nanoparticles (Kennedy et al., 2010). But the solubility of the particles, their state of aggregation, and their coatings are not always characterized in the studies.

For biomedical applications themselves, to obtain a stable dispersion of NPs in solution is, of course, one of the key parameters. In this chapter we will first consider the different approaches to obtain such dispersion before discussing the main characterization techniques for NPs.

Note that two characterization techniques are now used in most studies: Transmission electron microscopy (TEM; García-Alonso et al., 2011; Khan et al., 2011; Li et al., 2011) and dynamic light scattering (DLS), often coupled to TEM to characterize the size (Haase et al., 2012; Mukherjee et al., 2012); more rarely to scanning electron microscopy (SEM; Greulich et al., 2009; Griffitt et al., 2008) or X-ray diffraction (Chicea et al., 2012; Martínez-Castañón et al., 2008), or sometimes used alone (Lim et al., 2013).

Inductively coupled plasma mass spectroscopy (ICP-MS) and its derivatives are used, for example, for Ag NPs (Gaiser et al., 2009; Roh et al., 2009). The use of TEM to characterize the size (geometric diameter), shape (aspect ratio), and the state of aggregation of nanomaterials is now common in publications, but an isolated image is often unrepresentative of the nano–object size distribution. Some articles are now beginning to present a statistical analysis of TEM images. It may be added that the TEM grid preparation method can lead to several means of characterization: First, the frequent ultrasound dispersion before deposition on the grid, and the way to collect them, can lead one to observe only a particular category of particles; then, drying the sample on the grid generally leads to (re-) agglomeration. Therefore, it is very complex to produce a representative sample. A change in sample size may result from the preparation prior to analysis because of the need for suspending, dilution, drying, and dispersion of the particles.

It is important to note that measurement techniques give mean diameters depending on the physical principle of the analysis method used. Thus, DLS also provides information on the average particle size, but is different from those of MET as they relate to the hydrodynamic volume of the objects. That information is reliable in the case of unimodal distribution only. DLS also allows access to the size distribution of the particles, and the facilities often allow the coupled measurement of zeta potential. Some studies focus strictly to the question of size, differentiating the nominal size of the PDI (mean particle size), and the Z-average, and the intensity in% as given by the technique.

In addition or substitution of these techniques can be found also in Figure 2.1:

- UV-visible or X-ray absorption spectroscopy
- Environmental scanning electron microscopy (ESEM) with the use of energy-dispersive X-ray spectroscopy for chemical analysis (EDS or EDX for energy dispersive X-ray spectrometry; Fabrega et al., 2009)
- The X-ray diffraction (XRD) for measuring the average size of (nano) crystallites
- Atomic force microscopy (AFM) to "see" the nanoparticles on a surface
- XPS-UPS to get the composition and particle surface chemistry
- X-ray diffraction at small angles (SAXS)

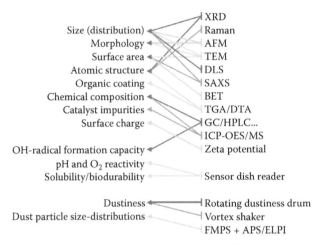

Abbreviations: XRD (X-ray diffraction); Raman (Raman spectroscopy); TEM (transmission electron microscopy); AFM (atomic force microscopy); DLS (dynamic light scattering); SAXS and uSAXS (small angle X-ray
scattering and ultrafine SAXS); BET (Brunauer, Emmett, and Teller gas adsorption); TGA (thermogravi-
metric analysis); DTA (differential thermal analysis); GC (gas-chromatography); HPLC (high-performance
liquid chromatography); ICP-MS (inductively coupled plasma mass spectrometry); FMPS (fast mobility
particle sizer); APS (aerodynamic particle sizer); ELPI (electrical low-pressure impactor).

FIGURE 2.1   Summary list of physicochemical parameters and measurement techniques
employed in Nanogenotox Final Report. (From Nanogenotox, Nanogenotox Final Report,
2013. With permission from Parimage.)

- The atomic absorption spectroscopy (AAS) for the concentration of metal-
  lic ions
- Fractionation coupling flux force (FFF) to particle size
- The BET method (Brunauer, Emmett, and Teller) for measuring specific
  surface area, which also makes it possible to give an average particle size
- Extended X-ray absorption fine structure
- Gamma spectrometry

One important question relates to the state of the nanoparticles to be characterized, and this may suppose three series of characterization. First, in the dry state,
which is usually the native state, as-synthetized or as-received from the fabricant.
Much of the physical properties, such as the crystallinity and the chemical purity,
may be characterized at this step. Electronic microscopies (TEM, SEM) and X-ray
diffraction, for instance, analyze dry samples. But at least a second step of characterization has to be performed on nanoparticles in aqueous solutions or suspensions.
Indeed, all surface properties exhibited by nanoparticles will depend on the media,
as well as the aggregation and agglomeration state. The DLS technique, for example,
is very useful at this step. The media may vary from (ultra) pure water to cell culture
solution by PBS solution, for example. A third step of characterization that is much
more difficult to achieve is those of nanoparticles interacting with living cells in
an *in vitro* or *in vivo* medium. Of course, this last characterization would be more
relevant for toxicity assessment, but few techniques give access to such information.

In this chapter, we will not deal with the subject of the nanoparticle synthesis, but we recall here the main techniques, which will lead to different physicochemical conditions: Hydrothermal methods, sol-gel methods, polyol methods, coprecipitation, thermal decomposition, emulsion-solvent evaporation method, emulsion-diffusion method, salting out method, etc.

2.2 DISPERSION OF NANOPARTICLES

Dispersing nanoparticles in liquids is the key step of sample preparation for biological/toxicological studies. For the particle in the nanometer size range, the high-stress intensity dispersion processes are especially required to overcome the adhesion forces. The micromechanical approach of ultrafine particle adhesion was reviewed in Tomas (2007) and the references therein. Briefly, particle adhesion can be divided into three categories (Figure 2.2):

- Surface and field forces in direct contact, like van der Waals, electrostatic, and magnetic
- Material bridges between particle surfaces:
  - Caused by organic macromolecules such as flocculants in suspensions

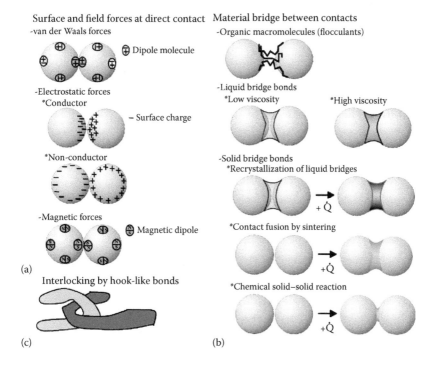

FIGURE 2.2 Particle adhesion and microprocesses of particle bond effects in contact. (a) Surface and field forces at direct contact. (b) Material bridge between contacts. (c) Interlocking by hook-like bonds. (Adapted from Tomas, J., *Chem. Eng. Sci.*, 62, 1997–2010, 2007. With permission from Elsevier.)

- Liquid bridges of wetting liquids by capillary pressure and surface tension
- Solid bridges due to contact fusion by sintering, chemical reactions with adsorbed surface layers, recrystallization of liquid bridges which contain solvents (salt)
- Interlocking by macromolecular (e.g., proteins) and particle shape effects, such as hook-like bonds of fibers

During synthesis processes and post-processes, primary particles often form large clusters. Depending on the bond strength between primary particles, clusters or secondary particles can be classified into two types: Aggregates and agglomerates. The definition of primary and secondary particles and their characteristics are given in Table 2.1. When introducing a liquid, the state of nanoparticles change. They can be in individual or agglomerated form, depending on the colloidal stability (Figure 2.3). Furthermore, nanoparticles may regroup back into several hundred nanometer clusters shortly after deagglomeration if the suspension is not stabilized enough against reagglomeration. Therefore, dispersion of nanoparticles in solutions requires both deagglomeration and stabilization.

2.2.1 Deagglomeration

A simple mechanical agitation is often used to improve the homogeneity of suspensions, but it is not enough to break up agglomerates and aggregates. Numerous

---

TABLE 2.1
List of the Definitions of Particle and Particle Clusters

Terms	Definition and Characteristics	Reference
Particle	Minute piece of matter with defined physical boundaries. Original individual particles are termed *primary particles*.	ISO 14644-6:2007
Aggregate	Particle comprising strongly bonded or fused particles where the resulting external surface area may be significantly smaller than the sum of calculated surface areas of the individual components. The forces holding an aggregate together are strong forces, for example, covalent bonds, or those resulting from sintering or complex physical entanglement. Aggregates are named secondary particles.	ISO/TS 27687:2008
Agglomerate	Collection of weakly bound particles or aggregates or mixtures of the two where the resulting external surface area is similar to the sum of the surface areas of the individual components. The forces holding agglomerate together are weak forces, for example van der Waals forces, or simple physical entanglement. Agglomerates are also called secondary particles.	ISO/TS 27687:2008

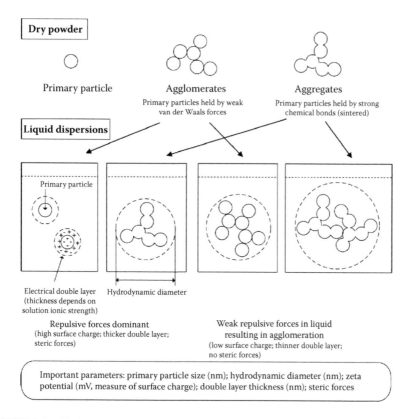

FIGURE 2.3 Various states and configurations of particles in dry state and when dispersed in liquids. (Adapted from Jiang, J., Oberdorster, G., and Biswas, P., *J. Nanoparticle Res.*, 11, 77–89, 2009. With permission from Springer.)

techniques are used for the fragmentation, such as ultrasonicator (Nguyen et al., 2014, 2011; Sato et al., 2008; Sauter et al., 2008), rotor–stator devices (Bałdyga et al., 2008), the ball mill (Zhou et al., 2013), or supercritical CO_2 systems like rapid expansion of supercritical CO_2 suspensions (RESS; Debenedetti et al., 1993; To et al., 2009; Wei et al., 2002). Among the commonly used techniques, ultrasonic dispersion is the most efficient in terms of specific energy (energy applied on a given liquid volume; see Figure 2.4). The ultrasonic dispersion mechanism in media involves acoustic streaming—inducing chaotic mixing and acoustic cavitation (formation, growth, and implosion of bubbles). The implosion of the cavitation bubbles creates high stresses on clusters, resulting in rupture of agglomerates. For a given vibration amplitude, the mean size of clusters often decreases exponentially with increasing ultrasonic time. The hard aggregates cannot be broken into individual nanoparticles, even at very high applied energy. However, an excess of specific energy using high vibration amplitude or prolonged ultrasonication shows no enhance in the breakage process, but can lead to reagglomeration of nanoparticles (Nguyen et al., 2011) and contaminate the suspension due to ultrasonic horn erosion (Mandzy et al., 2005).

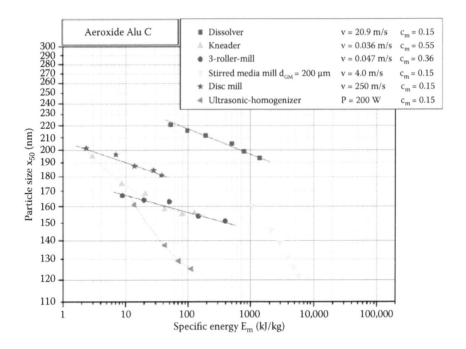

FIGURE 2.4 Evolution of mean alumina nanoparticle size versus specific energy for different dispersing techniques. (Adapted from Schilde, C., Mages-Sauter, C., Kwade, A., and Schuchmann, H. P., *Powder Technol.*, 207, 353–361, 2011. With permission from Elsevier.)

2.2.2 STABILIZATION

In suspensions, the total interparticle potential energy (V_{total}), which controls the colloidal stability is given by (Lewis, 2000):

$$V_{total} = V_{vdW} + V_{elect} + V_{steric} + V_{structural}$$

Where

V_{vdW} is the attractive potential energy resulting from van der Waals interaction between particles.

V_{elect} is the repulsive potential energy due to the electrostatic interaction between like-charged particle surfaces.

V_{steric} is the repulsive potential energy due to steric interaction induced from adsorbed organic species around the particle surface.

$V_{structural}$ is the potential energy resulting from the presence of non-adsorbed species in suspensions that may either increase or decrease suspension stability.

Therefore, to overcome the van der Waals attractive forces, the stabilization must be carried out with electrostatic, steric, and electrosteric effects.

2.2.2.1 Electrostatic Repulsion

The dissociation of surface groups induced from the interaction of suspended particles and liquid medium, especially in aqueous solution, generates electric charges resulting repulsive forces between colloidal particles (Figure 2.5a). The surface potential can be estimated from zeta potential or electrokinetic potential, which is described as the difference in electric potential between that at the slipping plane and that of the bulk liquid (ISO 13099-3:2014). Zeta potential depends not only on particles' surface properties but also on solution conditions, for example, pH, ionic strength (Greenwood, 2003). Therefore, by changing the pH or adding inert electrolytes or the adsorption of surfactants, polymers can alter the electrostatic interactions and, consequently, the stability of the suspensions. In high zeta potential (either positive or negative, ≥30 mV) suspensions, the particles are stabilized by electrostatic repulsion against agglomeration. Low zeta potential can lead to unstable suspension and agglomeration (Figure 2.6). The point where zeta potential is zero is called *isoelectric point* (IEP).

Zeta potential is not a directly measurable parameter but it can be determined using appropriate theoretical models and experimental parameters. Zeta potential of

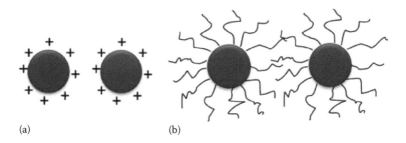

(a)   (b)

FIGURE 2.5 Schematic representation of (a) electrostatic stabilization and (b) steric stabilization of nanoparticles.

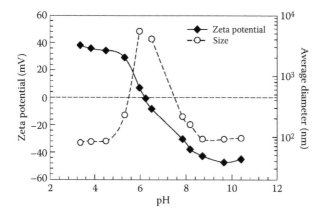

FIGURE 2.6 The influence of solution pH on the zeta potential and the hydrodynamic diameter of TiO_2 dispersions. (Adapted from Jiang, J., Oberdorster, G., and Biswas, P., *J. Nanoparticle Res.*, 11, 77–89, 2009. With permission from Springer.)

nanoparticles is usually determined by electrophoresis. By measuring the velocity of nanoparticles in an electric field, the zeta potential can be calculated from electrophoretic mobility or dynamic electrophoretic mobility using the Henry equation.

2.2.2.2 Steric Stabilization

Another method to prevent agglomeration of particles is adsorption of organic species, often surfactant or polymer, around the particle surface (Figure 2.5b). The adsorbed layer (adlayer) with sufficient thickness and density can stabilize the particles against the attractive van der Waals forces through mechanisms such as steric hindrance. The adsorbed species should possess a head group able to strongly anchor onto the nanoparticle surface and a long-chain alkyl to increase the adlayer thickness to prevent particles approach together. The conformation of the adlayer depends on not only molecular architecture and number of anchoring groups of adsorbed species but also solvent, density of active surface site of nanoparticle, and colloid and organic concentration in solution. The steric stabilization can be used in aqueous and organic suspensions.

2.2.2.3 Electrosteric Stabilization

The adsorption of polyelectrolytes onto the particle surface can modify both electrostatic and steric stabilization of suspensions. It is often referred to as *electrosteric stabilization*. Polyelectrolytes possess at least one ionizable group or segment, such as carboxylic, sulfuric, or their derivatives. On one hand, the adsorption of these charged molecules onto the particle surface modify strongly and even invert the surface charge and hence the zeta potential (Figure 2.7). At low concentrations,

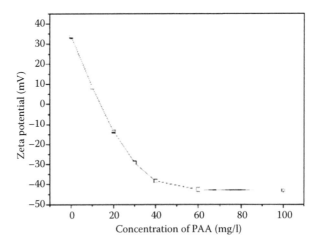

FIGURE 2.7 Influence of PAA concentration on zeta potential of alumina nanoparticles. (Adapted from Nguyen, V. S., Rouxel, D., Hadji, R., Vincent, B., and Fort, Y., *Ultrason. Sonochem.*, 18, 382–388. With permission from Elsevier.)

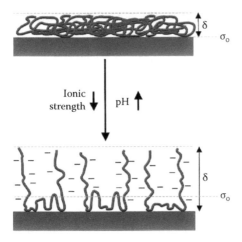

FIGURE 2.8 Schematic illustration of adsorbed anionic polyelectrolyte species on an particle surface as a function of pH and ionic strength (δ is the adlayer thickness and σ_o the plane of charge). (Adapted from Lewis, J. A., *J. Am. Ceram. Soc.*, 83, 2341–2359. With permission from Wiley.)

they neutralize the surface charge which can induce the agglomeration. However, at higher adsorbed amounts, the suspension stability increases thanks to electrostatic repulsion. On the other hand, by increasing the adlayer thickness, the steric hindrance increases and stabilizes the suspension. Like steric stabilization, the adsorption and conformation of polyelectrolytes can be modulated by tailoring their molecular weight, concentration, and suspension conditions, such as pH and ionic strength (Figure 2.8; Greenwood, 2003; Lewis, 2000). However, long polymer chains can adsorb simultaneously on two or more neighboring surfaces of particles, which combines them and forms agglomerates (Nguyen et al., 2011). An excess of surfactant or polyelectrolytes can also cause agglomeration due to a depletion effect resulting from the interaction between large colloidal particles in the presence of non-adsorbing, small species (Lewis, 2000).

2.2.2.4 Summary

- Dispersion = deagglomeration + stabilization
- Ultrasonication is the most efficient dispersion technique in terms of applied specific energy. Ultrasonication time and amplitude should be optimized
- Electrostatic stabilization: Measure of surface charge (zeta potential) by changing pH, adding salt (ionic strength)
- Steric stabilization: Adsorption of surfactant
- Electrosteric stabilization: Adsorption of polyelectrolytes

2.3   CHARACTERIZATION OF NANOPARTICLES SIZE

As explained in the introduction, size, morphology, and surface state are generally characterized to describe nanoparticles. A recent national study in France marks a standardization effort of the procedures and calibrations.

The main methods to obtain the size of nanoparticles include microscopic methods such as Transmission Electron Microscopy (TEM) and Scanning Electron Microscopy (SEM) and imply a description of average diameter and size distribution. An important point for TEM concerns the sample preparation. In standard conditions, a deposition of a diluted solution of nanoparticles is realized on grids. As a function of the nature of nanoparticles, a fixation of a sample with a negative staining material can prove necessary for organic or biological nanoparticles, for example. The most common negative staining materials are phosphotungstic acid and derivatives or uranyl acetate. This fixation by staining allows the use of standard TEM. If the use of cryo-TEM is possible, the staining will be unnecessary and the samples will be exposed to liquid nitrogen temperatures after embedding in vitreous ice to avoid damage to polymers or organic entities. For inorganic nanoparticles without interaction with biological media, a simple deposition on a standard grid will be sufficient to obtain a satisfying visualization. It is also possible to observe TEM inorganic nanoparticles embedded in an organic matrix (Houf et al., 2013; Mohan et al., 2015; Nguyen et al., 2013). For a one-size characterization of nanoparticles and particularly for an aggregation state characterization, the TEM technique which presents better resolution may be preferred to SEM as a vizualisation method. Nanoparticles 5 nm and smaller will be less well-visualized and the aggregation state will be characterized with difficulty. However, information about surface state can be obtained by emission of secondary electrons by nanoparticles. Concerning the work conditions, dry samples (powders) are generally used and should be conductive. If necessary to meet this requirement, a coating by a conductive material is possible by the deposition of a thin film of gold or carbon, for example, at the surface. For low conductivity materials, the use of carbon or copper tape may be sufficient to improve conductivity and reduce the preparation time of the samples. In standard conditions, SEM is a method best suited to inorganic materials. To overcome the difficulties in the organic or biological materials, work in several configurations is possible: High vacuum, low vacuum, and environmental scanning electron spectroscopy (ESEM), which can give some images of nanoparticles embedded in electrospun polymer nanofibers (Augustine et al., 2016). TEM may be coupled to energy-dispersive X-ray spectroscopy (EDS or EDX) for chemical analysis (Mohan et al., 2016). After characterization by TEM or SEM, the average diameter and size distribution can be determined with precision using software of image treatment from the size measurements of several hundred of nanoparticles. Currently, ImageJ is the software the most commonly used (Ferreira and Rasband, 2012).

Both methods are generally used with a complementary method on size particle: DLS. This technique, also known as photon correlation spectroscopy (PCS), is based on the Brownian movement of particles in colloidal suspension. The size is calculated considering the Doppler shift of a monochromatic light (laser or diode) by the particles. The resolution is in nano-micro ranges. In this model, all particles are assimilated as spheres. The technique doesn't allow access to the object's morphology. A size distribution can be determined considering intensity, number, and volume. Using the autocorrelation function of this technique and an evaluation in intensity will give information on the formation and proportion of aggregates or agglomerates in colloidal suspension. A distinction between aggregates and agglomerates is possible with a preliminary step of ultrasonication. With DLS equipment, detailed studies of the evolution of average hydrodynamic diameter as a function of external stimuli as pH and temperature are regularly reported (Chang et al., 2016), particularly for drug release applications. The comparison between the size determined by TEM or SEM measurements and the size obtained by DLS is regularly reported in literature now (Hall et al., 2007; Pichon et al., 2011) and considered an essential step in the characterization of nano-objects. At the same time, the comparison of size distribution calculated by these methods conducts an evaluation of the monodispersity of samples which allows for better control of properties. The exploitation of these complementary results implies a consideration of the nanoparticles' nature and analysis conditions. For example, whatever the shape of the nanoparticles, the DLS assimilates them as spheres while the manual image treatment of electronic microscopy micrographs are considered the morphology in their size determination. This may explain a first difference between the results. Another aspect relates to the nature of the nanoparticles. For example, as reported in a publication of Pichon et al. (2011), a surface functionalization of inorganic nanoparticles with organic molecules will lead to a difference in the evaluation of their average diameter. In this study (see Figure 2.9), the DLS provides access to the mean hydrodynamic diameter, which in this case corresponds to the addition of the inorganic core diameter and twice the thickness of the organic coating layer; the TEM measurements indicate the inorganic core only.

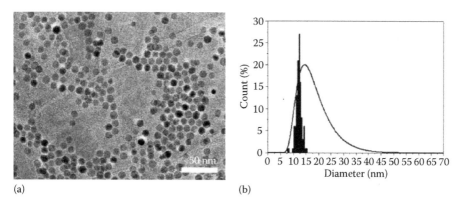

(a)   (b)

FIGURE 2.9   (a) TEM micrograph and (b) size distribution (histogram) and DLS measurements (line) of iron oxide nanoparticles with a surface coating. (From Pichon, B. P. et al., *Chem. Mater.*, 23, 2886–2900, 2011. With permission from the American Chemical Society.)

For functionalization of surface after synthesis with polymers, proteins, biological molecules, or antibodies, DLS technique will be a rapid first control of quality of surface functionalization, no-aggregation, and colloidal stability of samples considering the evolution of mean hydrodynamic diameter measured. An example was reported by Casals et al. (2010; see Figure 2.10). In this study of time evolution of the nanoparticle protein corona, the DLS allows the characterization of the stability and the surface state of the NPs. The conjugation of proteins to nanoparticles is evidenced by the increase of hydrodynamic diameter.

It is important to remember the influence of surface functionalization by these organic molecules on the Brownian motion of nanoparticles before an exploitation of DLS data. These entities are at the origin of a significant frictional drag, so an increase in their rate in suspension implies an increase of Brownian diffusion and an artificial increase of a measured hydrodynamic diameter. Viscosity, concentration, and temperature of suspension constitute essential parameters for DLS because they affect the Brownian motion of nanoparticles. A sample dilution should be preferred and the concentration of nanoparticles should be considered in light of recommendations specific to the used equipment. The sample temperature should be precisely controlled and the variation of the solvent viscosity with the temperature should be considered. Lim et al. (2013) provide a review of the use of DLS. The review focuses on the size study and the colloidal stability of iron oxide nanoparticles as an example. Methods of measurements and mathematical analysis, precautions, advantages, and limitations are reported and influences of surface coating, size differences, morphology, and concentration of particles are considered.

Concerning the size determination of crystallized inorganic nanoparticles, in numerous publications (Jang et al., 2013; Rao et al., 2009) these results are compared at a size determined by XRD. In this method of structural characterization,

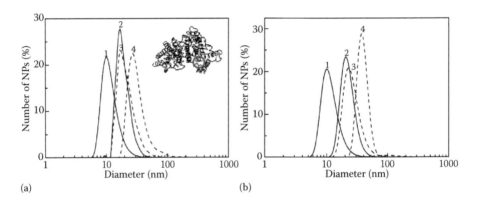

FIGURE 2.10 Analysis of the hard protein corona (PC) coating (a) and bovine serum albumin (BSA) conjugates (b) with BSA specific antibody and anti-IgG antibody. Increase of mean hydrodynamic diameter measured by DLS of (1) AuNPs, (2) AuNPs-hard PC, (3) AuNPs-hard PC _ IgG antibody, and (4) AuNPs-hard PC _ BSA-antibody. (From Casals, E., Pfaller, T., Duschl, A., Oostingh, G. J., and Puntes, V., *ACS Nano*, 4, 3623–3632, 2010. With permission from American Chemical Society.)

an exploitation of the width of the diffraction peak full width at half maximum (FWHM) allows the determination of a crystallite size considering the Scherrer equation (Monshi et al., 2012):

$$B(2\theta) = \frac{K\lambda}{L\cos\theta} \quad B(2\theta) = \frac{K\lambda}{L\cos\theta}$$

where L is the average crystallite size (nm), K is the shape factor, λ is the X-ray wavelength (nm), B is the diffraction peak FWHM corrected for instrumental broadening (radians), and θ is the Bragg angle of diffraction.

For a more accurate result, the FWHM can be corrected by taking into account the instrumental broadening characteristic of the used instrument as the X-ray wavelength λ. The shape factor K (the Scherrer constant) considered as a constant of proportionality depends on how the width is determined, the shape of the crystal, and the size distribution. The most common value for K is 0.94 for FWHM of spherical crystals with cubic crystalline symmetry and 0.89 for integral breadth of spherical crystals with other symmetry. The crystallite size is equal to the size determined by the TEM or SEM measurements if the nanoparticle is a perfect crystal. The crystallite size will be smaller than the size obtained by microscopy if defects are present. A nano-object may be composed of several crystallites and microstrains that are very common in nanocrystalline materials. For an evaluation of the relevance of the comparison between the results of microscopy and diffraction, it may be interesting to calculate the degree of crystallinity of samples (Pang and Bao, 2003).

In addition to these classical techniques of the characterization of nanoparticle size, a size measurement can be realized with a high resolution by atomic force microscopy (AFM). For a simple size determination, the AFM isn't the first method of choice. The results registered with this technique are generally reported in correlation with a study of specific properties or surface state and the determined size is compared with TEM or SEM micrographs. However, for a nonconductive material, AFM is an advantageous method compared with SEM because it is without special sample preparation. AFM can also provide a size measurement in different media and biological conditions without the constraints associated with type (crystalline or amorphous for example) of nanoparticles (Polakovic et al., 1999; Shi et al., 2003). Contrary to TEM, a fixation with staining will not be necessary and there is no requirement for high vacuum; contrary to SEM, the nature of samples (polymeric, organic, and biological nanoparticles) will involve no specific experimental conditions (high vacuum, low vacuum, or ESEM). Muhlen et al. (1996) reported studies of solid lipid nanoparticles by AFM with an ultra-high resolution in particle size measurement based on a physical scanning of samples at the sub-micron level using a probe tip of atomic scale. Dobrovolskaia et al. (2009) reported a gold nanoparticle size using AFM (Figure 2.11) before and after plasma incubation performing lateral interactions between the AFM tip, gold colloid, and plasma proteins with AFM measurements by

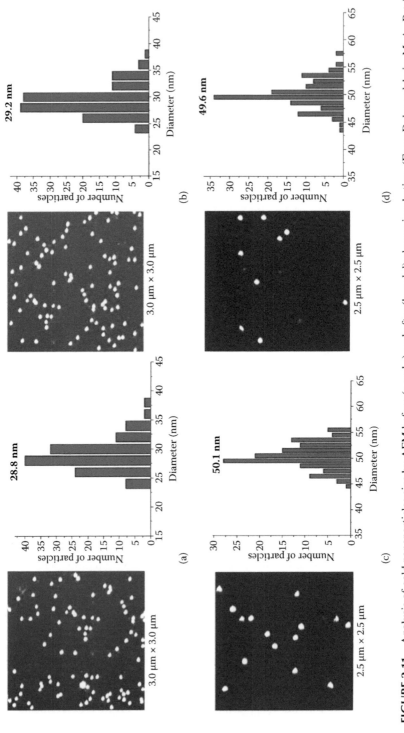

FIGURE 2.11 Analysis of gold nanoparticles size by AFM before (a and c) and after (b and d) plasma incubation. (From Dobrovolskaia, M. A., Patri, A. K., Zheng, J., Clogston, J. D., Ayub, N., Aggarwal, P., Neun, B. W., Hall, J. B., and McNeil, S. E. *Nanomedicine Nanotechnol. Biol. Med.*, 5, 106–117, 2009. With permission from Elsevier.)

tipping in-liquid mode. This analysis allowed a study of the plasma protein effect on nanoparticle size to determine the interactions between colloidal gold nanoparticles and human blood. In this work, AFM measurements have been compared with TEM and DLS analysis considering the complementarity of these techniques and precautions to be taken in interpreting the results as previously mentioned.

2.4 CHARACTERIZATION OF NANOPARTICLES MORPHOLOGY AND STRUCTURE

As for size determination, the morphology characterization of nano-objects is systematically realized with TEM (Figure 2.12a,c,e) or SEM (Figure 2.12b,d,f) in a first time. Considering the previously mentioned characteristics of the two techniques, TEM will allow characterization of isolated nanoparticles or dilution of samples with higher magnification by comparison with SEM. In Figure 2.12 (b,d,f), SEM images allow us to consider the samples' homogeneity for a great number of nanoparticles.

Crassous et al. (2006) demonstrated that cryogenic transmission electron microscopy (cryo-TEM) is the privileged method to characterize the morphology of microgels in situ (Figure 2.13). This microscopy method can be employed for different natures of nanoparticles with a visualization of a core–shell structure where organic entities are implied (Ballauff and Lu, 2007). At the core–shell interface, cryo-TEM can indicate defaults and inhomogeneities, for example, with a fluctuation of density resulting in non-homogenous chemical links. A characterization of nanomaterials/biological cell interaction can be optimized with cryo-TEM. This technique allows a direct investigation of morphology without staining (Nizri et al., 2009, 2004).

For microgel nanoparticles, light scattering techniques can be considered the methods of choice for structural analysis of microgel particles. Many investigations are performed on microgels using dynamic light scattering (DLS) or static light scattering (SLS; Saunders and Vincent, 1999). With the aim of a characterization of structural and phase behavior for nanoparticles with stimuli-responsive properties, for example, these techniques have been used in a complementary approach with NMR spectroscopy (Maherani et al., 2012; Nakabayashi et al., 2016) or small-angle neutron scattering (SANS) and small angle X-ray scattering (SAXS; Dingenouts et al., 2001, 1998).

AFM can be applied to investigate the morphology of nanoparticle in agreement with a study of their properties or as a function of nature and composition (Eschbach et al., 2007; Maherani et al., 2012). For example, in a work reported in 2009, morphology and the aggregation state of Chitosan–DNA complexes were investigated by AFM (Yuan et al., 2009). In the same work, the AFM technique was used to investigate the morphology of HeLa cells transfected with Chitosan–siRNA complexes and realize a study of cell surface with a three-dimensional map of the cell ultrastructure. In a previous work, Kumar et al. (2008) characterized the triangular morphology of gold nanoparticles well-dispersed on a mica surface (Figure 2.14). Distance between particles, size, surface height and length profile have been determined too and the heterogeneity of sample has been considered.

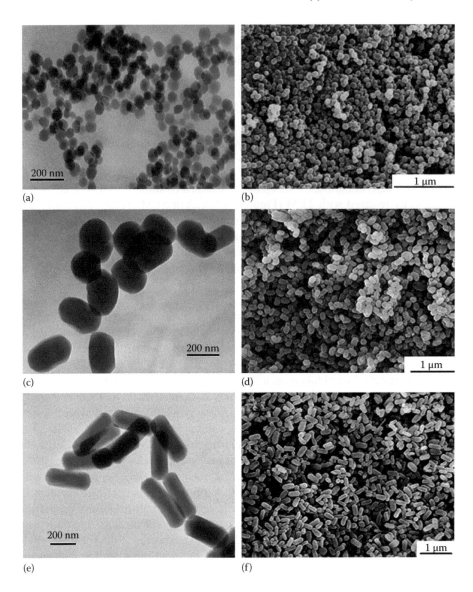

FIGURE 2.12 TEM and SEM images of three different-shaped mesoporous silica nanoparticles. (a, c, e) TEM images of sphere-shaped particles (a), short rod-shaped particles (c), and long rod-shaped particles (e). (b, d, f) SEM images of sphere-shaped particles (b), short rod-shaped particles (d), and long rod-shaped particles (f). (From Huang, X., Teng, X., Chen, D., Tang, F., and He, J., *Biomaterials*, 31, 438–448, 2010. With permission from Elsevier.)

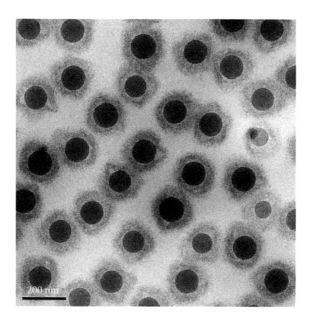

FIGURE 2.13   Cryo-TEM image of core-shell microgel particles. (From Crassous, J. J., Ballauff, M., Drechsler, M., Schmidt, J., and Talmon, Y., *Langmuir*, 22, 2403–2406, 2006. With permission from the American Chemical Society.)

With a more brightness of electron beam compared to SEM, TEM presents a higher resolution. Information can be provided at the atomic scale and on the crystalline structure (Baaziz et al., 2014; Pichon et al., 2011; Schneidewind et al., 2012; see Figure 2.15). Indeed, to obtain a better understanding and characterization of inorganic nanoparticles structure, a combination of techniques such as XRD (previously cited to obtain a crystallite size) and transmission electron microscopy (TEM) or high resolution–transmission electron microscopy (HR-TEM) can be used. In 2011, Pichon et al. exploited a combination of techniques to determine the morphology of iron oxide nanoparticles and the crystal structure of these nanoparticles since several iron oxides exist: FeO, Fe_3O_4, and Fe_2O_3. Spherical (Figure 2.15a) and cubic (Figure 2.15b,c) can be observed on HR-TEM images. A homogeneous contrast is observed for spherical-shaped nanoparticles. On the other hand, a non-homogeneous contrast is observed for cubic-shaped nanoparticles with a difference between the inner and the outer parts associated with different orientations of structure planes and characteristic of crystalline structure. In this study, the result of both HR-TEM and XRD analysis demonstrated a core–shell structure for cubic-shaped nanoparticles with a wüstite core and a spinel shell.

A structural investigation of nano-objects by Schneidewind et al. (2012) with a scanning transmission electron microscopy (STEM) demonstrated the crystal structure of individual silver nanoparticles with atomic planes of silver visible on high-resolution images and characterized by comparison with a reference diffraction pattern. In Figure 2.16, HR-TEM images of iron oxide nanoparticles in a study by

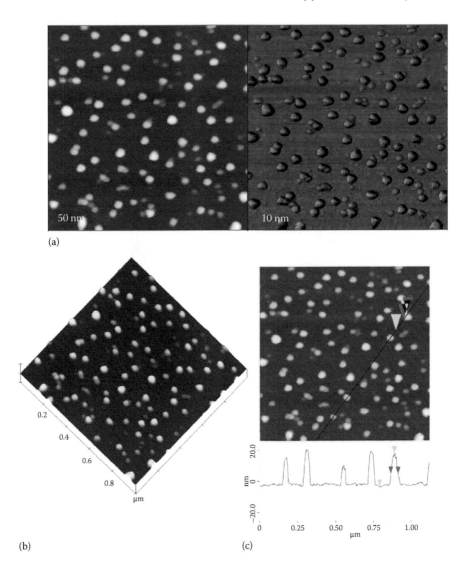

FIGURE 2.14 AFM images of the gold nanoparticles. (a) Topographical image. (b) Three-dimensional view. (c) Surface height and length profile of a selected set (black line) of the triangular nanoparticles seen in (b). (From Kumar, S. A., Peter, Y.-A., and Nadeau, J. L., *Nanotechnology*, 19, 495101, 2008. With permission from IOP Publishing.)

Baaziz et al. (2014) are presented. These images show different crystalline planes. The distance between planes has been determined and reported in Figure 2.16. These distances are characteristic of an orientation of nanoparticles and exhibit (422), (311), and (111) plans of a spinel structure (magnetite or maghemite for iron oxides) as reported. A complementary XRD analysis is able to confirm the crystalline nanoparticles composition.

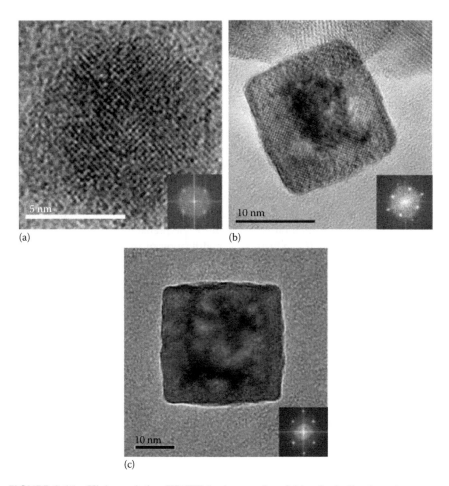

FIGURE 2.15 High resolution HR-TEM micrographs of (a) spherically shaped nanoparticles and (b,c) cubic-shaped nanoparticles. (From Pichon, B. P. et al., *Chem. Mater.*, 23, 2886–2900, 2011. With permission from the American Chemical Society.)

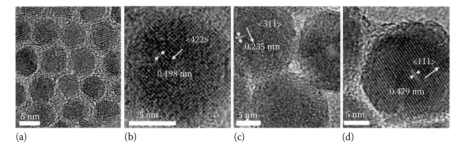

FIGURE 2.16 High-resolution TEM images of iron oxide nanoparticles of (a) 5 nm, (b) 11 nm, (c) 15 nm and (d) 20 nm. Crystalline planes and distances between planes are reported on (b), (c), and (d). (From Baaziz, W. et al., *J. Phys. Chem. C*, 118, 3795–3810, 2014. With permission from the American Chemical Society.)

2.5   PHYSICOCHEMICAL CHARACTERIZATION OF NANOPARTICLES

Other important parameters in the characterization of nanoparticles are the elemental composition and physicochemical characterization. The surface state of nanoparticles can evolve in interaction with the biological environment. Concerning physicochemical and chemical composition characterization of nanoparticles, TEM and SEM can be coupled with chemical analysis detectors (Schneidewind et al., 2012). But a limitation can be observed with the samples scale and the preparation methods, which could alter the physicochemical state of nanoparticles. TEM coupled with energy dispersion spectroscopy (EDS) or electron energy loss spectroscopy (EELS) is limited, considering the dispersion and thickness of analyzed samples. The high energy of a primary beam allowing penetration could be caused by artifacts. Another limitation is the result of the preparation of samples by fixation with staining, which conducts at a modification of the chemical composition and interactions. In good experimental conditions, the EELS will allow a differentiation of different forms of an element or the characterization of nanoparticle functionalization or encapsulation by an organic shell (Park et al., 2005). For SEM coupled with EDS, the excitation volume limits the information of chemical interactions for core–shell structures, for example. The registered results must be compared with other techniques for a complete chemical characterization of nanoparticles. The improvement of this characterization part leads to the development of original protocols in parallel with new nano-objects synthesis. For example, in a publication from 2015, Soulé et al. use two techniques in an original and complementary approach: X-ray photoelectron spectroscopy (XPS) and solution- and solid-state NMR to characterize thermoresponsive core–shell inorganic–organic nanoparticles and to allow the study of chemical interactions of hybrid interfaces at the nanoparticle surface. In a previous work (Ledeuil et al., 2014), the same team reports an original route to achieve a morphological and chemical characterization of a core–shell Ag–Au alloy/ SiO_2 nanostructures by a coupled study with SEM, XPS, and auger (known also AES auger electron spectroscopy) methods as high-resolution techniques to overcome the limits of detection.

Indeed, in this work, a chemical resolution of these core–shell nanostructures was carried out by the AES characterization of two characteristic points after a sample cross-cut as reported in Figure 2.17a; points 1 and 2 are characteristics of the core and shell, respectively. Both AES spectra presented in Figure 2.17b indicate the synthesis of an Ag–Au core and a SiO_2 shell for these nanoparticles.

In the same work, a high-resolution auger mapping was conducted on a single cross-cut nanoparticle (Figure 2.18) to show a ring of Ag–Au alloys with a shell of pure SiO_2.

In the complementary way, the chemical analysis of the components of the nanoparticles may be made by ICP-MS. A study using infrared spectroscopy will allow a better understanding of the surface state of nanoparticles, in particular. The interactions and the nanoparticles' nature can be characterized on powder or in various media by this method for a comparison with other analysis techniques (Raman, RMN, XPS, etc.).

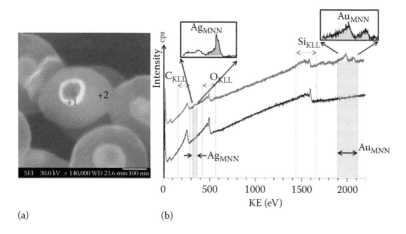

(a)   (b)

FIGURE 2.17   Analysis of point 1 and point 2 of a cross-cut Ag/Au@SiO$_2$ nanoparticle: (a) high magnification SEM image and (b) the corresponding wide energy range AES spectra. (From Ledeuil, J. B., Uhart, A., Soulé, S., Allouche, J., Dupin, J. C., and Martinez, H., *Nanoscale*, 6, 11130–11140, 2014. With permission from the Royal Society of Chemistry.)

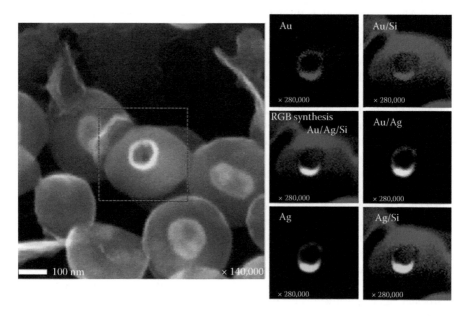

FIGURE 2.18   High resolution auger mapping (SAM) of a single cross-cut Ag/Au@SiO$_2$ nanoparticle (red-dotted square in the left SEM image)—RGB synthesis from element SAM overlays (right): Red (Au); green (Ag); and blue (Si). (From Ledeuil, J. B., Uhart, A., Soulé, S., Allouche, J., Dupin, J. C., and Martinez, H., *Nanoscale*, 6, 11130–11140, 2014. With permission from the Royal Society of Chemistry.)

2.6   CONCLUSION

The nanoparticle properties result from a combination of physicochemical parameters, including the size, chemical composition, shape, surface condition, and so on. To some extent, these properties can be modulated by varying one of these parameters: For the size, this is the case of optical properties in quantum dots (like CdSe nanoparticles), but also of magnetism in iron oxide nanocrystals (Fe_3O_4).

With this plurality of parameters defining a nanoparticle, it is clear that no characterization techniques described in this chapter may be used alone to characterize it efficiently. But this is even the case for a single specific parameter such as particle size: We showed in this chapter that only a combination of several measurement methods may lead to obtaining an accurate, reliable, and robust measure. In recent literature, more and more studies have incorporated the importance of combining multiple methods of characterization—at least TEM and DLS techniques for the nanoparticle size.

However, with our present state of knowledge, it is not yet possible to define a standard protocol adapted to the characterization of all nanomaterials; indeed, observed differences in behavior among nanomaterials are too important. Such a lack prevents, in particular, an ability to obtain predictive and strongly relevant toxicological studies. Necessary efforts are underway to try to harmonize procedures for studies, for example, through the recent European research projects Nanogenotox and NANoREG, as well as through several studies in United States (Bonner et al., 2013; Xia et al., 2013). These works aim at obtaining standard operating procedures, including a measurement uncertainty evaluation and a metrological traceability.

It should be noted also that by routine laboratory methods it is often difficult to produce nanomaterials in large quantities. Of course this is not the case for the few nanomaterials produced industrially, like silica SiO_2, carbon black (including carbon nanotubes), titanium dioxide TiO_2, and alumina Al_2O_3 (in tonnage, these four families represent 95 percent of the market), but these nanoparticles are generally not involved in biomedical applications. When NPs are produced in laboratory conditions, the low quantity available may be a limitation to toxicological studies that require enough material to perform both *in vitro* and *in vivo* studies, but also all the characterizations described in this chapter. In this context it may be interesting to select analytical techniques that consume few NPs (like DLS) or allow retrieving them after the analysis (such as XRD).

One of the challenges remains the physicochemical as well as toxicological characterization of nanomaterials in organs or in matrices close to biological media. The usual characterization techniques described in this chapter may rarely be used in complex organic media (the exceptions are environmental MEB and AFM dedicated to biological media, or specific applications like cryo-TEM). Aggregation or agglomeration state in particular can be greatly affected by the environment. And in a complex environment, nanoparticles are usually coated with an adsorption layer (for instance, the formation of a protein corona by interaction with endogenous proteins) that can evidently alter their chemical and biological reactivity and limit for instance the drug delivery.

Also, for biomedical applications of nanomaterials, it would be appropriate to make biokinetic studies prior to toxicological studies and parallel to physicochemical characterizations, in order to identify target organs and levels of internal dose. This would justify, in the toxicological study, the choice of specific cells and of the maximum concentrations which will be tested *in vitro* and *in vivo* (Anses, 2015).

REFERENCES

Anses. 2015. Assessment of the risks associated with nanomaterials: Issues and update of current knowledge.

Augustine, R., Sarry, F., Kalarikkal, N., Thomas, S., Badie, L., and Rouxel, D. 2016. Surface acoustic wave device with reduced insertion loss by electrospinning P(VDF–TrFE)/ZnO nanocomposites. *Nano-Micro. Lett.* 8:282–290. doi:10.1007/s40820-016-0088-2.

Baaziz, W., Pichon, B. P., Fleutot, S., Liu, Y., Lefevre, C., Greneche, J.-M., Toumi, M., Mhiri, T., and Begin-Colin, S. 2014. Magnetic iron oxide nanoparticles: Reproducible tuning of the size and nanosized-dependent composition, defects, and spin canting. *J. Phys. Chem. C* 118:3795–3810. doi:10.1021/jp411481p.

Bałdyga, J., Orciuch, W., Makowski, Ł., Malik, K., Özcan-Taşkin, G., Eagles, W., and Padron, G. 2008. Dispersion of nanoparticle clusters in a rotor–stator mixer. *Ind. Eng. Chem. Res.* 47:3652–3663. doi:10.1021/ie070899u.

Ballauff, M., and Lu, Y. 2007. "Smart" nanoparticles: Preparation, characterization and applications. *Polymer* 48:1815–1823. doi:10.1016/j.polymer.2007.02.004.

Bonner, J. C., Silva, R. M., Taylor, A. J., Brown, J. M., Hilderbrand, S. C., Castranova, V., Porter, D., Elder, A., Oberdörster, G., Harkema, J. R., Bramble, L. A., Kavanagh, T. J., Botta, D., Nel, A., and Pinkerton, K. E. 2013. Interlaboratory Evaluation of Rodent Pulmonary Responses to Engineered Nanomaterials: The NIEHS Nano GO Consortium. *Environ. Health Perspect.* 121:676–682. doi:10.1289/ehp.1205693.

Casals, E., Pfaller, T., Duschl, A., Oostingh, G. J., and Puntes, V. 2010. Time evolution of the nanoparticle protein corona. *ACS Nano* 4:3623–3632. doi:10.1021/nn901372t.

Chang, R., Tian, Y., Wang, Y., and Qin, J. 2016. pH-responsive vesicles with tunable membrane permeability and hydrodynamic diameters from a cross-linkable amphiphilic block copolymer. *Nanomater. Nanotechnol.* 1. doi:10.5772/6215.1.

Chicea, D., Indrea, E., and Cretu, C. M. 2012. Assesing Fe_3O_4 nanoparticle size by DLS, XRD and AFM. *J. Optoelectron. Adv. Mater.* 14:460.

Crassous, J. J., Ballauff, M., Drechsler, M., Schmidt, J., and Talmon, Y. 2006. Imaging the volume transition in thermosensitive core–shell particles by cryo-transmission electron microscopy. *Langmuir* 22:2403–2406. doi:10.1021/la053198f.

Debenedetti, P. G., Tom, J. W., Kwauk, X., and Yeo, S.-D. 1993. Rapid expansion of supercritical solutions (ress): Fundamentals and applications. *Fluid Phase Equilib.* 82:311–321. doi:10.1016/0378-3812(93)87155-T.

Dingenouts, N., Norhausen, C., and Ballauff, M. 1998. Observation of the volume transition in thermosensitive core–shell latex particles by small-angle x-ray scattering. *Macromolecules* 31:8912–8917. doi:10.1021/ma980985t.

Dingenouts, N., Seelenmeyer, S., Deike, I., Rosenfeldt, S., Ballauff, M., Lindner, P., and Narayanan, T. 2001. Analysis of thermosensitive core–shell colloids by small-angle neutron scattering including contrast variation. *Phys. Chem. Chem. Phys.* 3:1169–1174. doi:10.1039/b009104i.

Dobrovolskaia, M. A., Patri, A. K., Zheng, J., Clogston, J. D., Ayub, N., Aggarwal, P., Neun, B. W., Hall, J. B., and McNeil, S. E. 2009. Interaction of colloidal gold nanoparticles with human blood: Effects on particle size and analysis of plasma protein binding profiles. *Nanomedicine Nanotechnol. Biol. Med.* 5:106–117. doi:10.1016/j.nano.2008.08.001.

Eschbach, J., Rouxel, D., Vincent, B., Mugnier, Y., Galez, C., Le Dantec, R., Bourson, P., Krüger, J. K., Elmazria, O., and Alnot, P. 2007. Development and characterization of nanocomposite materials. *Mater. Sci. Eng. C* 27:1260–1264. doi:10.1016/j .msec.2006.07.035.

Fabrega, J., Renshaw, J. C., and Lead, J. R. 2009. Interactions of silver nanoparticles with *Pseudomonas putida* biofilms. *Environ. Sci. Technol.* 43:9004–9009. doi:10.1021 /es901706j.

Ferreira, T., and Rasband, W. 2012. *ImageJ User Guide.*

Gaiser, B. K., Fernandes, T. F., Jepson, M., Lead, J. R., Tyler, C. R., and Stone, V. 2009. Assessing exposure, uptake and toxicity of silver and cerium dioxide nanoparticles from contaminated environments. *Environ. Health* 8:S2. doi:10.1186/1476-069X-8-S1-S2.

García-Alonso, J., Khan, F. R., Misra, S. K., Turmaine, M., Smith, B. D., Rainbow, P. S., Luoma, S. N., and Valsami-Jones, E. 2011. Cellular internalization of silver nanoparticles in gut epithelia of the estuarine polychaete *Nereis diversicolor. Environ. Sci. Technol.* 45:4630–4636. doi:10.1021/es2005122.

Greenwood, R. 2003. Review of the measurement of zeta potentials in concentrated aqueous suspensions using electroacoustics. *Adv. Colloid Interface Sci.* 106:55–81. doi:10.1016 /S0001-8686(03)00105-2.

Greulich, C., Kittler, S., Epple, M., Muhr, G., and Köller, M. 2009. Studies on the biocompatibility and the interaction of silver nanoparticles with human mesenchymal stem cells (hMSCs). *Langenbecks Arch. Surg.* 394:495–502. doi:10.1007 /s00423-009-0472-1.

Griffitt, R. J., Luo, J., Gao, J., Bonzongo, J.-C., and Barber, D. S. 2008. Effects of particle composition and species on toxicity of metallic nanomaterials in aquatic organisms. *Environ. Toxicol. Chem.* 27:1972–1978.

Haase, A., Rott, S., Mantion, A., Graf, P., Plendl, J., Thunemann, A. F., Meier, W. P., Taubert, A., Luch, A., and Reiser, G. 2012. Effects of silver nanoparticles on primary mixed neural cell cultures: Uptake, oxidative stress and acute calcium responses. *Toxicol. Sci.* 126:457–468. doi:10.1093/toxsci/kfs003.

Hall, J. B., Dobrovolskaia, M. A., Patri, A. K., and McNeil, S. E. 2007. Characterization of nanoparticles for therapeutics. *Nanomed.* 2:789–803. doi:10.2217/17435889 .2.6.789.

Houf, L., Mugnier, Y., Rouxel, D., Le Dantec, R., Badie, L., Vincent, B., Coustal, C., Beauquis, S., Thevenet, C., and Galez, C. 2013. Preparation of transparent PMMA/ Fe(IO$_3$)$_3$ nanocomposite films from microemulsion polymerization. *J. Appl. Polym. Sci.* 130:1203–1211. doi:10.1002/app.39271.

Huang, X., Teng, X., Chen, D., Tang, F., and He, J. 2010. The effect of the shape of mesoporous silica nanoparticles on cellular uptake and cell function. *Biomaterials* 31:438–448. doi:10.1016/j.biomaterials.2009.09.060.

Jang, J.-H., Lee, E., Park, J., Kim, G., Hong, S., and Kwon, Y.-U. 2013. Rational syntheses of core-shell Fex@Pt nanoparticles for the study of electrocatalytic oxygen reduction reaction. *Sci. Rep.* 3. doi:10.1038/srep02872.

Jiang, J., Oberdorster, G., and Biswas, P. 2009. Characterization of size, surface charge, and agglomeration state of nanoparticle dispersions for toxicological studies. *J. Nanoparticle Res.* 11:77–89. doi:10.1007/s11051-008-9446-4.

Kennedy, A. J., Hull, M. S., Bednar, A. J., Goss, J. D., Gunter, J. C., Bouldin, J. L., Vikesland, P. J., and Stevens, J. A. 2010. Fractionating nanosilver: Importance for determining toxicity to aquatic test organisms. *Environ. Sci. Technol.* 44:9571–9577.

Khan, Z., Al-Thabaiti, S. A., Obaid, A. Y., and Al-Youbi, A. O. 2011. Preparation and characterization of silver nanoparticles by chemical reduction method. *Colloids Surf. B Biointerfaces* 82:513–517. doi:10.1016/j.colsurfb.2010.10.008.

Kumar, S. A., Peter, Y.-A., and Nadeau, J. L. 2008. Facile biosynthesis, separation and conjugation of gold nanoparticles to doxorubicin. *Nanotechnology* 19:495101. doi:10.1088/0957-4484/19/49/495101.

Ledeuil, J. B., Uhart, A., Soulé, S., Allouche, J., Dupin, J. C., and Martinez, H. 2014. New insights into micro/nanoscale combined probes (nanoAuger, µXPS) to characterize Ag/Au@SiO_2 core–shell assemblies. *Nanoscale* 6:11130–11140. doi:10.1039 /C4NR03211J.

Lewis, J. A. 2000. Colloidal processing of ceramics. *J. Am. Ceram. Soc.* 83:2341–2359. doi:10.1111/j.1151-2916.2000.tb01560.x.

Li, C., Li, D., Wan, G., Xu, J., and Hou, W. 2011. Facile synthesis of concentrated gold nanoparticles with low size-distribution in water: Temperature and pH controls. *Nanoscale Res. Lett.* 6:1–10.

Lim, J., Yeap, S. P., Che, H. X., and Low, S. C. 2013. Characterization of magnetic nanoparticle by dynamic light scattering. *Nanoscale Res. Lett.* 8:1–14.

Maherani, B., Arab-Tehrany, E., Kheirolomoom, A., Cleymand, F., and Linder, M. 2012. Influence of lipid composition on physicochemical properties of nanoliposomes encapsulating natural dipeptide antioxidant l-carnosine. *Food Chem.* 134:632–640. doi:10.1016/j.foodchem.2012.02.098.

Mandzy, N., Grulke, E., and Druffel, T. 2005. Breakage of TiO_2 agglomerates in electrostatically stabilized aqueous dispersions. *Powder Technol.* 160:121–126.

Martínez-Castañón, G. A., Niño-Martínez, N., Martínez-Gutierrez, F., Martínez-Mendoza, J. R., and Ruiz, F. 2008. Synthesis and antibacterial activity of silver nanoparticles with different sizes. *J. Nanoparticle Res.* 10:1343–1348. doi:10.1007/s11051-008-9428-6.

Mohan, S., Oluwafemi, O. S., Songca, S. P., George, S. C., Miska, P., Rouxel, D., Kalarikkal, N., and Thomas, S. 2015. Green synthesis of yellow emitting PMMA–CdSe/ZnS quantum dots nanophosphors. *Mater. Sci. Semicond. Process.* 39:587–595. doi:10.1016/j mssp.2015.05.070.

Mohan, S., Oluwafemi, O. S., Songca, S. P., Jayachandran, V. P., Rouxel, D., Joubert, O., Kalarikkal, N., and Thomas, S. 2016. Synthesis, antibacterial, cytotoxicity and sensing properties of starch-capped silver nanoparticles. *J. Mol. Liq.* 213:75–81. doi:10.1016/j .molliq.2015.11.010.

Monshi, A., Foroughi, M. R., and Monshi, M. R. 2012. Modified Scherrer equation to estimate more accurately nano-crystallite size using XRD. *World J. Nano Sci. Eng.* 2:154–160. doi:10.4236/wjnse.2012.23020.

Muhlen, A., Muhlen, E., Niehus, H., and Mehnert, W. 1996. Atomic force microscopy studies of solid lipid nanoparticles. *Pharm Res* 1411–1416.

Mukherjee, S. G., O'Claonadh, N., Casey, A., and Chambers, G. 2012. Comparative in vitro cytotoxicity study of silver nanoparticle on two mammalian cell lines. *Toxicol. In Vitro* 26:238–251. doi:10.1016/j.tiv.2011.12.004.

Nakabayashi, K., Noda, D., Takahashi, T., and Mori, H. 2016. Design of stimuli-responsive nanoparticles with optoelectronic cores by post-assembly cross-linking and self-assembly of functionalized block copolymers. *Polymer* 86:56–68. doi:10.1016/j.polymer.2016.01.029.

Nanogenotox. 2013. Nanogenotox Final Report.

Nguyen, V. S., Badie, L., Lamouroux, E., Vincent, B., Santos, F. D. D., Aufray, M., Fort, Y., and Rouxel, D. 2013. Nanocomposite piezoelectric films of P(VDF-TrFE)/$LiNbO_3$. *J. Appl. Polym. Sci.* 129:391–396. doi:10.1002/app.38746.

Nguyen, V. S., Rouxel, D., Hadji, R., Vincent, B., and Fort, Y. 2011. Effect of ultrasonication and dispersion stability on the cluster size of alumina nanoscale particles in aqueous solutions. *Ultrason. Sonochem.* 18:382–388. doi:10.1016/j.ultsonch.2010.07.003.

Nguyen, V. S., Rouxel, D., and Vincent, B. 2014. Dispersion of nanoparticles: From organic solvents to polymer solutions. *Ultrason. Sonochem.* 21:149–153. doi:10.1016/j .ultsonch.2013.07.015.

Nizri, G., Magdassi, S., Schmidt, J., Cohen, Y., and Talmon, Y. 2004. Microstructural characterization of micro- and nanoparticles formed by polymer–surfactant interactions. *Langmuir* 20:4380–4385. doi:10.1021/la0364441.

Nizri, G., Makarski, A., Magdassi, S., and Talmon, Y. 2009. Nanostructures formed by self-assembly of negatively charged polymer and cationic surfactants. *Langmuir* 1980–1985.

Pal, S. L., Jana, U., Manna, P. K., Mohanta, G. P., and Manavalan, R. 2011. Nanoparticle: An overview of preparation and characterization. *J. Appl. Pharm. Sci.* 1:228–234.

Pang, Y. X., and Bao, X. 2003. Influence of temperature, ripening time and calcination on the morphology and crystallinity of hydroxyapatite nanoparticles. *J. Eur. Ceram. Soc.* 23:1697–1704.

Park, S.-H., Oh, S.-G., Mun, J.-Y., and Han, S.-S. 2005. Effects of silver nanoparticles on the fluidity of bilayer in phospholipid liposome. *Colloids Surf. B Biointerfaces* 44:117–122. doi:10.1016/j.colsurfb.2005.06.002.

Pichon, B. P., Gerber, O., Lefevre, C., Florea, I., Fleutot, S., Baaziz, W., Pauly, M., Ohlmann, M., Ulhaq, C., Ersen, O., Pierron-Bohnes, V., Panissod, P., Drillon, M., and Begin-Colin, S. 2011. Microstructural and magnetic investigations of wüstite-spinel core-shell cubic-shaped nanoparticles. *Chem. Mater.* 23:2886–2900. doi:10.1021/cm2003319.

Polakovic, M., Gorner, T., Gref, R., and Dellacherie, E. 1999. Lidocaine loaded biodegradable nanospheres II. Modelling of drug release. *J Control Release* 60(2–3):169–77

Rao, Y., Antalek, B., Minter, J., Mourey, T., Blanton, T., Slater, G., Slater, L., and Fornalik, J. 2009. Organic solvent-dispersed TiO_2 nanoparticle characterization. *Langmuir* 25:12713–12720. doi:10.1021/la901783g.

Roh, J., Sim, S. J., Yi, J., Park, K., Chung, K. H., Ryu, D., and Choi, J. 2009. Ecotoxicity of silver nanoparticles on the soil nematode *Caenorhabditis elegans* using functional eco-toxicogenomics. *Environ. Sci. Technol.* 43:3933–3940. doi:10.1021/es803477u.

Sato, K., Li, J., Kamiya, H., and Ishigaki, T. 2008. Ultrasonic dispersion of TiO_2 nanoparticles in aqueous suspension. *J. Am. Ceram. Soc.* 91:2481–2487. doi:10.1111/j.1551-2916.2008 .02493.x.

Saunders, B. R., and Vincent, B. 1999. Microgel particles as model colloids: Theory, properties and applications. *Adv. Colloid Interface Sci.* 80:1–25.

Sauter, C., Emin, M. A., Schuchmann, H. P., and Tavman, S. 2008. Influence of hydrostatic pressure and sound amplitude on the ultrasound induced dispersion and de-agglomeration of nanoparticles. *Ultrason. Sonochem.* 15:517–523. doi:10.1016/j.ultsonch.2007.08.010.

Schilde, C., Mages-Sauter, C., Kwade, A., and Schuchmann, H. P. 2011. Efficiency of different dispersing devices for dispersing nanosized silica and alumina. *Powder Technol.* 207:353–361. doi:10.1016/j.powtec.2010.11.019.

Schneidewind, H., Schüler, T., Strelau, K. K., Weber, K., Cialla, D., Diegel, M., Mattheis, R., Berger, A., Möller, R., and Popp, J. 2012. The morphology of silver nanoparticles prepared by enzyme-induced reduction. *Beilstein J. Nanotechnol.* 3:404–414. doi:10.3762 /bjnano.3.47.

Shi, H., Farber, L., Michaels, J., Dickey, A., Thompson, K., Shelukar, S., Hurter, P., Reynolds, S., and Kaufman, M. 2003. Characterization of crystalline drug nanoparticles using atomic force microscopy and complementary techniques. *Pharm Res* 479–484.

Soulé, S., Allouche, J., Dupin, J.-C., Courrèges, C., Plantier, F., Ojo, W.-S., Coppel, Y., Nayral, C., Delpech, F., and Martinez, H. 2015. Thermoresponsive gold nanoshell@ mesoporous silica nano-assemblies: An XPS/NMR survey. *Phys Chem Chem Phys* 17:28719–28728. doi:10.1039/C5CP04491J.

To, D., Dave, R., Yin, X., and Sundaresan, S. 2009. Deagglomeration of nanoparticle aggregates via rapid expansion of supercritical or high-pressure suspensions. *AIChE J.* 55:2807–2826. doi:10.1002/aic.11887.

Tomas, J. 2007. Adhesion of ultrafine particles—A micromechanical approach. *Chem. Eng. Sci.* 62:1997–2010. doi:10.1016/j.ces.2006.12.055.

Wei, D., Dave, R., and Pfeffer, R. 2002. Mixing and characterization of nanosized powders: An assessment of different techniques. *J. Nanoparticle Res.* 4:21–41. doi:10.1023/A:1020184524538.

Xia, T., Hamilton, R. F., Bonner, J. C., Crandall, E. D., Elder, A., Fazlollahi, F., Girtsman, T. A., Kim, K., Mitra, S., Ntim, S. A., Orr, G., Tagmount, M., Taylor, A. J., Telesca, D., Tolic, A., Vulpe, C. D., Walker, A. J., Wang, X., Witzmann, F. A., Wu, N., Xie, Y., Zink, J. I., Nel, A., and Holian, A. 2013. Interlaboratory evaluation of in vitro cytotoxicity and inflammatory responses to engineered nanomaterials: The NIEHS Nano GO Consortium. *Environ. Health Perspect.* 121:683–690. doi:10.1289/ehp.1306561.

Yuan, Y., Tan, J., Wang, Y., Qian, C., and Zhang, M. 2009. Chitosan nanoparticles as non-viral gene delivery vehicles based on atomic force microscopy study. *Acta Biochim. Biophys. Sin.* 515–526.

Zhou, L., Zhang, H., Zhang, H., and Zhang, Z. 2013. Homogeneous nanoparticle dispersion prepared with impurity-free dispersant by the ball mill technique. *Particuology, Nanoscale Particuology* 11:441–447. doi:10.1016/j.partic.2013.01.001.

3 Nanomedicine Clinical and Preclinical Use
A Status Report

Roudayna Diab, Sanghoon Kim, Ileana-Alexandra Pavel, Nadia Canilho, Fernanda Bianca Haffner, Sijin Li, Alain Celzard, Mihayl Varbanov, Emmanuel Lamouroux, and Andreea Pasc

CONTENTS

3.1 INTRODUCTION

As said Albert Einstein in 1929, "Imagination is more important than knowledge." Numerous inventions and technologies have been made possible thanks to researchers' ambitious dreams or imaginations. Indeed, nanomedicines were inspired from Paul Ehrlich's imagination of a "magic" vehicle for drugs directing its cargo to the targeted site of action while avoiding the counterproductive widespread biodistribution and off-target adverse effects, as well. It is easy to understand that this "magic" vehicle or carrier would display a size that matches its cellular or molecular target, and thus would vary between several hundreds of nanometers and a few nanometers (Kreuter, 1994). Since then, researchers' attention has been directed toward nanotechnologies as a unique strategy that embodies the dream of an ideal drug carrier.

Early research works implementing nanotechnologies in medical applications were in the domains of vaccination, cancer, and infectious diseases (Kreuter, 2007). Because of their sustained release properties, nano-carried vaccines were intended to produce a sufficient immune response while using a unique injection rather than often needed multiple injections (Birrenbach and Speiser, 1976). Anticancer agents, with their large volume of distribution, short half-lives, and severe cytotoxicity, were excellent candidates for nanoencapsulation, as a way to circumvent these drawbacks. In addition, drug transport through "impassable" blood–brain barriers (BBB) was made possible, accompanied by an enhanced survival of rats bearing glioblastoma (Gulyaev et al., 1999). Later, lysosomotropic effects of nanoparticles (NPs) based on polyalkylcyanoacrylate was discovered by Couvreur et al. (1977). Henceforth, subcellular targeting was feasible, holding hopes to fight intracellular infections. In fact, nanoencapsulation enables anti-infective agents to be delivered inside the cell and hence to readily interact with intracellular bacteria (Abed and Couvreur, 2014).

Despite the tremendous efforts and the great progress being made for half a century, Paul Ehrlich's dream remains challenging. There are only a few nanomedicines that have entered the clinical practice. The first nanomedicine to be marketed was Doxil® (OrthoBiotech) in 1995, an FDA-approved drug containing a liposomal nanoformulation of doxorubicin, an anticancer agent. Afterwards, other liposomal nanoformulations of doxorubicin were approved: in Europe, Evacet® (The Liposome Company, Inc.) and Myocet® (Zeneus Pharma Sopherion Therapeutics) and in Asia, Lipo-Dox® (Taiwan Liposomal Company). Other drugs containing amphotericin, an antifungal agent, such as AmBisome® (Gilead Sciences), and Abelect® (Elan Corporation), were also developed using lipid-based nanoformulation technologies, and were marketed by Elan Corporation and then by Enzon Pharmaceuticals. Furthermore, Abraxis Biosciences developed and marketed Abraxane®, which consists of albumin-based NPs loaded with paclitaxel, an anticancer agent.

Global nanomedicine market was valued at \$214.2 billion in 2013 and \$248.3 billion in 2014 (BCC Research, 2015). The total market is projected to grow at a compound annual growth rate (CAGR) of 16.3 percent from 2014 through 2019 and reach \$528 billion by 2019 (BCC Research, 2015).

It is noteworthy that the current definition of NPs limits the particle size in the range of 10 and 100 nm, as stipulated by various organizations, e.g., International Organization for Standardization, American Society for Testing and Materials, National Institute of Occupational Safety and Health, etc. NPs are synthetized starting from different organic or inorganic materials and designed using a variety of physicochemical synthesis and functionalization methods leading to a wide battery of nanostructures.

This chapter provides a concise overview of the different types of micro- and nanoparticulate delivery systems used for therapeutic or diagnostic purposes. Emphasis will be placed on the most important findings in terms of clinical or preclinical assessments of recently developed nanomedicines.

3.2 MICRO- AND NANOPARTICULATE DELIVERY SYSTEMS

3.2.1 LIPID-BASED NANOPARTICLES

Lipid-based NPs are nanosized carrier systems based on solid lipid matrix stabilized by a biocompatible emulsifier (Schwarz et al., 1994). Solid lipid NPs (SLNs) were introduced at the beginning of the 1990s as an alternative to traditional colloidal carriers. They can be cheaply produced at the industrial scale by high-pressure homogenization or at the laboratory scale by various techniques such as microencapsulation, solvent emulsification–evaporation, ultrasonication, or solvent injection method (Geszke-Moritz and Moritz, 2016).

The main SLNs advantages as drug delivery systems lie in their biodegradability and biocompatibility altogether with the physical protection of entrapped drug against environmental attacks and the targeted release in the site of action (Geszke-Moritz and Moritz, 2016). Besides, SLNs fit well for different administration routes, oral, dermal, parenteral, ocular, pulmonary, intranasal, or rectal delivery and thus were used for the treatment of various diseases (Müller et al., 2000). For instance, it was found that clonazepam (CLZ)-loaded SLNs was superior to CLZ-loaded micelles or to the free drug when orally administrated to rats (Leyva-Gómez et al., 2014). In the case of Parkinson's disease treatment, Tsai et al. demonstrated that the poor oral bioavailability of apomorphine (<2%) could be remarkably increased via its encapsulation in SLNs (Tsai et al., 2011).

SLNs were found to be versatile for gene delivery. A wise choice of cationic lipids allows nucleic acids to be complexed inside a well-tolerated lipid matrix (Tabatt et al., 2004). Severino et al. showed that SLNs cytotoxicity depends on applied concentrations (Severino et al., 2015). More importantly, SLNs conjugated with tamoxifen and lactoferrin were found to be able to cross the BBB and thus to deliver its cargo to targeted malignant cells, suggesting its promising use for the treatment of glioblastoma (Kuo and Cheng, 2016).

3.2.2 SELF-ASSEMBLED NANOSYSTEMS

Self-assembled nanoparticulate systems include a wide variety of spontaneously-organized molecules or polymers in aqueous media, forming supramolecular structures. For instance, phospholipids self-assemble in water, forming a variety of liquid crystalline phases, for example, lamellar (liposomes; see Figure 3.1), inverted hexagonal (micelles), or inverted cubic phases (cubosomes). This self-assembly tendency is mainly explained by their very low critical micelle concentration (CMC), for instance, in the sub-nanomolar range (Monnard and Deamer, 2002).

Likewise, amphiphilic co-polymers composed of hydrophobic and hydrophilic blocks form in water polymeric micelles characterized by a core–shell structure (Gaucher et al., 2005); the core is composed by the self-assembled hydrophobic chains while the hydrophilic blocks are exposed at the surface, forming a "brush." When the hydrophilic moiety is longer, the micelles have a spherical shape, while cylindrical or lamellar structures are formed when the hydrophobic moiety are longer than hydrophilic counterparts (see Figure 3.1; Gaucher et al., 2005).

The common feature of these systems is their versatility for drug delivery using different administration routes, being based on naturally-occurring components (for liposomes) or biocompatible and biodegradable polymers (for polymeric micelles) and sizing less than 100 nm (aside from giant liposomes). In addition, both systems are suitable for loading hydrophilic (inside liposomal aqueous core or at the micellar surface) and hydrophobic drugs (within the liposomal membrane or inside the hydrophobic micellar core; Allen and Cullis, 2013; Gaucher et al., 2005).

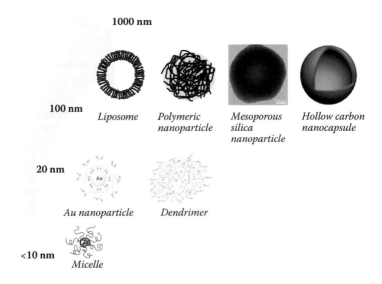

FIGURE 3.1 Illustration of micro- and nanoplatforms for the delivery of therapeutic or diagnostic agents. (Dendrimers illustration is reprinted with permission from Bhadra, D., Bhadra, S., Jain, S., and Jain, N. K., *Int J Pharm*, 257, 111–124, 2003. Copyright Elsevier 2003. Silica mesoporous nanoparticles illustration is reprinted with permission from Kim, S., Diab, R., Joubert, O., Canilho, N., and Pasc, A., *Colloids Surf B Biointerfaces*, 140, 161–188, 2016. Copyright Elsevier 2016.)

Today, numerous marketed nanomedicines or those undergoing clinical trials are based on liposomal formulations, such as DaunoXome®, Myocet®, Doxil®, or micelles ones, such as Genexol-PM®, NK911, and NC4016.

A new generation of nanoassemblies has been proposed by Couvreur's research team in 2006 on the basis of drug squalenoylation (Couvreur et al., 2006). By covalent linkage to squalene, drug molecules are converted into amphiphilic derivatives that self-organize in water as nanoassemblies of 100–300 nm. This approach was first applied on nucleoside analogs (NA), anticancer and anti-HIV agents displaying poor therapeutic indexes and resistance induction. Nanoassemblies formed by squalenoylated NA showed higher *in vitro* and *in vivo* effectiveness against cancerous cells and HIV-infected lymphocytes (Couvreur et al., 2006). The main reasons behind this, as suggested by the authors, are the enhanced stability of nanoassemblies in plasma beside the prolonged intracellular release of NA molecules occurring upon the intracellular cleavage of squalene moiety (Couvreur et al., 2006).

Since then, squalenoylation was successfully applied on other therapeutic classes, for example, paclitaxel (Dosio et al., 2010), siRNA (Ali et al., 2014), and antibiotics (Sémiramoth et al., 2012), as well as diagnostic agents, such as gadolinium (Othman et al., 2011) and ruthenium (Dosio et al., 2013).

3.2.3 POLYMERIC MICRO- AND NANOPARTICLES

Emerged during the 1960s, biodegradable polymeric particles showed higher *in vitro* and *in vivo* stability compared to liposomes and other self-assembled delivery systems, which makes them versatile for several administration routes (Singh and Lillard, 2009). In addition, drug encapsulation in polymeric particles is an interesting approach enabling to overcome issues related to drug poor solubility or stability, to tune drug release and absorption kinetics, to achieve a passive or active targeting using particle surface functionalization, and so on (Singh and Lillard, 2009).

Biodegradable polymeric particles are prepared starting from monomers, for example, polyalkylcyanoacrylates MPs and NPs, or using preformed polymers, for example, MPs and NPs composed from polycaprolactone (PCL), polylactic acid (PLA), or poly(lactide-co-glycolide) (PLGA) copolymers or starting from biopolymers, for example, albumin, alginate, and cellulose derivatives (Singh and Lillard, 2009). All the currently known preparation processes are based on the bottom-up principle. Briefly, preformed polymers are solubilized (molecularly dispersed) in a volatile organic solvent and then the obtained solution is dispersed in a surfactant-containing aqueous phase. MPs and NPs are formed following polymer precipitation in the micro- or nano-droplets after organic solvent removal or rapid diffusion toward the external aqueous phase. According to the miscibility of the used organic solvent, the process is called *nanoprecipitation* (Fessi and Devissaguet, 1987), *emulsification–diffusion* (Leroux et al., 1995), or *emulsion–solvent extraction method* (Vanderhoff et al., 1979) for miscible, semi-miscible, or non-miscible solvents, respectively.

Similarly, MPs or NPs prepared by polymerization are performed by dispersing the monomer-containing solution in a non-solvent. Then, polymerization is triggered within dispersed micro- or nano-droplets which finally turn into MPs or NPs, respectively (Couvreur et al., 1982). Biopolymer-based particles, being composed of hydrophilic polymers, are prepared starting from aqueous solutions. Afterward, polymer aqueous solutions will be either injected in cross-linker cation solution leading to droplet rapid gelation, the method is called then ionic gelation or dispersed in oils followed by droplets hardening by coacervation or covalent crosslinking (Joye and McClements, 2016).

The famous example of polymeric NPs-based nanomedicines is Abraxane®, composed albumin–based NPs loaded with paclitaxel and approved for the treatment of breast cancer.

3.2.4 INORGANIC NANOPARTICLES

3.2.4.1 Silica Nanoparticles

The major advantage of silica NPs is their safety. Amorphous silica is approved as additives for animal and human food. Moreover, silica materials with a special molecular arrangement forming hexagonal or cubic nanopores, ranging from 2 to 50 nm, are of great interest because of their high surface area and high loading capacity (Simovic et al., 2011). Drugs could be adsorbed or covalently attached to pores by virtue of exposed silanol groups (Tang and Cheng, 2013).

Mesoporous silica NPs (MSNs) are generally synthesized by hydrolysis of an alkoxysilane silica source, typically tetraethyl orthosilicate, in acidic (pH 0–2) or alkaline (pH 8–12) solutions in the presence of a surfactant at concentrations > CMC. Hydrolyzed silica precursors polymerize around micelles which play the role of organic templates. The porous structure is then obtained after removal of surfactant by calcination (Wu et al., 2013). Accordingly, the pore size and geometry depend upon the type of the organic template.

Silica NPs and MSNs were extensively studied as nanoplatforms for therapeutic agents with the aim to enhance the oral bioavailability of pH-sensitive or poorly soluble drugs (Simovic et al., 2010) to enable its loaded drug to cross the BBB (Cui et al., 2013; Mo et al., 2016), boost the immune response to administered antigens (Skrastina et al., 2014), carry contrast agents in order to enhance the imaging outcome (Santra, 2010), and enhance tissue regeneration (Zhou et al., 2014).

3.2.4.2 Metal and Metal Oxides Nanoparticles

Metal-based NPs are mainly made of d-block elements of the periodic table. Elements of the block-p can be incorporated in the NPs lattice to form different types of compounds, such as metal oxide or metal sulfide. Since the surface-to-volume ratio is dramatically increased in NPs, the properties of nanosized materials will differ from the ones of bulk one (i.e., electronic, optic, magnetic, and catalytic properties; Mody et al., 2010). These properties are of particular interest for biomedical applications, such as imaging and hyperthermia therapy, as previously reviewed (Chen et al., 2016). NPs could be classified as a function of their physical properties used for biomedical applications: (1) plasmonic NPs, (2) magnetic NPs, and (3) quantum dots (QDs). Moreover, metal-based NPs are widely used as antibacterial agents.

3.2.4.2.1 *Plasmonic Nanoparticles*

Upon illumination, plasmonic NPs exhibit a *localized surface plasmon resonance* (LSPR), that is, a collective oscillation of conductive electrons. This resonant oscillation occurs when the frequency of an incident electromagnetic wave matches the oscillation frequency of conduction band electrons present on the surface of a metallic NP. Then, these oscillations induce charge separation on the surface and hence the creation of large electric fields near the NPs surface (Figure 3.2; Ghosh and Pal, 2007). For instance, spherical gold (Au) NPs with a diameter of 10–20 nm show a typical LSPR at around 530 nm (Li et al., 2014). However, LSPR wavelength is sensitive to the NP size and shape and also to the nature of the NP stabilizer and the surrounding dielectric environment. Thanks to the surrounding sensitivity of LSPR plasmonic, NPs can be used as sensors (Abadeer and Murphy, 2016; Saha et al., 2012). Moreover, in anisotropic NPs, LSPR signal can be separated in different peaks corresponding to the axis of each NP. Thus, LSPR of gold nanorods (AuNRs) which is characterized by an aspect ratio (length/width) will be composed of two different signals, that is, a transversal and a longitudinal one. If their aspect ratios range from 1.1 to 4.4, the λ_{max} of the longitudinal peak will be shifted from 640 nm to 850 nm (Abadeer and Murphy, 2016).

Spherical plasmonic NPs can be easily prepared using the Turkevich (Turkevich et al., 1951) or Shiffrin–Brust (Brust et al., 1994) methods. For *in vivo* biomedical applications, anisotropic NPs such as nanorods are preferred because they exhibit LSPR signals within the near-infrared "biological window" (Huang et al., 2009). Following the bottom-up approach, AuNRs can be prepared by template, electrochemical, or seed-mediated growth method (Martin, 1994; Yu et al., 1997). It is worth noting that the seed-mediated growth method also allows the preparation of various shapes, such as platonic solids or nanoplates, with different metals (e.g., silver, gold, or palladium; Xia et al., 2009).

During the Raman experiment in the presence of plasmonic NPs, the LSPR phenomenon induces a local electromagnetic enhancement leading to an enhancement up to 10^{14} of the Raman scattering intensity. Hence, plasmonic NPs are perfect candidate for *surface enhanced raman scattering* (SERS)–based sensors (Saha et al., 2012). For example, AuNPs have been used in SERS-based assays of proteins for diagnostics of rheumatoid arthritis (Chon et al., 2015). Liang et al. introduced aggregated silver (Ag) NPs-based SERS into an ELISA (enzyme–linked immunosorbent assay) signal generation system for prostate specific antigen and the adrenal stimulant ractopamine assays (Liang et al., 2015). Thanks to the presence of AgNPs, ultralow concentrations were detected, that is, 10^{-9} and 10^{-6} ng/mL, respectively.

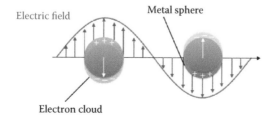

FIGURE 3.2 Schematic representation of surface plasmon resonance.

Another biomedical application of plasmonic NPs is in plasmonic photothermal therapy. Indeed, non-radiative dissipation (heat) subsequent to strong optical absorption (i.e., LSPR) is transferred to the lattice of NPs through phonon–phonon interaction and then to the surrounding of NPs (Link and El-Sayed, 2000).

Anisotropic plasmonic NPs are also capable of controlled drug delivery taking advantage of this plasmonic photothermal property (Lal et al., 2014). For example, Zhang et al. (2012) prepared mesoporous silica-coated AuNRs with doxorubicin hydrochloride loaded as theranostic platform for cancer treatment. This theranostic agent combined two light-mediated therapeutic modes; low power density laser-triggered DOX release for chemotherapy, and high-power density laser-induced photothermal therapy, that is, hyperthermia.

Currently, only AuroShell® particles are used for clinical trials. The AuroLase® therapy consists of using AuroShell for photothermal therapeutics ablation of solid tumors. AuroShell particles consist of a silicon core of around 120 nm in diameter covered by a gold shell which is protected by thiol-polyethylene glycol and exhibit λmax from 780 to 820 nm, depending on gold shell thickness (Anselmo and Mitragotri, 2016; Abadeer and Murphy, 2016). These PEGylated particles are injected intravenously and then are accumulated in tumors thanks to enhanced permeability and retention effect of tumor tissues. Up to now, AuroLase therapy has been used for two human clinical trials. The first trial began in April 2008 and ended in August 2014 (ClinicalTrials.gov Identifier:NCT00848042). This pilot study of AuroLase concerned the treatment of patients with refractory or recurrent tumors of the head and neck. The patients received a single dose of particles followed by interstitial illumination and then they were observed for six months after this treatment. Only partial results were posted dealing with adverse device effects attributable to gold nanoshell administration and shown excellent human tolerability. The second clinical trial dealt with AuroLase therapy of primary or metastatic lung tumors. During this trial, patients were given a systemic infusion of AuroShell and subsequent escalating doses of laser radiation. This study started in October 2012 and ended in June 2016, but no study results have yet been posted (ClinicalTrials.gov Identifier: NCT01679470).

3.2.4.2.2   Magnetic Nanoparticles

Among them, iron oxide NPs are the best known as biomedical application is concerned. They are relatively easy to prepare, non-toxic, chemically stable, and can be superparamagnetic (Hervault and Thanh, 2014). Superparamagnetic iron oxide NPs (SPION), the two main forms of iron oxide are Fe_3O_4 and $\gamma\text{-}Fe_2O_3$, can be easily prepared by thermal decomposition of iron complexes in an organic solvent, the microemulsion process, or the co-precipitation technique (Laurent et al., 2008), (Reddy et al., 2012). Chemical co-precipitation consists in hydrolysis of a stoichiometric mixture of ferrous and ferric salts in aqueous medium under inert atmosphere (Equation 3.1).

$$Fe^{2+} + 2Fe^{3+} + 8HO^- \rightarrow Fe_3O_4 + 4H_2O \tag{3.1}$$

Under aerobic conditions, magnetite (Fe_3O_4), which is not thermodynamically stable, can be transformed in maghemite (γ-Fe_2O_3). Another way to achieve the formation of maghemite is to use acidic media under anaerobic conditions (Equation 3.2).

$$Fe_3O_4 + 2H^+ \rightarrow \gamma Fe_2O_3 + Fe^{2+} + H_2O \qquad (3.2)$$

However, particle size and size distribution are hardly controlled during co-precipitation process. An alternative consists in using organometallics precursors such as iron pentacarbonyl, iron oleate, or iron acetylacetonate (Woo et al., 2004; Bronstein et al., 2007; Wang et al., 2012). The decomposition of such precursors in organic solvent in presence of appropriate stabilizers allows obtaining monodispersed iron oxide NPs of controlled size.

Superparamagnetic phenomenon occurs when the NPs size is small enough to be assimilated to a macrospin, that is, a single-domain, and has two equivalent easy magnetic directions. Applying a high-frequency magnetic field to superparamagnetic NPs results in the conversion from magnetic energy to thermal energy. This phenomenon is used for treatment of tumors by hyperthermia using SPION, such as iron-oxide NPs, called Magnablate, which have been approved for a Phase 0 clinical trial about dose escalation safety and evaluation of the retention of magnablate NPs in the prostate (ClinicalTrials.gov identifier: NTC02033447). Another aspect of such a trial was the study of influence of the injection site on the anatomical distribution of NPs, taking advantage of magnetic properties for imaging purposes.

Magnetic hyperthermia can also be combined with drug delivery which did not require high T as high for hyperthermia therapy (Ward and Georgiou, 2011). Magnetic hyperthermia has also been used for on-demand drug release triggered. Che Rose et al. demonstrated that a micro-carrier consisting of 10 wt% iron oxide NPs eicosane coated capsule exposed to an alternative magnetic field activates drug release (Che Rose et al., 2016).

Beside hyperthermia applications, magnetic NPs are also used as magnetic resonance imaging (MRI) agents (Shin et al., 2015). For T_1 contrast agents, the corresponding effect comes from magnetic disorder at the surface of the magnetic NPs. Indeed, when the environments of core atoms and surface ones of magnetic NPs are compared, it appears atoms localized at the NPs surface have more unpaired electrons. Hence, the smaller the magnetic NPs, the stronger the T_1 contrast effect. Theoretically strong T_1 contrast effects can be obtained with magnetic NPs smaller than 10 nm (Roch et al., 1999). For strong T_2 contrast agents, it is better to exhibit a high magnetization saturation (M_S) value, which is usually the case with SPION-doped or un-dopted (Tong et al., 2010).

It is worth underlining that five different SPION have been designed and clinically tested as MRI contrast agents: Feridex®, Resovist®, Combidex®, Sinerem®, and Clariscan® (Wang, 2015). They differ by their coating materials and hydrodynamic diameter. The development of Combidex and Sinerem was stopped due to a lack of significant benefit for sensitivity. Clariscan did not receive regulatory approval. Feridex has been withdrawn from the market and Resovist is only available in some countries.

3.2.4.2.3   Quantum Dots

Quantum dots (QDs) are fluorescent semiconductor NPs of few nanometers, typically below 10 nm. QDs for biomedical application consist of elements from groups II to VI (e.g., Cadmium-Selenium: CdSe) or III to V (e.g., Gallium-Arsenic and Gallium-Indium-Arsenide-Phosphide: GaAs and GaInAsP, respectively; Fang et al., 2012). Their optical and electronic properties are an intermediate between bulk materials and molecules, that is, a set of discrete energy states instead of energy bands or levels. Excited by light, QDs absorb photons and then re-emit radiation (fluorescence), the "color" (wavelength) of which depends on the size of the nanocrystal. This is a direct result of "quantum confinement" due to their small size. For a defined QD, band gap (E_{gap}) increases as NPs size decreases. Therefore, as adsorbed photon energy and fluorescence wavelength are directly related to E_{gap}, a fine tuning of QDs composition and size allows making them suitable for *in vivo* imaging (i.e., fluorescence in near-infrared).

Different technique can be used to prepare QDs, such as lithography, chemical vapor deposition, or hot injection process. Among them, the hot injection process appears the most popular way to synthesize QDs for biomedical applications (Qu and Peng, 2002). QDs are mainly used as biomedical imaging and photodynamic therapy agent (Fang et al., 2012). The major issue associated with QD use lies in the toxicity of metal, such as cadmium or lead. To circumvent it, researchers tried to replace cadmium with a zinc compound or to make core–shell NPs with cadmium in the inner part. For instance, PbS@CdS@ZnS QDs are a typical example of core@ inner-shell@shell. These QDs, with a diameter of 4 nm and an emission band at around 1270 nm, that is, in the near-infrared region, have been tested on mice for photothermal treatment of malignant tumors. Results demonstrated the possibility to use QDs for tumor ablation in mice models. Moreover, as QDs fluorescence is thermos-sensitive, it is possible to monitor the evolution of intratumoral temperature during photothermal treatment.

3.2.4.2.4   Metal-Based NPs as Antibacterial Agents

It is worth noting that bulk metals such as Ag, Cu, or Au were used for centuries for their antibacterial activities (Dizaj et al., 2014). Then it is not surprising that the use of NPs made of such metals did not cease growing these last years for antibacterial application. For instance, AgNPs prepared by photo-irradiation of $AgNO_3$ solution in Triton X-100 have been tested as antibacterial agent on *E. coli*.

Recent studies confirm that AgNPs surface atoms can be oxidized and then Ag^+ ions are released, which act as antimicrobial agents (Le Ouay and Stellacci, 2015). Antibacterial activity of gelatin-stabilized Cu NPs on *E. coli* has also been studied (Chatterjee et al., 2012). Similarly, Cu^{2+} ions originated from NPs oxidation showed antibacterial activity. The semiconductor NPs (e.g., TiO_2 or ZnO NPs) are assumed to act as photocatalyst for the formation of reactive oxygen species (ROS; Hajipour et al., 2012; Sirelkhatim et al., 2015).

3.2.5 CARBON NANOCARRIERS

3.2.5.1 Carbon Nanocapsules and Nanospheres

Carbon nanocapsules (CNs) refer to hollow-structured carbon particles of nanometer size with thin shells (as illustrated in Figure 3.1). These materials are presently attracting great attention due to their unique properties, such as encapsulation ability, controllable permeability, surface functionality, high surface-to-volume ratios, and excellent chemical and thermal stabilities (Li et al., 2016). In many aspects, CNs are therefore superior to their polymer- or metal-based counterparts. There are two main synthetic strategies, hard-templating and soft-templating routes for synthesis CNs (Li et al., 2016).

CNs are used as protective shells for metal or metal oxide NPs. Indeed, NPs composed of pure metals such as Fe, Co, and Ni display a main concern arising from their instability towards oxidation in air, which becomes easier as the particle size decreases. One chemical stabilization approach is the formation of protective shells around the nanoparticle surface, which thus prevents the reaction of oxygen with the metal surface atoms (Kim et al., 2008). The carbon coating of metals indeed induces an effective protection method against environmental degradation due to the excellent adhesive bonding with the surface of metal particles. These carbon shells are airtight and protect the entrapped materials from oxidation. Such CNs were proposed as a new approach for preparing magnetic carriers designed for the administration of drugs and vaccines (Kim et al., 2008). One of the prospective medical applications of CNs is the drug delivery to specific targets, controlled by an external magnetic field. For this purpose, the carrier particles themselves must be biologically inert and biodegradable. Moreover, they must also have a high sorption capacity for the drug, and the rate of drug desorption in the organism needs to be slow enough so that the high concentration of the cytostatic drug can be maintained in the tumor area for a prolonged period of time.

Since the particles must be controlled by the applied magnetic field, both their magnetic properties and their dispersity and agglomeration degree are important (Kim et al., 2008). For example, nanocapsules (100–200 nm in size) wrapping iron carbide particles were successfully obtained and tested as drug delivery systems (Kim et al., 2008). Peapod-like hollow carbon nanospheres (HCNSs) exhibited ultra-high drug loading capacity above 98.4 percent for doxorubicin hydrochloride due to the high specific surface area, porous shell, and unique nanostructure (Guo et al., 2015).

Carbon nano- and microspheres with surface-engineered functional groups have great potential for bioimaging labels (Guo et al., 2008). In 2012, Fang et al. proposed an ingenious synthetic method for the production of aggregated hollow fluorescent carbon NPs (HFCNs) by simply mixing acetic acid, water, and diphosphorus (Fang et al., 2012). Abundant small oxygenous graphite domains endowed the HFCNs with fluorescent properties. After simple post-treatments, the crosslinked HCNSs could be used for cell imaging applications. Compared to traditional dyes and to CdTe QDs, these materials were better fluorescent bio-imaging agents according to their low toxicity, good stability, and resistance to photo-bleaching, and were also successfully applied as watermark ink and fluorescent powder, showing their promising potentials for further uses (Fang et al., 2012).

Contrast agents based on micron-size bubbles have been employed to greatly expand the scope of sonography applications in medical imaging by providing enhanced backscattering from blood or tissue. The application of Cu-doped HCSs as ultrasound contrast agents was investigated (Jia et al., 2013). Obvious gray-scale imaging enhancement was detected, suggesting the good contrast-enhancing ability of this material.

3.2.5.2 Carbon Nanotubes

Carbon nanotubes (CNTs) are cylindrical tubes of one (single-walled) or multiple layers (multiple-walled) of graphite with a diameter of few nanometers and length of several millimeters (Szabó et al., 2010). CNTs are prepared by arc-discharge method, laser ablation method (using graphite), and chemical vapor deposition (Szabó et al., 2010).

The major advantages of CNTs are (1) high specific surface area, which makes them versatile for drug loading; (2) high electrical and thermal conductivity, which is particularly interesting for thermal therapy and theranostics applications; and (3) high mechanical strength and fibrous structure, which make them potential candidates for tissue engineering (Szabó et al., 2010). CNTs were found to interact with mammalian cells via cytoplasmic translocation (Lacerda et al., 2012); which lead to potential applications in intracellular delivery of macromolecules, including proteins, nucleic acids, and being loaded by attachment to CNTs (Boyer et al., 2016).

The major issues inherent to the use of CNTs is their low biodegradability, immunogenicity, and genotoxicity, following their systemic administration (Kim et al., 2016). If inhaled, CNTs can be more toxic than carbon black or as toxic as quartz (Lam et al., 2006). The cytotoxicity of CNTs has been attributed to the cellular oxidative stresses induced by this material. However, other research papers reported that CNTs have limited toxicity on endothelial cells *in vitro* (Albini et al., 2010).

Obviously there is controversy about the toxic effects of CNTs, which explains why no CNTs-based product for medical use has been marketed till now. Yet innovative CNTs in therapy and diagnosis for life-threatening diseases, for example, cancer and neurodegenerative diseases, are expected to enter clinical use in the near future.

3.2.6 DENDRIMERS

Dendrimers or arborols belongs to the fourth class of polymer architecture (Tomalia and Fréchet, 2002). Thus, dendrimers are highly branched globular macromolecules with symmetric tree-like arms and precise distribution of functional groups from the core to the periphery. This monodisperse chemical architecture is completely artificial. Indeed, Tomalia et al. (1985), Fritz Vögtle (Friedhofen and Vögtle, 2006), and George R. Newkome (Hwang et al., 2008) discovered the synthetic route in early 1980s from independent investigations. At that time, Tomalia and Newkome worked on poly(amidoamine) (PAMAM), a dendrimer still largely used in medical applications today.

In general, dendrimer chemical architecture built up by generation is composed of three components: core, branches, and end groups (Figure 3.1). Initially, Tomalia investigated the divergent synthetic route on PAMAM (Tomalia, 1996). But in early 1990s through the research work of Jean Fréchet and coworkers, the convergent methodology itself has become more efficient and flexible than the divergent methodology (Hawker and Fréchet, 1990). Indeed, the convergent approach affords a remarkable control on the growth, the chemical structure, and the functionality (Fréchet, 2003). The divergent approach expands the dendritic chemical structure from a short chemical group being the core to the peripheral shell carrying the functionalized end groups. This type of structural growth leads to an increase in the number of end groups as a function of the generation. Conversely, in the convergent synthesis, the dendrimer is growing up from the required peripheral shell molecules to the core, also called focal point in this case. Since then and to 2003, with the work reported by Caminade et al. on phosphorous dendrimers, the divergent approach was associated with "lego" chemistry (Maraval et al., 2003). This way of proceeding allows synthesis of dendrimers in one step per generation and facilitates the synthetic conditions (less solvent and only water and nitrogen as byproducts) and reduces the purification steps. Almost simultaneously, Fréchet et al. produced dendrimers by using "click" chemistry applied to convergent methodology, with high purity and excellent yield (Wu et al., 2004).

These synthetic methodologies, well mastered now, offer the possibility to design a dendrimer with a specific molecular weight, possessing compositionally different interiors (i.e., carbon, nitrogen, silicon, sulfur, phosphorus, or metals) and multiplicity values (Enciso et al., 2016). Over these last almost 30 years, it has been possible to establish that dendritic polymers to which category belongs dendrimers, are defined by six nanoscale features called *critical nanoscale design parameters* (CNDPs). The parameters to be considered are the size, shape, surface chemistry, flexibility/rigidity, architecture and elemental composition (Tomalia, 2016).

The synthetic route is so fine that nowadays, by varying the CNDPs, it is possible to produce new dendrimers and to predict the properties of the dendrimer with respect to the intended application (Menjoge et al., 2010; Kannan et al., 2014). The behavior understanding is particularly needed in biomedical applications regarding biocompatibility and pharmacokinetics.

Thereby, investigations on the syntheses of dendrimers for nanomedicine (Lee et al., 2005) is still of great interest since dendritic macromolecules possess similar topologies, function, and dimensions fitting with a wide variety of biological polymers. For example, PAMAM dendrimers of generations 3, 4, and 5, have, respectively, the same size of insulin (3 nm), cytochrome C (4 nm), and hemoglobin (5.5 nm). Recently, a PAMAM generation 13, as synthesized, reaches the size of a small virus (30 nm; Lim et al., 2013).

Thus, dendrimers are widely studied as platforms for drugs against cancer, bacteria, or viruses, for tissue repair scaffolds, targeted carriers of chemotherapeutics, gene transfection, MRI imaging or for the development of theranostic devices (Kannan et al., 2014).

As presented in a recent review written by R.M. Kannan et al. (2014), some dendrimers are involved in clinical trials. A dendrimer-based nanomedicine labeled

VIVAGel®SPL7013 recently entered Phase III of clinical trials with indication in the treatment of bacterial vaginosis. Another dendrimer-based nanomedicine, DEP™-Docetaxel, is being investigated during Phase I of clinical trials with indication in the treatment of advanced or metastatic cancer. PAMAM-based dendrimers, grafted PAMAM, and phosphorous- or PEG-based dendrimers are currently undergoing preclinical evaluations in the treatment of inflammation and neurodegenerative diseases, respectively (Fruchon et al., 2015; Sousa-Herves et al., 2014).

In fact, their tuned chemical topology from the core to the shell allows their use as a container (free space in between the shells) or as a nano-scaffold through the multivalent surface opportunities. Therefore, such monodisperse macromolecules are highly polyvalent. Inventiveness of synthesis methods is continuously evolving to emerge new functional dendritic polymers with specific nano-periodic properties.

3.2.7 NANOCRYSTALS

Drug nanocrystals, as their name suggests, are nanosized particles composed only of the active substance, in a crystalline state. No excipient or carrier materials are used for the preparation of nanocrystals, in contrast to the above mentioned nanoparticulate systems.

Nanonization of drug powders to sizes below 1 micron has emerged when micronization failed to overcome bioavailability issues of some BCS class II and IV drugs. According to the Noyes–Whitney equation, the reduction in particle size increases the specific surface area in contact with the diffusion media (Noyes and Whitney, 1897). Consequently, a considerable increase in the dissolution velocity could be obtained by nanonization. Moreover, when the particle size is reduced below 1 micron, the saturation solubility becomes a variable parameter that increases with particle size decreasing.

According to the literature, the highest increase in saturation solubility could be reached for particle sizes below 50 nm. Indeed, the optimal size depends upon the required pharmacokinetic profile and the administration route (Junghanns and Müller, 2008). Too fast a dissolution could result in fast absorption and thus abruptly leading to high plasma peaks.

NanoCrystal technology could be achieved by pearl milling, high pressure homogenization, and supercritical fluid methods (Junghanns and Müller, 2008). Interestingly, some methods could produce drug NPs in an amorphous state, which are then referred to "nanocrystals in the amorphous state." After nanonization, drug nanocrystals are introduced in conventional dosage forms, for example, tablets, capsules, pellets, and injectable suspensions.

Today, numerous nanocrystal-based drug products are marketed, such as Rapamune® (oral tablet), Emend® (oral capsule), Megace ES® (oral suspension), Invega® Sustenna™ (intramuscular suspension), and so on. Indeed, nanonization led to enhanced bioavailability of a poorly soluble drug (e.g., Rapamune®), with a narrow absorption window (e.g., Emend®) and independently of fed/fast state (e.g., Megace ES®; U.S. FDA, 2000; Wu et al., 2004). In addition, thanks to NanoCrystal technology, drug nanosuspension could be prepared in a small volume, with low viscosity suitable for parenteral administration along with a sustained plasma level (e.g., Invega® Sustenna™).

3.3   NANOPARTICLE USE IN THERAPY

3.3.1   CANCER

Cancer chemotherapy is the widest medical field to use nanotechnologies. Numerous anticancer agents have received the benefit of nanotechnologies aiming to improve their poor therapeutic indexes to overcome drug resistance or to target metastasis; namely nucleosides analogs (Diab et al., 2007), anthracyclines (Ma and Mumper, 2013), taxus alkaloids (Ma and Mumper, 2013), platinum derivatives (Xue et al., 2013), and so on.

Recent researches are focused on the development of smart nano-platforms that are responsive to external or internal stimuli. These smart delivery systems enable the anticancer agent to be selectively delivered to the tumor interstitial matrix and/ or to cancerous cells. For instance, Xu et al. (2016) designed a sophisticated dual pH-responsive micelle achieving a selective sequential delivery of axitinib to tumor extracellular microenvironment and doxorubicin to intracellular lysosome compartments. In this system, doxorubicin was covalently conjugated to amphiphilic hydroxypropyl methacrylamide polymers using pH sensitive hydrazone linkage. Afterward, axitinib was encapsulated into the self-assembly micelles. Finally, obtained micelles were stabilized using benzoic-imine cross-linking. The benzoic-imine bond is sensitive to tumor microenvironment's pH (6.5). Therefore, crosslinking would be broken down in the vicinity of tumor cells. Axitinib is then released and could readily interact with its extracellular target, that is, tyrosine kinase receptors. Once taken up by endocytosis, micelles would release doxorubicin following the hydrolysis of hydrazone linkage in the lysosomal low pH (5). Doxorubicin is then accumulated inside cancerous cells and could readily interact with its intracellular targets.

Tagami et al. (2011) developed heat-responsive liposomes for the delivery of doxorubicin. Accordingly, drug release depends on an external stimulus, that is, tumor-localized heating at $\approx 42°C$. The thermosensitive liposomal formulation is based on phospholipids with phase transition temperature around 41–42°C. After reaching this temperature, pores in liposomal membranes are formed resulting in rapid drug release. It is noteworthy that the thermosensitive formulation was found to be stable at 37–38°C. Recently, this formulation, called ThermoDox®, was used in boosting tumor ablation by radiofrequency in a porcine model (Swenson et al., 2015).

Active and passive targeting based on NPs surface functionalization with a specific ligand and hydrophilic polymeric shell, respectively, are old approaches that have been developed over the last few decades and led to nanotherapeutics that recently entered clinical trials stages. Passive targeting is based on the enhanced permeation of cancerous tissues with large inter-endothelial gaps and retention effect which results from the defective lymphatic drainage (Lammers et al., 2012). For this purpose, several hydrophilic polymers were used, for example, polyethylene glycol (PEG), polyethylene–polypropylene copolymers (Pluronic®), cyclodextrines, poly(L-glytamic), etc. Hydrophilic shells help NPs to evade clearance by the reticuloendothelial system and thus to behave as stealth particles in the general circulation. Genexol-PM® (Kim et al., 2015), NK911® (Matsumura et al., 2004), and SPI-77® (Seetharamu et al., 2010) are examples of PEG-based polymeric NPs, micelles, and liposomes, respectively, that are currently undergoing Phase II of clinical trials.

Active targeting is based on the recognition of a specific NP-attached ligand by a biological target overexpressed at the cancerous cell membrane. The main objective is to enhance NPs internalization in the target cells. A variety of targeting ligands were used in the literature, namely peptides, monoclonal antibodies (mAb) or their fragments, aptamers, and small molecules (Sanna et al., 2014). To date, only a few nanoplatforms based on active targeting have reached clinical trials stages. The reasons behind this are multiple: (1) the failure of ligand-bearing NPs to overcome the biological barriers, (2) the early clearance and immunogenicity, especially in the case of mAb-bearing NPs, and (3) development and scaling-up difficulties (Lammers et al., 2012).

MCC-465® and C225-ILS-DOX® are formulations of doxorubicin using PEG-liposomes that are undergoing Phase I of clinical trials. In the former, PEG-liposomes bear the fragment F(ab')2 of human mAb GAH directed to cancerous stomach tissues (Matsumura et al., 2004) and in the latter, PEG-liposomes are functionalized with cetuximab, an anti-epithelial growth factor receptor (EGFR) and used for the treatment of EGFR-overexpressing solid tumors (Mamot et al., 2012).

3.3.2 Neurodegenerative Diseases

Neurodegenerative diseases (NDs) are characterized by a serious disorder of the central nervous system. Alzheimer's disease (AD) and Parkinson's disease (PD) are the most common NDs, especially since according to the National Institute on Aging (2016) more than five million American people are affected by AD. Although the cause of these diseases has not been clearly elucidated, it is generally believed that cholinergic deficit, aggregation of the amyloid-beta (Aβ), and oxidation stress could be the main factors responsible for AD disorders.

In the field of NDs, many efforts have been focused on the development of efficient active ingredients and delivery systems for diagnostic and therapeutic purposes, including functional nanocarriers that are able to pass through the BBB (Roney et al., 2005). Indeed, the assay of acetylcholine (ACh) or acetylcholinesterase activity (AChE) is the most important factor to determine in order to assess treatment effectiveness. In general, ACh concentration in human blood is about 9 nM and its detection and quantification is not a simple task. Traditional methods, like chromatography, are still being widely used despite being expensive and time consuming. Metallic NPs have been used for Ach assay, and their results are promising, even if they are still at lab scale. For instance, AuNPs have been used for continuous colorimetric assay for AChE activity (Wang et al., 2009). AChE catalyses the hydrolysis of acetylthiocoline into thiocoline. In turn, thiocoline causes aggregation of AuNPs resulting in a red-shift of the plasmon absorption. The shift of the plasmon absorption of AuNPs is significant, even with the small change of thiocholine concentration. Accordingly, AChE activity could be assayed at AChE concentration as low as 0.6 mU/mL.

The accumulation of the amyloid-beta (Aβ) plaques is considered a major pathological feature of AD. In a general consensus, the self-assembly of Aβ into a cross β-sheeted fibril can affect molecular signaling pathways (neuron system), including mitochondria L dysfunction. For this reason, the inhibition of Aβ fibrillation using NPs or small molecules could be an efficient strategy for AD treatment. Palmal et al. studied the effectiveness of surface-functionalized AuNPs for delaying or inhibiting Aβ fibril growth (Palmal et al., 2014). Cationic AuNPs coated with a histidine-based polymer were shown to efficiently inhibit amyloid fibrillation in a concentration-dependent manner, whereas Aβ fibrils remained undisturbed in the presence of histidine monomers even at a concentration as high as 10 mM.

In addition, as Aβ induced the neuronal dysfunction which is often combined with abnormal production of ROS, NPs decorated with antioxidant molecules have been intensively investigated. Recently, mitochondria-targeting ceria (CeO_2) NPs have been developed as an antioxidant for AD treatment. Indeed, CeO_2 NPs have already been used to protect cells from ROS as ceria NPs show excellent oxygen radical scavenger ability through redox cycle Ce^{3+}/Ce^{4+} on the surface (Kwon et al., 2016). In this work, CeO_2 NPs were then decorated with triphenylphosphonium (TTP) with the aim to target mitochondria (Figure 3.3). TPP-CeO_2 NPs sized 22 nm and bearing a zeta potential of 45 mV were shown to efficiently penetrate mitochondria and to inhibit Aβ-induced mitochondrial ROS in both *in vitro* and *in vivo* studies (Kwon et al., 2016). It is noteworthy that *in vivo* tests showed that TPP-CeO_2 NPs were not able to disturb the aggregation of Aβ, which is not in good agreement with the previously reported *in vitro* test results (Palmal et al., 2014).

In this field, it is important to mention curcumin whose benefits were highlighted not only for its excellent antioxidant and anti-inflammatory properties but

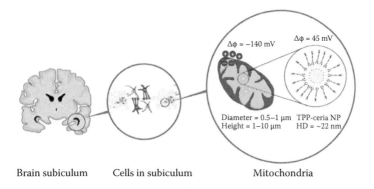

Brain subiculum   Cells in subiculum   Mitochondria

FIGURE 3.3 TPP-ceria nanoparticles inside mitochondria of subicular cells. (Reprinted with permission from Kwon, H. J., Cha, M., Kim, D., Kim, D. K., Soh, M., Shin, K., Hyeon, T., and Mook-Jung, I., *ACS Nano*, 10, 2860–2870, 2016. Copyright 2016 American Chemical Society.)

also for its good binding ability to Aβ plaques as demonstrated both *in vitro* and *in vivo* studies (Park and Kim, 2002; Yang et al., 2005; Garcia-Alloza et al., 2007; Fiala et al., 2007). Moreover, computational calculation using ab-inito methods showed that curcumin electronic and structural features, especially charge delocalization, can facilitate its penetration into the BBB along with binding to Aβ plaques (Balasubramanian, 2006). The main drawback of this "silver bullet" molecule is its low solubility in aqueous solutions, which lowers also its bioavailability. Thus, loading curcumin into nanocarriers could be a good strategy to address this issue. Among currently reported nanocarriers, PLGA NPs conjugated with Tet-1 peptide as a target ligand have been developed for curcumin delivery in AD treatment (Mathew et al., 2012). Curcumin conjugated-magnetic NPs have also been proved to be efficient for reducing Aβ plaques (Cheng et al., 2015). However, up till now, these promising results are based only on *in vitro* tests. Thus, *in vivo* studies should be performed before further consideration of practical use of these curcumin delivery platforms.

In summary, although nanocarriers in ND treatment could afford a number of promising possibilities, the use of these nanocarriers is still far from being widely adopted because of the lack of sufficient and reliable clinical or even preclinical studies.

3.3.3 AUTOIMMUNE DISEASES

An ideal therapeutic against autoimmune diseases counteracts the harmful inflammatory responses without impairing the immune homeostasis. Indeed, traditional treatment is based on immunosuppressive drugs that down-regulate the global immune response leading to increased susceptibility to infections and decreased tumor cell suppression. Besides, severe adverse effects inherent to treatment are also observed, for example, hematological toxicities, especially for antimetabolite agents, as well as difficulty in treatment management because of the narrow therapeutic range and low bioavailability, especially for calcineurin and mTOR inhibitors. In addition, mAb-based therapy may induce a life-threatening anaphylactic shock.

Nano- and microencapsulation enable immunosuppressive drugs to be delivered with spatiotemporal precisions along with limiting the off-target side effects. As a result, systemic doses could be reduced leading to reduced toxicity. For instance, cyclosporine A-lipid NPs oral formulation developed by Guada et al. showed a better pharmacological response in the treatment of inflammatory bowel disease (Guada et al., 2016). Moreover, the well-known nephrotoxicity related to cyclosporine was countered, according to histopathological evaluations (Guada et al., 2016). Tacrolimus-loaded albumin NPs recently developed by Thao et al. (2016) showed *in vitro* selective antiproliferative activity on activated T cells without affecting normal cell proliferation. Preclinical studies showed an enhanced anti-arthritic activity of the developed NPs administered intravenously when compared to tacrolimus solution or suspension administered intravenously and orally, respectively (Thao et al., 2016). Importantly, tacrolimus-albumin NPs showed targetability to inflamed joints which could be explained by the increased permeability of the blood–joint barrier in arthritic animals.

Polymeric NPs were found to be preferentially taken up by macrophages and dendritic cells, that is, antigen-presenting cells (APCs) that play a key role in induction of inflammation or tolerance responses. Accordingly, several reasearch studies suggested the use of polymeric NPs for delivery of tolerogenic molecules to APCs. Maldonado et al. (2015) developed PLGA NPs loaded with auto-antigen and a tolerogenic immunomodulatory molecule, rapamycin. NPs were found to inhibit the activation of antigen-specific CD4+ and CD8+ T cells and B cells while inducing antigen-specific Tregs and Bregs. It is of note that NPs containing only rapamycin had no regulatory effect on APCs. The authors concluded that "the co-delivery of antigen and rapamycin provide an instruction set that could allow for the conditioning of tolerogenic dendritic cells capable of inducing CD4+ Treg."

In short, the advent of nanotechnologies feed the hope of a treatment based on specific-antigen tolerance induction rather than generalized immunosuppression.

3.3.4 Metabolic Disorders

In this section, two examples of metabolic disorders will be discussed: diabetes mellitus type 1, a serious metabolic disease of growing incidence and prevalence levels all over the world; and lactose intolerance, a burgeoning problem with socioeconomic impacts since it is often accompanied with other comorbidities (Schiffner et al., 2016).

3.3.4.1 Diabetes Mellitus Type 1

Diabetes mellitus type 1 is the most common metabolic disease. Replacement therapy is based on multiple daily subcutaneous injections of insulin, associated with multiple drawbacks. Apart from the burden of frequent injections on patients, lipodystrophy and lipohypertrophy in the injection site are frequent complications. Moreover, subcutaneous injections fail to mimic the physiological secretion of insulin, in which insulin undergoes hepatic first pass effect, resulting in a concentration gradient between portal and systemic circulations. Consequently, insulin subcutaneous administration may lead to hyperinsulinemia and thus predisposes to hypoglycemia and overweight.

Oral administration of insulin remains the desirable noninvasive alternative. Beside the ease of administration, orally delivered insulin could reproduce the physiological concentration gradient between portal and peripheral blood. Indeed, oral administration of insulin is highly challenging. Obstacles, such as the gastric acidity, proteolytic enzymes, efflux-pumps, etc., jeopardize its oral bioavailability, which is less than 1 percent.

Engineered NPs and MPs were found to be versatile vehicles for oral drug delivery (Diab et al., 2012). Encapsulation advantages are multiple, for example, enhanced apparent water solubility, enhanced permeation through intestinal epithelium, and physicochemical protection during gastrointestinal transition (Diab et al., 2012). Accordingly, a huge number of researches dealing with insulin encapsulation in polymeric and lipid-based NPs have been conducted and reviewed (Kaklotar et al., 2016).

Unfortunately, to date no oral formulation of insulin is marketed. Oral formulations featured limitations, such as low cost-effectiveness, lower bioavailability when compared to subcutaneous formula, and consequently higher doses were needed to produce an equivalent insulinemia. Nevertheless, recently the use of inorganic NPs was found to be promising for insulin oral delivery. Guha et al. (2016) designed an oral nanoparticulate platform for insulin with an encouraging relative bioavailability of about 73 percent. The formulation is based on MSNs coated with a pH-responsive shell of poly(methacrylic acid-co-vinyl triethoxysilane). Preclinical studies showed that animals displayed a stabilized glycaemia effect over 16 h after a single oral dose of insulin-loaded NPs (Guha et al., 2016).

Furthermore, Cho et al. (2014) prepared AuNPs stabilized with a shell of chondroitin sulfate. Insulin was adsorbed onto the NPs surface post synthesis. *In vivo* studies showed a significant lowering in glycaemia up to 32 percent when compared to the basal level in diabetic rats (Cho et al., 2014). These results indicate that the structural and functional integrity of insulin was maintained during processing but also during gastrointestinal transition. Chondroitin sulfate is thought to enhance the uptake of NPs by intestinal epithelial cells via CD44 receptor-mediated endocytosis (Fujimoto et al., 2001).

3.3.4.2 Lactose Intolerance

Lactose is the main disaccharide present in milk and derivatives, in different food products and as pharmaceutical excipient in drugs. Lactose intolerance is the inability to digest lactose. The brush-border enzymes, that is, β-galactosidases hydrolyze lactose in galactose and glucose that are easily absorbed in the intestine. Lactose intolerance appears when the enzyme activity decreases. Consequently, lactose persists in the intestine lumen, causing digestive disorders such as diarrhea, bloating, flatulence, and abdominal pain (Mattar et al., 2012).

Almost 70 percent of the world population has lactose intolerance as intestinal β-galactosidases lose their activities during lifetime. There is no treatment for lactose intolerance, but there are a couple of solutions. One of them will be to take medications/food loaded with β-galactosidases, or to eat only lactose-free products.

The development of food containing β-galactosidases is challenging, since enzymes can lose their activity through pH and temperature changes, during processing, but also after ingestion over gastrointestinal transit. Recently, encapsulation of β-galactosidases within hydrogel microbeads was proposed as an alternative to protect it in different pH and thermal conditions (Zhang et al., 2016). MSNs were also suggested as a protective matrix for β-galactosidases (Wu et al., 2010). Unfortunately, neither porous hydrogel microbeads nor mesoporous silica particles were able to give an efficient protection in low pH media (<2.5).

In addition, to date no biosensor is available on the market that can estimate lactose amount in food products. However, ongoing researches are looking to develop such biosensors. For instance, AuNPs were used to chemisorb β-galactosidases with a spacer arm (cysteamine-glutaraldehyde). The developed nanoprobes were found to enhance the enzyme kinetics parameters, stability, and reusability (Dwevedi et al., 2009). β-Galactosidases from *E. coli* were entrapped in silica NPs and then immobilized in a three-dimensional (3D) network on the sensor silicon surface, leading to a 3.5-fold increase in enzyme loading compared with the direct immobilization with glutaraldehyde (Betancor et al., 2008). The 3D structure offered the possibility of increasing the biosensor sensitivity. Moreover, the 3D-structured biosensor was found to preserve more than 80 percent of the initial enzymatic activity over 10 days at 24°C (Betancor et al., 2008).

3.3.5 CARDIOVASCULAR DISEASES

Cardiovascular diseases (CVD) represent the first cause of death in the world. Micro- and nanotechnologies hold promises for the improvement of CVD management through potential advances in diagnosis, drug delivery systems, and cardiovascular implantable devices.

Selective drug delivering to the pathological sites is a major advantage of micro- and nanotherapeutics. Functionalized NPs with collagen IV ligands were found to enable targeting of the sites of vascular injury (Chan et al., 2010). Indeed, collagen IV, a main component of vascular basement membrane, is exposed at sites of vascular inflammation or injury. Accordingly, collagen IV polymeric NPs were loaded with an anti-inflammatory peptide Ac2-26 and used to enhance resolution of inflammatory responses in a preclinical study using a hind-limb ischemia-reperfusion murine model (Kamaly et al., 2013). Injection of developed NPs were found to decrease neutrophils recruitment by 56 percent and to significantly block tissue damage by 30 percent in comparison to animals treated with the free Ac2-26 peptide (Kamaly et al., 2013).

Furthermore, passive targeting is likely to be possible because of the increased permeability at the sites of vascular lesions. In a clinical study, long-circulating liposomal prednisolone demonstrated an efficient targeting of atherosclerotic plaque macrophages upon their intravenous administration (van der Valk et al., 2015). Clinical evaluations are currently pursued on Nanocort® (PEG-liposomal prednisolone sodium phosphate) with the hope to produce selective anti-inflammatory effect on atherosclerotic plaques along with avoiding a general immunosuppression.

Recently, Thaxton et al. (2009) reported an interesting approach for the prevention and treatment of hypercholesterolaemia-associated diseases. The researchers designed synthetic cholesterol nanocarriers mimicking high density lipoprotein (HDL). NPs were composed of AuNP core surrounded with multiple phospholipid layers and at last with a protein layer of apolipoprotein A1, the main component of physiological HDL. Importantly, these synthetic NPs were shown to be able to reversely bind cholesterol in solution (Thaxton et al., 2009). Moreover, NPs biomimetic behavior, that is, the ability to bind to cholesterol and to efflux cholesterol from macrophages, could be modified by adjusting NPs size, shape, and surface properties (Luthi et al., 2012).

Nanotechnology-based approaches were also implemented for the improvement of cardiovascular implantable devices. Stents are widely used to support a segment of blood vessel despite the potential risk of in-stent restenosis. This occurs because of vascular smooth muscle cell (VSMC) migration, deposition on stent surface, and proliferation in addition to platelet activation, which finally leads to thrombus formation (Rymer et al., 2016). In order to prevent restenosis, stents were covered with biodegradable polymers releasing anti-angiogenic drugs such as paclitaxel and sirolimus. The obtained stents are so-called drug-eluting stents. Nevertheless, polymer biodegradation causes inflammation and thus increases the risk of restenosis and delays restoration of vascular lesions (Nakamura et al., 2016).

As alternatives to drug-eluting stents, NP-coated and nanostructured stents were proposed. In the former, covering NPs are thought to be released and then to be taken up by the damaged tissues exerting an effective inhibition of VSMC proliferation without affecting vascular re-endothelialization (Luderer et al., 2011). Nanostructured stents are polymer-free drug-eluting, designed by the way of surface topography using hydrothermal treatment in alkaline conditions (Jia et al., 2011). Nanostructured stents exhibit nanoporous surfaces mimicking the topography of endogenous tissues and thus enhancing compatibility with blood. Moreover, they were found to suppress VSMC proliferation along with enhancing vascular healing (Jia et al., 2011).

Recently, Liang et al. (2016) designed stents exhibiting VSMC-biomimetic patterned surfaces. These stents were fabricated on 316L stainless steel stent using a femtosecond laser and then coated with PLGA/rapamycin. They were found to be pro-healing by promoting re-endothelialization of damaged vessels (Liang et al., 2016).

Furthermore, combination of nanotechnologies and tissue engineering opened the way for a new generation of vessel prosthesis with a good mechanical performance and hemo- and cytocompatibility. Stefani and Cooper-White (2016) reported a composite tubular biomaterial scaffold composed of core-shell fibers with PCL forming the core and acrylate-L-lactide-co-trimethylene carbonate forming the shell. Accordingly, elastic nanofibrous scaffolds were obtained exhibiting *in vitro* burst pressures and suture retention strengths comparable to native vessels. The composite biomaterial displayed increased toughness when compared to tubes composed of PCL alone. Incubation of sterilized fibers with human mesenchymal stem cells over fourteen days showed progressive cell attachment to, and proliferation on, the 3D fibrous network (Stefani and Cooper-White, 2016).

3.3.6 VACCINATION AND INFECTIOUS DISEASES

Antibiotic resistance in the treatment of bacteria is currently one of the foremost issues in the medical world. The issue is further exacerbated by the cessation of development of new antimicrobials and the immense impact that antimicrobial resistance has on medical funds (Wang et al., 2016). In a single year in Europe, nearly 400,000 known infections of multiple drug resistant bacteria were recorded, with 25,000 cases causing death. More than €1.5 billion is spent annually on extra hospital costs associated with antibiotic resistance (Bush et al., 2011).

Indeed, antibiotic activity could be hampered by bacteria's destructive enzymes, or by their incapacity to cross complex matrixes, for example, biofilms, or to permeate through bacterial walls. Nanotechnologies represent a promising approach to overcome bacterial barriers and thus to reverse bacterial resistance to antibiotics. NPs help to bypass bacterial resistance through several mechanisms (Diab et al., 2015) such as (1) altering the bacterial efflux pump activity, (2) down-regulating the oxidative-stress resistance genes, (3) offering a protective barrier of the entrapped antibiotic against enzymatic inactivation, and (4) enhancing permeation through bacterial biofilm and wall.

Moreover, it is currently believed that the development of NP-based vaccinations could be extremely beneficial in fighting infections and potentially in overcoming antibiotic resistance (Wang et al., 2016). NPs have a unique shape, size, structure, and chemical composition that enable them to overcome biological barriers and to target specific cell types, such as APCs. NPs act as immunomodulators or adjuvants. For instance, soluble antigens, although generally poorly immunogenic, elicit a strong immune response when encapsulated in NPs (Renukaradhya et al., 2015; Vela Ramirez et al., 2016). NP-based vaccines conjugated with toll-like receptor ligands were shown to produce long-lasting T cell specific response altogether with neutralizing antibodies (Kasturi et al., 2011).

AuNPs show promise as a means of bacterial treatment, in particular their application for vaccine design, because of their ease of synthesis, biocompatibility, and their ability to enhance vaccine stability and Ag presentation on NPs surface, as well as their site-directed release of Ag (Renukaradhya et al., 2015; Marasini et al., 2016). AuNPs have shown specific potential in creating a vaccine against Glanders disease, which is produced by non-motile Gram negative bacteria *Burkholderia mallei*. Glanders is an epidemic disease in many parts of the world, in particular Asia and the Middle East (Torres et al., 2015). The development of a vaccine for this bacterium is specifically important due to (1) its ability to be weaponized, (2) the small number of organisms needed to cause infection, and (3) its high mortality rate and the current lack of effective treatment (Gregory et al., 2015; Torres et al., 2015).

In a study performed by Gregory et al. (2015), it was shown that mice immunized with AuNPs had a significantly greater survival time than mice that did not received AuNPs vaccine. AuNPs glycoconjugate vaccines, which conjugate polysaccharides from bacterial wall to a carrier protein (Torres et al., 2015), have also shown strong evidence of being immunogenic and protective against Glanders disease in a murine model.

The delivery of NP-based vaccines to mucosal sites is another mechanism being developed to combat bacterial infection. The main advantage is their ability to mimic the delivery pathway of bacterial pathogens. Mucosal NPs vaccines show further potential since approximately 80 percent of immune cells are located at the mucosal surface. However, there are numerous factors that may limit the success of NPs mucosal vaccines, such as mucociliary clearance, extremes of pH, and deteriorating enzymes. One way to overcome these problems is to design mucoadhesive polymeric NPs that are able to enhance NPs persistence at the mucosal site (Renukaradhya et al., 2015).

3.3.7 NUTRITION

It is widely recognized that well-balanced nutrition has a direct benefit in the prevention of chronic diseases and help to guarantee health or well-being. Even more, some spices such as curcumin were found to be active against several serious diseases. In this context, in the mid-1980s, *functional foods* were introduced in Japan. Hence, "functional" components, such as omega-3 fatty acids, vegetable fibers, vitamins, digestive enzymes or probiotics, are incorporated in the food matrix (Hasler, 2002).

Micro- and nanotechnologies were also implemented in food delivery in order to insure an effective intake of functional ingredients suffering from instability during food processing, storage, or gastrointestinal transit (Singh, 2016).

This section offers a special focus on micro- and nanoencapsulation of two types of functional ingredients, that is, curcumin and probiotics.

3.3.7.1 Curcumin

Curcumin is a hydrophobic natural polyphenolic molecule, extracted from *Curcuma longa*, which has been considered as food additive and traditional herbal remedy for wound care treatment as is well-documented in ancient literature, especially in some Asian countries. Recent studies have shown that curcumin has not only anti-inflammatory activities, but also a wide range of pharmacological properties such as antioxidant, anti-Alzheimer's, antitumor, and antimicrobial effects (Yallapu et al., 2012). Curcumin has also shown to be effective against a variety of cancer including skin, breast, lung cancers, and so on (Aggarwal et al., 2003). However, despite promising pharmaceutical properties, the main drawbacks of curcumin are its poor bioavailability due to low solubility at physiological pH and its rapid hydrolysis along with poor absorption. Various types of curcumin delivery systems have been elaborated to overcome the aforementioned problems, like polymeric NPs (Rabanel et al., 2015), metal oxide NPs (Yallapu et al., 2012), or MSNs (Kim et al., 2015, 2016). In this part, we will only focus on some remarkable works together with some recent studies including *in vivo*, and (pre-) clinical test results.

Among various delivery systems, lipid-based NPs has been, in particular, highlighted as they show very limited toxicity (Müller et al., 2000). Recently, a study dealing with curcumin-loaded SLN showed prolonged antitumor activity and cellular uptake. According to pharmacokinetic studies, the oral bioavailability of SLN-loaded curcumin was improved up to 125 percent, compared to the free molecule (Sun et al., 2013).

Polymeric NPs were also found to be good candidates for curcumin oral delivery for the treatment of inflammatory bowel disease. PLGA- and polymethacrylate-based NPs significantly enhanced cell uptake of curcumin in Caco-2 cells line and reduced TNF-α secretion by LPS-activated macrophages. These results were also supported by *in vivo* tests in which the decrease of neutrophil infiltration and TNF-α was clearly observed (Beloqui et al., 2014).

Noble metallic, silica, and metal oxide–based NPs have also been widely investigated for curcumin delivery, owing to their stability and facile functionalization as well as tuneable size, up to real nano-scale (less than 10 nm; Yang et al., 2016; Dey and Sreenivasan, 2015; Kim et al., 2015).

Some papers have dealt with curcumin-loading on carbon nanotubes or graphene; among them, single-walled carbon nanotubes were functionalized with curcumin and tested for *in vitro* inhibiting PC-3 cell growth (Li et al., 2014). The result would be promising; however, no further study has been done to support wide use of carbon nanocarriers.

Curcumin loaded self-assembled systems such as micelles or vesicles are already commercialized in the global market (Douglass and Clouatre, 2015). They are mostly classified as food additives and their efficiency is based on some fragmented data sets. Some scientific research data showed highly effective activities of curcumin-loaded micelles when tested for cancer therapy compared to free or other nanocarriers (Prasad et al., 2014); therefore, it could be said that micelle- or vesicle-based curcumin formulations are now mostly closed to "real" clinical applications, as all (or most) ingredients of micelle or vesicles have already been approved by the U.S. FDA and European EMA.

3.3.7.2 Probiotics

In past years, there have been extensive efforts to understand and prove the positive effects of the use of probiotic bacteria for different types of health issues, spanning from oral to topical formulated products and to treat conditions ranging from gastric diseases to atopic dermatitis (Iannitti and Palmieri, 2010). An estimation of about 10^{14} viable cells from probiotics to potentially harmful bacteria are harbored in the gastrointestinal tract of an adult (Holzapfel et al., 1998), and their harmonic relationship is dictated by the host's diet, medication intake, hygiene habits, and diseased state. Consequently, an individual's microbiome holds a unique diverse community implying in its health maintenance (Woting and Blaut, 2016).

Recent evidences evoke the considerable role played by the gut microbiota in the predisposition to different disease phenotypes, which are often accompanied by dysbiosis and are of major public health issues, for example, obesity, diabetes, and intestinal syndromes (Woting and Blaut, 2016). In this context, probiotics play a role in modification of the gene expressions, which are involved in immunomodulation, nutrient absorption, suppression of pathogens, energy metabolism, and intestinal barrier function such as stimulation of epithelial cell proliferation or induction of mucin secretion (Cani et al., 2009; Maynard et al., 2012). Yet the positive health benefits provided by these probiotic cells are essentially strain-dependent as well as disease-dependent.

To restore an imbalance in the microbiota, the oral intake of probiotics is a practice. In this case, cell microencapsulation is oftentimes necessary in order to provide external protection to the load that must arrive viable to the intestines after going through the harsh conditions of the gastrointestinal passage, for example, low pH and the presence of bile salts and enzymes. Currently the four main technologies used in microcapsule formation are extrusion, emulsion, spray-drying, and freeze-drying (Haffner et al., 2016) along with ionic polysaccharides (alginate and chitosan), microbial exopolysaccharides (gellan and xanthan gums), and milk proteins as examples of most commonly used encapsulating agents (Corona-Hernandez et al., 2013). Assuming that single microbes are of about a few μm in length, the final micro-cargo size should fall in the μm range and can contain single or multiple strains.

Few recent studies report not only the formulation of loaded-microparticles, but as well their probiotic effect in *in vitro* or *in vivo* models. For instance, entrapped *L. rhamnosus* GG in hydrogel beads formulated with pectin, glucose, and calcium chloride showed enhanced production of p40 in mice, a known LGG-derived protein involved in preventing and treating experimental colitis (Li et al., 2016). A system encapsulating *L. rhamnosus* PBS070, *L. plantarum* PBS067, and

B. animalis subsp. *lactis* in chitosan-coated alginate microcapsules containing glucose and β-glucan Pleuran revealed a symbiotic effect of the probiotic mixture despite the presence or the absence of Pleuran. Moreover, the strains modulated the release of the interleukins IL-4, IL-10, and TNF-α on HT-29 human colon cells going through inflammatory stress *in vitro*, predicting the potential *in vivo* probiotic activity of the system (D'Orazio et al., 2015). In the case of alcoholic liver injury, *L. plantarum* encapsulated in chitosan-alginate has been reported as able to attenuate ALD in mice, inflammatory molecules released in alcohol-related disorders (Arora et al., 2014).

A magnitude of studies lacking animal testing, supposedly due to their high cost, report however relevant encapsulating systems every year. Co-encapsulation of probiotics and drugs is a promising approach envisioning a superior therapeutic effect for ulcerative colitis, Crohn's disease, and recurrent *Clostridium difficile–* associated diarrhea. In this context, Pandey et al. (2016) developed an oil-in-water emulsion gel for the controlled release of metronidazole, an antimicrobial drug, along with *L. plantarum* 299v in an oil-in-water emulsion gel composed by xanthan and guar gum.

In a formulation point of view alone, alginate-based materials are by far the most explored due to their biodegradation, very good cytocompatibility, and mucoadhesive properties (Sosnik, 2014). Another class of materials is the protein-based, which may combine polysaccharides or non-digestible fibers known as prebiotics (Dong et al., 2013). In the interest of ameliorating the alginate or protein protection during simulated gastrointestinal passage, few recent strategies can be exemplified:

1. Alginate with polymerized whey protein coating. The protein's microstructure uniformity and enclosing structure formed after freeze-drying explained the better performance (Jiang et al., 2016).
2. Chitosan-coated alginate containing prebiotics, herein inulin and galactooligosaccharide. Chitosan confers an extra wall protection to the encapsulated cells while the prebiotics can have a synergetic effect increasing the number of cells or their activity (Krasaekoopt and Watcharapoka, 2014).
3. Sweet whey and skim milk encapsulating *L. acidophilus* La-5[21].
4. A prebiotic, fructo-oligosaccharides, and whey protein isolate in the case of *L. plantarum* (Rajam and Anandharamakrishnan, 2015). The compartmentalization of probiotic bacteria in more sophisticated approaches, such as using hydrophobized silica NPs to stabilize a Pickering emulsion has been reported by van Wijk et al. (2014) and it opens up novel pathways in bacteria encapsulation.

The effectiveness of probiotic intake in some clinical cases is already accepted, for example, in acute gastroenteritis (Passariello et al., 2014). On the other hand, the use of probiotics as a daily basis supplementation for health maintenance and nutrition is still debatable in the scientific community. Some of the reasons lie behind delicate definitions, such as: What is a healthy microbiome at first, or even, how can an individual become healthier? How badly does a poor individual diet influence the diversity of its microbiome?

The frontiers of microbiome knowledge are far from being completely understood since this domain is still in its early childhood. To the present day, only a few papers report complete studies, that is, from the synthesis of the encapsulated cargo with further animal testing on the beneficial effects of the entrapped probiotics. Nevertheless, ongoing and future research will unravel the paths for promising newer health treatments and functional foods. Perhaps one day the microbiome will become a sort of a "gutprint," a medical indicator of our state of health.

3.4 NANOPARTICLE USE FOR THERAPEUTIC AND DIAGNOSTIC PURPOSES

While NPs are usually designed for target drug delivery, they can also simultaneously provide diagnostic information by a variety of *in vivo* imaging methods, such as magnetic resonance imaging (MRI), single photon emission computed tomography (SPECT), positron emission tomography (PET), or fluorescent optical imaging. Herein, are presented several approaches of these "multifunctional" NPs (Figure 3.4).

3.4.1 MAGNETIC NANOPARTICLES

Magnetic nanoparticles (MNP) offer a versatile platform for theranostic (therapeutic and diagnostic) applications. Their use as contrast agents for MRI is already approved (Cole et al., 2011). In addition to their biocompatibility, their small size (10–50 nm)

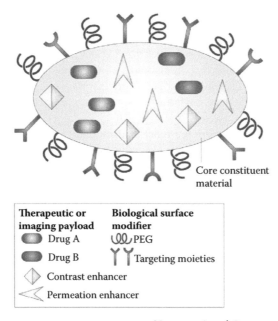

Core constituent material

Therapeutic or imaging payload	Biological surface modifier
Drug A	PEG
Drug B	Targeting moieties
Contrast enhancer	
Permeation enhancer	

Nature reviews | Cancer

FIGURE 3.4 Multifunctional nanoparticles. (Reprinted with permission from Ferrari, M., *Nat Rev Cancer*, 5, 161–171, 2005. Copyright 2005 Nature Publishing Group.)

enables them to reach specific targets in the human body and remarkably enhances their magnetic properties as contrast agents. Indeed, MNPs feature a superparamagnetic behavior as expressed by a high M_S and zero remanence ($M_R = 0$). A direct result of high M_S is the high responsiveness to external magnetic fields. Accordingly, MNP movement could be ordered by a moderate magnetic field. On the other hand, the zero remanence means that magnetization vanishes after the external magnetic field removal. As a consequence, particles could remain in circulation while avoiding vessel embolism.

The superparamagnetic behavior is mainly related to the particle size. Consistently, magnetic properties of MNP could easily be tuned (Xuan et al., 2009). SPION is a good example of MNP-based contrast agents for MRI. Based on nanosized (less than 20 nm) magnetite (Fe_3O_4) or its derivatives, obtained by doping with other metals like Mn and Zn, SPION show high M_S of around 100 emu g^{-1}, which cannot be obtained for their bulk counterparts. Nowadays, MNP-based contrast agents are extensively investigated in preclinical studies, as previously reviewed (Jin et al., 2014).

MNP are clinically used for cancer tissue ablation by hyperthermia (Thiesen and Jordan, 2008). Under an applied magnetic field, MNP causes tissues to heat up to $\approx 43°C$. Overheating is avoided thanks to the loss of particle magnetic properties above a critical temperature, called *Curie point*. When combined to chemotherapeutic agents, a synergistic cytotoxic effect is expected, as previously demonstrated (Hamoudeh et al., 2008).

For an effective hyperthermia therapy, the specific loss power that combines both M_S and anisotropy constant (K) should be high enough to give a good ratio between the applied magnetic field and the generated heat. For this purpose, iron oxide NPs doped with Zn or Mn seem to be suitable as they can give M_S values as high as 170 emu g^{-1}, which is three times higher than Feridex®, a previously commercialized agent (Li et al., 2013). The most remarkable clinical trials of MNP-induced hyperthermia were reported by the Maier-Hauff group, claiming improved survival time (up to two times) for patients suffering from glioblastoma multiforme (Maier-Hauff et al., 2007, 2011).

MNP could be used for surface-functionalization of porous materials like mesoporous silica, playing the role of pore-keeping gates and thus achieving a controlled release of co-loaded drugs. By applying an external magnetic field, local heating is generated inducing the gate opening (Thomas et al., 2010).

Finally, because of their ease of surface functionalization, MNPs were proposed as new platforms for gene delivery. For this purpose, MNPs are coupled with the nucleic acid, stabilized by a coating agent such as PEG, and then "decorated" with a targeting peptide, chosen as a function of the cancer tissues in question (Figure 3.5). NP location could be monitored by MRI and delivery of nucleic acids could be triggered using hyperthermia effect (Yang et al., 2010).

3.4.2 Photosensitizer Nanoparticles

Photosensitizer-loaded NPs are considered as promising theranostics based on targeted photodynamic destruction of diseased tissues. For cell destruction by photodynamic therapy, three ingredients are required: irradiated light (visible or

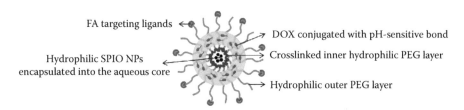

FA targeting ligands
Hydrophilic SPIO NPs encapsulated into the aqueous core
DOX conjugated with pH-sensitive bond
Crosslinked inner hydrophilic PEG layer
Hydrophilic outer PEG layer

FIGURE 3.5 Schematic representation of the SPIO/DOX-loaded vesicles with cross-linked inner hydrophilic PEG layers. (Reprinted with permission from Yang, X., Grailer, J. J., Rowland, I. J., Javadi, A., Hurley, S. A., Matson, V. Z., Steeber, D. A., and Gong, S., *ACS Nano*, 4, 6805–6817. Copyright 2010 American Chemical Society.)

near-infrared), molecular oxygen in the tissue, and photosensitizer molecules that are able to absorb light energy and move to an excited state, for example, 5-aminolevulinic acid and meso-tetra-hydroxyphenyl-chlorin, which are approved for clinical use. Briefly, irradiation of photosensitizer molecules leads to ROS generation and cell damage.

In order to spare normal tissues, targeting is achieved by encapsulating photosensitizer drug in nanoparticulate delivery systems, as previously reviewed (Chatterjee et al., 2008). Some types of inorganic NPs display photosensitizing properties by themselves, such as QDs, AuNPs, and AgNPs, as discussed in Section 3.2.4.

3.4.3 Radiolabeled Nanoparticles

Radionuclides-loaded NPs (RNPs) are of growing interest as a novel approach aiming to improve both radiotherapy and imaging outcomes. Indeed, following intratumoral or even systemic administrations, RNPs could accumulate within cancerous tissues while avoiding surrounding normal ones. Hence, low doses of radionuclides, even at trace level, could be monitored. A wide variety of micro- and nanoparticulate systems were formulated for radionuclide targeted delivery, as previously reviewed (Hamoudeh et al., 2008). The efficacy of RNP is dictated by the selectivity of the targeting ligand and by the radionuclide radiation properties, for example, physical half-life, decay mode, and emission properties.

The early clinical trials on RNP were conducted using ^{111}In-loaded liposomes and SPECT imaging for the detection of solid tumors (Presant et al., 1988) and Kaposi sarcoma and lymphoma in AIDS-suffering patients (Presant et al., 1990). Unfortunately, FDA approval was not obtained for this formulation, as the detection rate of malignant tissues (about 70 percent) was judged insufficient.

Silica ultra-small NPs (3–5 nm) containing fluorescent dye, called cornel-dots, were recently introduced in Phase I clinical trial stage using PET imaging (ClinicalTrials. gov identifier: NCT01266096). Silica NPs were functionalized with [124]I-labelled cRGD peptide, as a targeting ligand directed against $\alpha_v\beta_3$ integrin-expressing melanoma (Benezra et al., 2011). Pharmacokinetic studies showed that these NPs are fully removed from the body by renal clearance. Currently, these multifunctional particles are undergoing clinical evaluation for imaging of diseased lymph nodes during the surgical procedure in head and neck melanoma, breast cancer, and uterine cancer patients (ClinicalTrials.gov identifier: NCT02106598). The advantages of multifunctional NPs are discussed in the following sections.

3.4.4 BI- AND MULTIMODAL NANOPARTICLES

Being evaluated by only one imaging modality, NPs cannot provide enough and precise information in the human body with respect to anatomical, physiological, or molecular information. Therefore, to date, most NPs could not be translated from cell or *in vivo* small animal experiments to clinical applications. In this respect, multimodality imaging approaches can provide much more information by combining advantages and compensating for limitations from a single imaging modality to visualize the effects of the NPs. There are many possible combinations for dual-modal, trimodal, or other imaging modalities, including MR–optical, MR–PET, PET–CT, optical–PET, MR–CT, and MR–PET–optical.

Among them, the combination of MR–optical or MR–PET dual-modality imaging could provide the highest promising strategies in the near future. Indeed, MRI can provide anatomical and physiological images inside the human body with high spatial resolution (10–100 μm), but MRI agents are not currently of sufficient sensitivity (10^{-9}–10^{-6} moles of label detected). On the other side, optical or radionuclide imaging provide physiological and molecular information with high sensitivity (10^{-12} and 10^{-15} moles of label detected for optical imaging and for PET, respectively), but they have poor spatial resolutions for good anatomical images (>0.3 μm for optical imaging and 1–2 mm for PET).

3.4.4.1 MR–Optical Dual-Modality *in Vivo* Imaging

Optically active components include fluorescent dyes and QDs. The dyes can be physically or chemically bound to MNP. In order to avoid fluorescence quenching arising from energy transfer between the fluorescent molecules and the MNP, NPs can be coated either with long chemical linkers or with thick silica surfaces (Ow et al., 2005).

QDs ensure a high fluorescence signal, owing to their exceptional photostability, large extinction coefficients, and tunable absorption properties. One example is the assembly of multiple near-infrared (NIR) emitting QDs on Fe_3O_4 NPs (Shibu et al., 2013). NIR fluorescence offers deep tissue penetration capability, which allows high fluorescence sensitivity in deeply located organs such as the bladder. More recently, MRI-optical probes utilize NIR-to-visible up-conversion NPs composed of lanthanide-doped rare-earth elements (Cheng et al., 2011). The use of NIR light as an excitation source prevents auto-fluorescence in up-conversion NP-based optical imaging, which frequently arises from endogenous aromatic amino acid molecules (e.g., tryptophan, tyrosine, and phenylalanine) when short-wavelength (e.g., ultraviolet) radiation is used as an excitation source.

3.4.4.2 MR–PET Dual-Modality *in Vivo* Imaging

Torres Martin de Rosales et al. (2011) synthesized $^{64}Cu(II)$–Bis (dithiocarbamate-bisphosphonate) conjugated with dextran-coated SPION to image lymph nodes. Choi et al. (2008) used coated Mn-doped Fe_2O_4 conjugated to PET radionuclide ^{124}I via the coating. Those NPs were injected into the rat forepaw, and the position of the brachial lymph nodes was colocalized in MRI and PET, providing anatomical and physiological information from two imaging modalities (Choi et al., 2008). Uppal et al. (2011) synthesized and used NPs of Gd conjugates and ^{64}Cu to evaluated the fibrin imaging effect in the rat right internal carotid artery. Yang et al. (2011) demonstrated MRI–PET dual-modality NPs, adding the function of drug delivery to treat tumors. They synthesized the NPs using cyclo(Arg-Gly-Asp-d-Phe-Cys) peptides as tumor-targeting ligands, ^{64}Cu with a macrocyclic chelating agent for PET imaging, and doxorubicin-conjugated SPIOs for tumor treatment and MRI (Yang et al., 2011).

3.4.4.3 Other Multimodality Imaging

Among the imaging techniques, ultrasound (US) is the safest and it is currently used for pregnant women or infants. However, it has some limitations, such as penetration depth (e.g., several centimeters), bad sensitivity, and working poorly in air-containing organs. The image quality of US can be enhanced by combination with another imaging modality. John et al. (2012) reported the microsized particles for cancer imaging in MRI, magnetomotive optical coherence tomography, and US. Their particles consisted of protein–shell microspheres that were filled with iron oxide NPs in oil, and also the microspheres were functionalized with RGD peptides (John et al., 2012). Kim et al. (2011) demonstrated microsized capsules that contained Au, iron oxide, and islet cells for immunoprotection and CT–MR–US trimodality imaging. They injected the capsules into the mouse abdomen and evaluated the contrast effects in the three modalities (Kim et al., 2011).

REFERENCES

Abadeer, N. S., and Murphy, C. J. 2016. Recent progress in cancer thermal therapy using gold nanoparticles. *J Phys Chem* 120:4691–4716.

Abed, N., and Couvreur, P. 2014. Nanocarriers for antibiotics: A promising solution to treat intracellular bacterial infections. *Int J Antimicrob Agents* 43:485–496.

Aggarwal, B. B., Kumar, A., and Bharti, A. C. 2003. Anticancer potential of curcumin: Preclinical and clinical studies. *Anticancer Res* 23:363–398.

Albini, A., Mussi, V., Parodi, A., Ventura, A., Principi, E., Tegami, S., Rocchia, M., Francheschi, E., Sogno, I., Cammarota, R., Finzi, G., Sessa, F., Noonan, D. M., and Valbusa, U. 2010. Interactions of single-wall carbon nanotubes with endothelial cells. *Nanomedicine* 6:277–288.

Ali, H. M., Maksimenko, A., Urbinati, G., Chapuis, H., Raouane, M., Desmaële, D., Yasuhiro, H., Harashima, H., Couvreur, P., and Massaad-Massade, L. 2014. Effects of silencing the RET/PTC1 oncogene in papillary thyroid carcinoma by siRNA-squalene nanoparticles with and without fusogenic companion GALA-cholesterol. *Thyroid* 24:327–338.

Allen, T. M., and Cullis, P. R. 2013. Liposomal drug delivery systems: From concept to clinical applications. *Adv Drug Deliv Rev* 65:36–48.

Anselmo, A. C., and Mitragotri, S. 2016. Nanoparticles in the clinic: Nanoparticles in the clinic. *Bioengin Trans Medicine* 1:10–29.

Arora, S., Kaur, I. P., Chopra, K., and Rishi, P. 2014. Efficiency of double layered microencapsulated probiotic to modulate proinflammatory molecular markers for the management of alcoholic liver disease. *Mediators Inflamm* 2014:715130.

Balasubramanian, K. 2006. Molecular orbital basis for yellow curry spice curcumin's prevention of Alzheimer's disease. *J Agric Food Chem* 54:3512–3520.

BCC Research 2015. Nanotechnology in medical applications: The global market. Accessed from http://www.bccresearch.com/market-research/healthcare/nanotechnology-medical-applications-market-hlc069c.html.

Beloqui, A., Coco, R., Memvanga, P. B., Ucakar, B., des Rieux, A., and Préat, V. 2014. PH-sensitive nanoparticles for colonic delivery of curcumin in inflammatory bowel disease. *Int J Pharm* 473:203–212.

Benezra, M., Penate-Medina, O., Zanzonico, P. B., Schaer, D., Ow, H., Burns, A., DeStanchina, E., Longo, V., Herz, E., Iyer, S., Wolchok, J., Larson, S. M., Wiesner, U., and Bradbury, M. S. 2011. Multimodal silica nanoparticles are effective cancer-targeted probes in a model of human melanoma. *J Clin Invest* 121:2768–2780.

Betancor, L., Luckarift, H. R., Seo, J. H., Brand, O., and Spain, J. C. 2008. Three-dimensional immobilization of beta-galactosidase on a silicon surface. *Biotechnol Bioeng* 99:261–267.

Bhadra, D., Bhadra, S., Jain, S., and Jain, N. K. 2003. A pegylated dendritic nanoparticulate carrier of fluorouracil. *Int J Pharm* 257:111–124.

Birrenbach, G., and Speiser, P. P. 1976. Polymerized micelles and their use as adjuvants in immunology. *J Pharm Sci* 65:1763–1766.

Boyer, P. D., Ganesh, S., Qin, Z., Holt, B. D., Buehler, M. J., Islam, M. F., and Dahl, K. N. 2016. Delivering single-walled carbon nanotubes to the nucleus using engineered nuclear protein domains. *ACS Appl Mater Interfaces* 8:3524–3534.

Bronstein, L. M., Huang, X., Retrum, J., Schmucker, A., Pink, M., Stein, B. D., and Dragnea, B. 2007. Influence of iron oleate complex structure on iron oxide nanoparticle formation. *Chem Mater* 19:3624–3632.

Brust, M., Walker, M., Bethell, D., Schiffrin, D. J., and Whyman, R. 1994. Synthesis of thiol-derivatised gold nanoparticles in a two-phase liquid-liquid system. *J Chem Soc, Chem Comm* doi: 10.1039/C39940000801:801.

Bush, K., Courvalin, P., Dantas, G., Davies, J., Eisenstein, B., Huovinen, P., Jacoby, G., Kishony, R., Kreiswirth, B., Kutter, E., Lerner, S., Levy, S., Lewis, K., Lomovskaya, O., Miller, J., Mobashery, S., Piddock, L., Projan, S., Thomas, C., Tomasz, A., Tulkens, P., Walsh, T., Watson, J., Witkowski, J., Witte, W., Wright, G., Yeh, P., and Zgurskaya, H. 2011. Tackling antibiotic resistance. *Nat Rev Microbiol* 9:894–896.

Cani, P. D., Possemiers, S., Van de Wiele, T., Guiot, Y., Everard, A., Rottier, O., Geurts, L., Naslain, D., Neyrinck, A., Lambert, D. M., Muccioli, G. G., and Delzenne, N. M. 2009. Changes in gut microbiota control inflammation in obese mice through a mechanism involving GLP-2-driven improvement of gut permeability. *Gut* 58:1091–1103.

Chan, J. M., Zhang, L., Tong, R., Ghosh, D., Gao, W., Liao, G., Yuet, K. P., Gray, D., Rhee, J., Cheng, J., Golomb, G., Libby, P., Langer, R., and Farokhzad, O. C. 2010. Spatiotemporal controlled delivery of nanoparticles to injured vasculature. *Proc Natl Acad Sci U S A* 107:2213–2218.

Chatterjee, A. K., Sarkar, R. K., Chattopadhyay, A. P., Aich, P., Chakraborty, R., and Basu, T. 2012. A simple robust method for synthesis of metallic copper nanoparticles of high antibacterial potency against *E. coli*. *Nanotechnology* 23:085103.

Chatterjee, D. K., Fong, L. S., and Zhang, Y. 2008. Nanoparticles in photodynamic therapy: An emerging paradigm. *Adv Drug Deliv Rev* 60:1627–1637.

Che Rose, L., Bear, J. C., McNaughter, P. D., Southern, P., Piggott, R. B., Parkin, I. P., Qi, S., and Mayes, A. G. 2016. A spion-eicosane protective coating for water soluble capsules: Evidence for on-demand drug release triggered by magnetic hyperthermia. *Sci Rep* 6:20271.

Chen, G., Roy, I., Yang, C., and Prasad, P. N. 2016. Nanochemistry and nanomedicine for nanoparticle-based diagnostics and therapy. *Chem Rev* 116:2826–85.

Cheng, K. K., Chan, P. S., Fan, S., Kwan, S. M., Yeung, K. L., Wáng, Y. J., Chow, A. H. L., Wu, E. X., and Baum, L. 2015. Curcumin-conjugated magnetic nanoparticles for detecting amyloid plaques in Alzheimer's disease mice using magnetic resonance imaging (MRI). *Biomaterials* 44:155–172.

Cheng, L., Yang, K., Li, Y., Chen, J., Wang, C., Shao, M., Lee, S., and Liu, Z. 2011. Facile preparation of multifunctional upconversion nanoprobes for multimodal imaging and dual-targeted photothermal therapy. *Angew Chem Int Ed Engl* 50:7385–7390.

Cho, H., Oh, J., Choo, M., Ha, J., Park, Y., and Maeng, H. 2014. Chondroitin sulfate-capped gold nanoparticles for the oral delivery of insulin. *Int J Biol Macromol* 63:15–20.

Choi, J., Park, J. C., Nah, H., Woo, S., Oh, J., Kim, K. M., Cheon, G. J., Chang, Y., Yoo, J., and Cheon, J. 2008. A hybrid nanoparticle probe for dual-modality positron emission tomography and magnetic resonance imaging. *Angew Chem Int Ed Engl* 47:6259–6262.

Chon, H., Wang, R., Lee, S., Bang, S., Lee, H., Bae, S., Hong, S. H., Yoon, Y. H., Lim, D. W., deMello, A. J., and Choo, J. 2015. Clinical validation of surface-enhanced Raman scattering-based immunoassays in the early diagnosis of rheumatoid arthritis. *Anal Bioanal Chem* 407:8353–8362.

Cole, A. J., Yang, V. C., and David, A. E. 2011. Cancer theranostics: The rise of targeted magnetic nanoparticles. *Trends Biotechnol* 29:323–332.

Corona-Hernandez, R., Álvarez-Parrilla, E., Lizardi-Mendoza, J., Islas-Rubio, A., de la Rosa, L., and Wall-Medrano, A. 2013. Structural stability and viability of microencapsulated probiotic bacteria: A review. *Compr Rev Food Sci F* 12:614–662.

Couvreur, P., Kante, B., Grislain, L., Roland, M., Speiser, P. 1982. Toxicity of polyalkyl-cyanoacrylate nanoparticles ii: Doxorubicin-loaded nanoparticles. *J Pharm Sci* 71: 790–792.

Couvreur, P., Stella, B., Reddy, L. H., Hillaireau, H., Dubernet, C., Desmaële, D., Lepêtre-Mouelhi, S., Rocco, F., Dereuddre-Bosquet, N., Clayette, P., Rosilio, V., Marsaud, V., Renoir, J., and Cattel, L. 2006. Squalenoyl nanomedicines as potential therapeutics. *Nano Lett* 6:2544–2548.

Couvreur, P., Tulkens, P., Roland, M., Trouet, A., and Speiser, P. 1977. Nanocapsules: A new type of lysosomotropic carrier. *FEBS Lett* 84:323–326.

Cui, Y., Xu, Q., Chow, P. K., Wang, D., and Wang, C. 2013. Transferrin-conjugated magnetic silica PLGA nanoparticles loaded with doxorubicin and paclitaxel for brain glioma treatment. *Biomaterials* 34:8511–8520.

Dey, S., and Sreenivasan, K. 2015. Conjugating curcumin to water soluble polymer stabilized gold nanoparticles via pH responsive succinate linker. *J Mater Chem* 3:824–833.

Diab, R., Degobert, G., Hamoudeh, M., Dumontet, C., and Fessi, H. 2007. Nucleoside analogue delivery systems in cancer therapy. *Expert Opin Drug Deliv* 4:513–531.

Diab, R., Jaafar-Maalej, C., Fessi, H., and Maincent, P. 2012. Engineered nanoparticulate drug delivery systems: The next frontier for oral administration? *AAPS J* 14:688–702.

Diab, R., Khameneh, B., Joubert, O., and Duval, R. 2015. Insights in nanoparticle-bacterium interactions: New frontiers to bypass bacterial resistance to antibiotics. *Curr Pharm Des* 21:4095–4105.

Dizaj, S. M., Lotfipour, F., Barzegar-Jalali, M., Zarrintan, M. H., and Adibkia, K. 2014. Antimicrobial activity of the metals and metal oxide nanoparticles. *Mater Sci Eng C* 44:278–284.

Dong, Q., Chen, M., Xin, Y., Qin, X., Cheng, Z., Shi, L., and Tang, Z. 2013. Alginate-based and protein-based materials for probiotics encapsulation: A review. *Int J Food Sci Tech* 48:1339–1351.

D'Orazio, G., Di Gennaro, P., Boccarusso, M., Presti, I., Bizzaro, G., Giardina, S., Michelotti, A., Labra, M., and La Ferla, B. 2015. Microencapsulation of new probiotic formulations for gastrointestinal delivery: In vitro study to assess viability and biological properties. *Appl Microbiol Biotechnol* 99:9779–9789.

Dosio, F., Reddy, L. H., Ferrero, A., Stella, B., Cattel, L., and Couvreur, P. 2010. Novel nano-assemblies composed of squalenoyl-paclitaxel derivatives: Synthesis, characterization, and biological evaluation. *Bioconjug Chem* 21:1349–1361.

Dosio, F., Stella, B., Ferrero, A., Garino, C., Zonari, D., Arpicco, S., Cattel, L., Giordano, S., and Gobetto, R. 2013. Ruthenium polypyridyl squalene derivative: A novel self-assembling lipophilic probe for cellular imaging. *Int J Pharm* 440:221–228.

Douglass, B., and Clouatre, D. 2015. Beyond yellow curry: Assessing commercial curcumin absorption technologies. *J Am Coll Nutr* 34:347–358.

Dwevedi, A., Singh, A. K., Singh, D. P., Srivastava, O. N., and Kayastha, A. M. 2009. Lactose nanoprobe optimized using response surface methodology. *Biosens Bioelectron* 25:784–790.

Enciso, A. E., Neun, B., Rodriguez, J., Ranjan, A. P., Dobrovolskaia, M. A., and Simanek, E. E. 2016. Nanoparticle effects on human platelets in vitro: A comparison between PAMAM and triazine dendrimers. *Molecules* 21:428.

Fang, M., Peng, C., Pang, D., and Li, Y. 2012. Quantum dots for cancer research: Current status, remaining issues, and future perspectives. *Cancer Biol Med* 9:151–163.

Fang, Y., Guo, S., Li, D., Zhu, C., Ren, W., Dong, S., and Wang, E. 2012. Easy synthesis and imaging applications of cross-linked green fluorescent hollow carbon nanoparticles. *ACS Nano* 6:400–409.

Fessi, H., and Devissaguet, F. 1987. Procédé de preparation de systèmes colloidaux dispersibles d'une substance sous forme de nanocapsules. *European Patent* 274 961.

Fiala, M., Liu, P. T., Espinosa-Jeffrey, A., Rosenthal, M. J., Bernard, G., Ringman, J. M., Sayre, J., Zhang, L., Zaghi, J., Dejbakhsh, S., Chiang, B., Hui, J., Mahanian, M., Baghaee, A., Hong, P., and Cashman, J. 2007. Innate immunity and transcription of mgat-iii and toll-like receptors in Alzheimer's disease patients are improved by bisdemethoxycurcumin. *Proc Natl Acad Sci USA* 104:12849–12854.

Fréchet, J. 2003. Dendrimers and other dendritic macromolecules: From building blocks to functional assemblies in nanoscience and nanotechnology. *J Polym Sci Pol Chem* 41:3713–3725.

Friedhofen, J., and Vögtle, F. 2006. Detailed nomenclature for dendritic molecules. *New J Chem* 30:32–43.

Fruchon, S., Mouriot, S., Thiollier, T., Grandin, C., Caminade, A., Turrin, C., Contamin, H., and Poupot, R. 2015. Repeated intravenous injections in non-human primates demonstrate preclinical safety of an anti-inflammatory phosphorus-based dendrimer. *Nanotoxicology* 9:433–441.

Fujimoto, T., Kawashima, H., Tanaka, T., Hirose, M., Toyama-Sorimachi, N., Matsuzawa, Y., and Miyasaka, M. 2001. CD44 binds a chondroitin sulfate proteoglycan, aggrecan. *Int Immunol* 13:359–366.

Garcia-Alloza, M., Borrelli, L. A., Rozkalne, A., Hyman, B. T., and Bacskai, B. J. 2007. Curcumin labels amyloid pathology in vivo, disrupts existing plaques, and partially restores distorted neurites in an Alzheimer mouse model. *J Neurochem* 102:1095–1104.

Gaucher, G., Dufresne, M., Sant, V. P., Kang, N., Maysinger, D., and Leroux, J. 2005. Block copolymer micelles: Preparation, characterization and application in drug delivery. *J Control Release* 109:169–188.

Geszke-Moritz, M., and Moritz, M. 2016. Solid lipid nanoparticles as attractive drug vehicles: Composition, properties and therapeutic strategies. *Mater Sci Eng C Mater Biol Appl* 68:982–994.

Ghosh, S. K., and Pal, T. 2007. Interparticle coupling effect on the surface plasmon resonance of gold nanoparticles: From theory to applications. *Chem Rev* 107:4797–4862.

Gregory, A., Judy, B., Qazi, O., Blumentritt, C., Brown, K., Shaw, A., Torres, A., and Titball, R. 2015. A gold nanoparticle-linked glycoconjugate vaccine against *Burkholderia mallei*. *Nanomedicine* 11:447–456.

Guada, M., Lana, H., Gil, A. G., Dios-Viéitez, M. D. C., and Blanco-Prieto, M. J. 2016. Cyclosporine a lipid nanoparticles for oral administration: Pharmacodynamics and safety evaluation. *Eur J Pharm Biopharm* 101:112–118.

Guha, A., Biswas, N., Bhattacharjee, K., Sahoo, N., and Kuotsu, K. 2016. PH responsive cylindrical msn for oral delivery of insulin-design, fabrication and evaluation. *Drug Deliv* 1–30.

Gulyaev, A. E., Gelperina, S. E., Skidan, I. N., Antropov, A. S., Kivman, G. Y., and Kreuter, J. 1999. Significant transport of doxorubicin into the brain with polysorbate 80-coated nanoparticles. *Pharm Res* 16:1564–1569.

Guo, J., Zhang, H., Geng, H., Mi, X., Ding, G., and Jiao, Z. 2015. Efficient one-pot synthesis of peapod-like hollow carbon nanomaterials for ultra high drug loading capacity. *J Colloid Interface Sci* 437:90–96.

Guo, S., Gong, J., Jiang, P., Wu, M., Lu, Y., and Yu, S. 2008. Biocompatible, luminescent silver@phenol formaldehyde resin core/shell nanospheres: Large-scale synthesis and application for in vivo bioimaging. *Adv Funct Mater* 18:872–879.

Haffner, F., Diab, R., and Pasc, A. 2016. Encapsulation of probiotics: Insights into academic and industrial approaches. *AIMS Mater Sci* 3:114–136.

Hajipour, M. J., Fromm, K. M., Akbar Ashkarran, A., Jimenez de Aberasturi, D., Larramendi, I. R. D., Rojo, T., Serpooshan, V., Parak, W. J., and Mahmoudi, M. 2012. Antibacterial properties of nanoparticles. *Trends Biotechnol* 30:499–511.

Hamoudeh, M., Diab, R., Fessi, H., Dumontet, C., and Cuchet, D. 2008. Paclitaxel-loaded microparticles for intratumoral administration via the TMT technique: Preparation, characterization, and preliminary antitumoral evaluation. *Drug Dev Ind Pharm* 34:698–707.

Hamoudeh, M., Kamleh, M. A., Diab, R., and Fessi, H. 2008. Radionuclides delivery systems for nuclear imaging and radiotherapy of cancer. *Adv Drug Deliv Rev* 60:1329–1346.

Hasler, C. 2002. Functional foods: Benefits, concerns and challenges—A position paper from the american council on science and health. *J Nutr* 132:3772–3781.

Hawker, C., and Fréchet, J. 1990. Preparation of polymers with controlled molecular architecture. A new convergent approach to dendritic macromolecules. *J Am Chem Soc* 112:7638–7647.

Hervault, A., and Thanh, N. T. K. 2014. Magnetic nanoparticle-based therapeutic agents for thermo-chemotherapy treatment of cancer. *Nanoscale* 6:11553–11573.

Holzapfel, W. H., Haberer, P., Snel, J., Schillinger, U., and Huis in't Veld, J. H. 1998. Overview of gut flora and probiotics. *Int J Food Microbiol* 41:85–101.

Huang, X., Neretina, S., and El-Sayed, M. 2009. Gold nanorods: From synthesis and properties to biological and biomedical applications. *Adv Mater* 21:4880–4910.

Hwang, S., Moorefield, C., and Newkome, G. 2008. Dendrimers in the spotlight. *Phys Chem Chem Phys* 10:T87.

Iannitti, T., and Palmieri, B. 2010. Therapeutical use of probiotic formulations in clinical practice. *Clin Nutr* 29:701–725.

Jia, B., Qin, M., Zhang, Z., Chu, A., Zhang, L., Liu, Y., Lu, H., and Qu, X. 2013. One-pot synthesis of Cu-Carbon hybrid hollow spheres. *Carbon* 62:472–480.

Jia, H., Liu, H., Kong, J., Hou, J., Wu, J., Zhang, M., Tian, J., Liu, H., Ma, L., Hu, S., Huang, X., Zhang, S., Zhang, S., Yu, B., and Jang, I. 2011. A novel polymer-free paclitaxel-eluting stent with a nanoporous surface for rapid endothelialization and inhibition of intimal hyperplasia: Comparison with a polymer-based sirolimus-eluting stent and bare metal stent in a porcine model. *J Biomed Mater Res A* 98:629–637.

Jiang, Y., Zheng, Z., Zhang, T., Hendricks, G., and Guo, M. 2016. Microencapsulation of *lactobacillus acidophilus* NCFM using polymerized whey proteins as wall material. *Int J Food Sci Nutr* 67:670–677.

Jin, R., Lin, B., Li, D., and Ai, H. 2014. Superparamagnetic iron oxide nanoparticles for MR imaging and therapy: Design considerations and clinical applications. *Curr Opin Pharmacol* 18:18–27.

John, R., Nguyen, F. T., Kolbeck, K. J., Chaney, E. J., Marjanovic, M., Suslick, K. S., and Boppart, S. A. 2012. Targeted multifunctional multimodal protein-shell microspheres as cancer imaging contrast agents. *Mol Imaging Biol* 14:17–24.

Joye, I. J., and McClements, D. J. 2016. Biopolymer-based delivery systems: Challenges and opportunities. *Curr Top Med Chem* 16:1026–1039.

Junghanns, J. A. H., and Müller, R. H. 2008. Nanocrystal technology, drug delivery and clinical applications. *Int J Nanomedicine* 3:295–309.

Kaklotar, D., Agrawal, P., Abdulla, A., Singh, R. P., Mehata, A. K., Singh, S., Mishra, B., Pandey, B. L., Trigunayat, A., and Muthu, M. S. 2016. Transition from passive to active targeting of oral insulin nanomedicines: Enhancement in bioavailability and glycemic control in diabetes. *Nanomedicine (Lond)* 11:1465–1486.

Kamaly, N., Fredman, G., Subramanian, M., Gadde, S., Pesic, A., Cheung, L., Fayad, Z. A., Langer, R., Tabas, I., and Farokhzad, O. C. 2013. Development and in vivo efficacy of targeted polymeric inflammation-resolving nanoparticles. *Proc Natl Acad Sci USA* 110:6506–6511.

Kannan, R. M., Nance, E., Kannan, S., and Tomalia, D. A. 2014. Emerging concepts in dendrimer-based nanomedicine: From design principles to clinical applications. *J Intern Med* 276:579–617.

Kasturi, S., Skountzou, I., Albrecht, R., Koutsonanos, D., Hua, T., Nakaya, H., Ravindran, R., Stewart, S., Alam, M., Kwissa, M., Villinger, F., Murthy, N., Steel, J., Jacob, J., Hogan, R., Garcia-Sastre, A., Compans, R., and Pulendran, B. 2011. Programming the magnitude and persistence of antibody responses with innate immunity. *Nature* 470:543–547.

Kim, H. S., Lee, J. Y., Lim, S. H., Sun, J., Lee, S. H., Ahn, J. S., Park, K., Moon, S. H., and Ahn, M. 2015. A prospective phase II study of cisplatin and cremophor el-free paclitaxel (Genexol-PM) in patients with unresectable thymic epithelial tumors. *J Thorac Oncol* 10:1800–1806.

Kim, J., Arifin, D. R., Muja, N., Kim, T., Gilad, A. A., Kim, H., Arepally, A., Hyeon, T., and Bulte, J. W. M. 2011. Multifunctional capsule-in-capsules for immunoprotection and trimodal imaging. *Angew Chem Int Ed Engl* 50:2317–2321.

Kim, J. S., Song, K. S., and Yu, I. J. 2016. Multiwall carbon nanotube-induced DNA damage and cytotoxicity in male human peripheral blood lymphocytes. *Int J Toxicol* 35:27–37.

Kim, S., Diab, R., Joubert, O., Canilho, N., and Pasc, A. 2016. Core–shell microcapsules of solid lipid nanoparticles and mesoporous silica for enhanced oral delivery of curcumin. *Colloids Surf B Biointerfaces* 140:161–168.

Kim, S., Philippot, S., Fontanay, S., Duval, R., Lamouroux, E., Canilho, N., and Pasc, A. 2015. Ph- and glutathione-responsive release of curcumin from mesoporous silica nanoparticles coated using tannic acid–Fe(III) complex. *RSC Adv* 5:90550.

Kim, S., Shibata, E., Sergiienko, R., and Nakamura, T. 2008. Purification and separation of carbon nanocapsules as a magnetic carrier for drug delivery systems. *Carbon* 46:1523–1529.

Krasaekoopt, W., and Watcharapoka, S. 2014. Effect of addition of inulin and galactooligosaccharide on the survival of microencapsulated probiotics in alginate beads coated with chitosan in simulated digestive system, yogurt and fruit juice. *LWT-Food Sci Technol* 57:761–766.

Kreuter, J. 1994. Nanoparticles, in *Encyclopedia of Pharmaceutical Technology*, eds. J. Swarbrick and J. C. Boylan, pp. 165–190. New York: M. Dekker.

Kreuter, J. 2007. Nanoparticles: A historical perspective. *Int J Pharm* 331:1–10.

Kuo, Y., and Cheng, S. 2016. Brain targeted delivery of carmustine using solid lipid nanoparticles modified with tamoxifen and lactoferrin for antitumor proliferation. *Int J Pharm* 499:10–19.

Kwon, H. J., Cha, M., Kim, D., Kim, D. K., Soh, M., Shin, K., Hyeon, T., and Mook-Jung, I. 2016. Mitochondria-targeting ceria nanoparticles as antioxidants for Alzheimer's disease. *ACS Nano* 10:2860–2870.

Lacerda, L., Russier, J., Pastorin, G., Herrero, M. A., Venturelli, E., Dumortier, H., Al-Jamal, K. T., Prato, M., Kostarelos, K., and Bianco, A. 2012. Translocation mechanisms of chemically functionalised carbon nanotubes across plasma membranes. *Biomaterials* 33:3334–3343.

Lal, S., Verma, J., and Van Noorden, C. J. 2014. Nanoparticles for hyperthermic therapy: Synthesis strategies and applications in glioblastoma. *Int J Nanomedicine* 9:2863.

Lam, C., James, J. T., McCluskey, R., Arepalli, S., and Hunter, R. L. 2006. A review of carbon nanotube toxicity and assessment of potential occupational and environmental health risks. *Crit Rev Toxicol* 36:189–217.

Lammers, T., Kiessling, F., Hennink, W. E., and Storm, G. 2012. Drug targeting to tumors: Principles, pitfalls and (pre-) clinical progress. *J Control Release* 161:175–187.

Laurent, S., Forge, D., Port, M., Roch, A., Robic, C., Vander Elst, L., and Muller, R. N. 2008. Magnetic iron oxide nanoparticles: Synthesis, stabilization, vectorization, physicochemical characterizations, and biological applications. *Chem Rev* 108: 2064–2110.

Le Ouay, B., and Stellacci, F. 2015. Antibacterial activity of silver nanoparticles: A surface science insight. *Nanotoday* 10:339–354.

Lee, C. C., MacKay, J. A., Fréchet, J. M. J., and Szoka, F. C. 2005. Designing dendrimers for biological applications. *Nat Biotechnol* 23:1517–1526.

Leroux, J., Allémann, E., Gurny, R., and Doelker, E. 1995. New approach for the preparation of nanoparticles by a modified emulsification-diffusion method. *Eur J Pharm Biopharm* 41:14–18.

Leyva-Gómez, G., González-Trujano, M. E., López-Ruiz, E., Couraud, P., Wekslerg, B., Romero, I., Miller, F., Delie, F., Allémann, E., and Quintanar-Guerrero, D. 2014. Nanoparticle formulation improves the anticonvulsant effect of clonazepam on the pentylenetetrazole-induced seizures: Behavior and electroencephalogram. *J Pharm Sci* 103: 2509–2519.

Li, H., Zhang, N., Hao, Y., Wang, Y., Jia, S., Zhang, H., Zhang, Y., and Zhang, Z. 2014. Formulation of curcumin delivery with functionalized single-walled carbon nanotubes: Characteristics and anticancer effects in vitro. *Drug Deliv* 21:379–387.

Li, L., Jiang, W., Luo, K., Song, H., Lan, F., Wu, Y., and Gu, Z. 2013. Superparamagnetic iron oxide nanoparticles as MRI contrast agents for non-invasive stem cell labeling and tracking. *Theranostics* 3:595–615.

Li, N., Zhao, P., and Astruc, D. 2014. Anisotropic gold nanoparticles: Synthesis, properties, applications, and toxicity. *Angew Chem Int Edit* 53:1756–1789.

Li, R., Zhang, Y., Polk, D. B., Tomasula, P. M., Yan, F., and Liu, L. 2016. Preserving viability of *Lactobacillus rhamnosus* GG in vitro and in vivo by a new encapsulation system. *J Control Release* 230:79–87.

Li, S., Pasc, A., Fierro, V., and Celzard, A. 2016. Hollow carbon spheres, synthesis, and applications: A review. *J Mater Chem A* 4:12686–12713.

Liang, C., Hu, Y., Wang, H., Xia, D., Li, Q., Zhang, J., Yang, J., Li, B., Li, H., Han, D., and Dong, M. 2016. Biomimetic cardiovascular stents for in vivo re-endothelialization. *Biomaterials* 103:170–182.

Liang, J., Liu, H., Huang, C., Yao, C., Fu, Q., Li, X., Cao, D., Luo, Z., and Tang, Y. 2015. Aggregated silver nanoparticles based surface-enhanced Raman scattering enzyme-linked immunosorbent assay for ultrasensitive detection of protein biomarkers and small molecules. *Anal Chem* 87:5790–5796.

Lim, J., Kostiainen, M., Maly, J., da Costa, V. C. P., Annunziata, O., Pavan, G. M., and Simanek, E. E. 2013. Synthesis of large dendrimers with the dimensions of small viruses. *J Am Chem Soc* 135:4660–4663.

Link, S., and El-Sayed, M. A. 2000. Shape and size dependence of radiative, non-radiative and photothermal properties of gold nanocrystals. *Int Rev Phys Chem* 19:409–453.

Luderer, F., Löbler, M., Rohm, H. W., Gocke, C., Kunna, K., Köck, K., Kroemer, H. K., Weitschies, W., Schmitz, K., and Sternberg, K. 2011. Biodegradable sirolimus-loaded poly(lactide) nanoparticles as drug delivery system for the prevention of in-stent restenosis in coronary stent application. *J Biomater Appl* 25:851–875.

Luthi, A. J., Zhang, H., Kim, D., Giljohann, D. A., Mirkin, C. A., and Thaxton, C. S. 2012. Tailoring of biomimetic high-density lipoprotein nanostructures changes cholesterol binding and efflux. *ACS Nano* 6:276–285.

Ma, P., and Mumper, R. J. 2013. Anthracycline nano-delivery systems to overcome multiple drug resistance: A comprehensive review. *Nano Today* 8:313–331.

Ma, P., and Mumper, R. J. 2013. Paclitaxel nano-delivery systems: A comprehensive review. *J Nanomed Nanotechnol* 4:1000164.

Maier-Hauff, K., Rothe, R., Scholz, R., Gneveckow, U., Wust, P., Thiesen, B., Feussner, A., von Deimling, A., Waldoefner, N., Felix, R., and Jordan, A. 2007. Intracranial thermotherapy using magnetic nanoparticles combined with external beam radiotherapy: Results of a feasibility study on patients with glioblastoma multiforme. *J Neurooncol* 81:53–60.

Maier-Hauff, K., Ulrich, F., Nestler, D., Niehoff, H., Wust, P., Thiesen, B., Orawa, H., Budach, V., and Jordan, A. 2011. Efficacy and safety of intratumoral thermotherapy using magnetic iron-oxide nanoparticles combined with external beam radiotherapy on patients with recurrent glioblastoma multiforme. *J Neurooncol* 103:317–324.

Maldonado, R. A., LaMothe, R. A., Ferrari, J. D., Zhang, A., Rossi, R. J., Kolte, P. N., Griset, A. P., O'Neil, C., Altreuter, D. H., Browning, E., Johnston, L., Farokhzad, O. C., Langer, R., Scott, D. W., von Andrian, U. H., and Kishimoto, T. K. 2015. Polymeric synthetic nanoparticles for the induction of antigen-specific immunological tolerance. *Proc Natl Acad Sci U S A* 112:E156–165.

Mamot, C., Ritschard, R., Wicki, A., Stehle, G., Dieterle, T., Bubendorf, L., Hilker, C., Deuster, S., Herrmann, R., and Rochlitz, C. 2012. Tolerability, safety, pharmacokinetics, and efficacy of doxorubicin-loaded anti-EGFR immunoliposomes in advanced solid tumours: A phase 1 dose-escalation study. *Lancet Oncol* 13:1234–1241.

Marasini, N., Khalil, Z. G., Giddam, A. K., Ghaffar, K. A., Hussein, W. M., Capon, R. J., Batzloff, M. R., Good, M. F., Skwarczynski, M., and Toth, I. 2016. Lipid core peptide/poly(lactic-co-glycolic acid) as a highly potent intranasal vaccine delivery system against group a streptococcus. *Int J Pharm* 513:410–420.

Maraval, V., Caminade, A., Majoral, J., and Blais, J. 2003. Dendrimer design: How to circumvent the dilemma of a reduction of steps or an increase of function multiplicity? *Angew Chem Int Ed Engl* 42:1822–1826.

Martin, C. 1994. Nanomaterials: A membrane-based synthetic approach. *Science* 266: 1961–1966.

Mathew, A., Fukuda, T., Nagaoka, Y., Hasumura, T., Morimoto, H., Yoshida, Y., Maekawa, T., Venugopal, K., and Kumar, D. S. 2012. Curcumin loaded-PLGA nanoparticles conjugated with tet-1 peptide for potential use in Alzheimer's disease. *PLoS One* 7:e32616.

Matsumura, Y., Gotoh, M., Muro, K., Yamada, Y., Shirao, K., Shimada, Y., Okuwa, M., Matsumoto, S., Miyata, Y., Ohkura, H., Chin, K., Baba, S., Yamao, T., Kannami, A., Takamatsu, Y., Ito, K., and Takahashi, K. 2004. Phase I and pharmacokinetic study of mcc-465, a doxorubicin (DXR) encapsulated in peg immunoliposome, in patients with metastatic stomach cancer. *Ann Oncol* 15:517–525.

Matsumura, Y., Hamaguchi, T., Ura, T., Muro, K., Yamada, Y., Shimada, Y., Shirao, K., Okusaka, T., Ueno, H., Ikeda, M., and Watanabe, N. 2004. Phase I clinical trial and pharmacokinetic evaluation of NK911, a micelle-encapsulated doxorubicin. *Br J Cancer* 91:1775–1781.

Mattar, R., de Campos Mazo, D. F., and Carrilho, F. J. 2012. Lactose intolerance: Diagnosis, genetic, and clinical factors. *Clin Exp Gastroenterol* 5:113–121.

Maynard, C. L., Elson, C. O., Hatton, R. D., and Weaver, C. T. 2012. Reciprocal interactions of the intestinal microbiota and immune system. *Nature* 489:231–241.

Menjoge, A. R., Kannan, R. M., and Tomalia, D. A. 2010. Dendrimer-based drug and imaging conjugates: Design considerations for nanomedical applications. *Drug Discov Today* 15:171–185.

Mo, J., He, L., Ma, B., and Chen, T. 2016. Tailoring particle size of mesoporous silica nano-system to antagonize glioblastoma and overcome blood-brain barrier. *ACS Appl Mater Interfaces* 8:6811–6825.

Mody, V. V., Siwale, R., Singh, A., and Mody, H. R. 2010. Introduction to metallic nanoparticles. *J Pharm Bioallied Sci* 2:282–289.

Monnard, P., and Deamer, D. W. 2002. Membrane self-assembly processes: Steps toward the first cellular life. *Anat Rec* 268:196–207.

Müller, R. H., Mäder, K., and Gohla, S. 2000. Solid lipid nanoparticles (SLN) for controlled drug delivery—A review of the state of the art. *Eur J Pharm Biopharm* 50:161–177.

Nakamura, D., Attizzani, G. F., Toma, C., Sheth, T., Wang, W., Soud, M., Aoun, R., Tummala, R., Leygerman, M., Fares, A., Mehanna, E., Nishino, S., Fung, A., Costa, M. A., and Bezerra, H. G. 2016. Failure mechanisms and neoatherosclerosis patterns in very late drug-eluting and bare-metal stent thrombosis. *Circ Cardiovasc Interv* 9: pii: e003785.

National Institute on Aging. 2016. Alzheimer's disease education and referral center. Accessed from https://www.nia.nih.gov/alzheimers/publication/alzheimers-disease-fact-sheet.

Noyes, A., and Whitney, W. 1897. The rate of solution of solid substances in their own solutions. *J Am Chem Soc* 19:930–934.

Othman, M., Desmaële, D., Couvreur, P., Vander Elst, L., Laurent, S., Muller, R. N., Bourgaux, C., Morvan, E., Pouget, T., Lepêtre-Mouelhi, S., Durand, P., and Gref, R. 2011. Synthesis and physicochemical characterization of new squalenoyl amphiphilic gadolinium complexes as nanoparticle contrast agents. *Org Biomol Chem* 9:4367–4386.

Ow, H., Larson, D. R., Srivastava, M., Baird, B. A., Webb, W. W., and Wiesner, U. 2005. Bright and stable core-shell fluorescent silica nanoparticles. *Nano Lett* 5:113–117.

Palmal, S., Jana, N., and Jana, N. 2014. Inhibition of amyloid fibril growth by nanoparticle coated with histidine-based polymer. *J Phys Chem* 118:21630–21638.

Pandey, S., Senthilguru, K., Uvanesh, K., Sagiri, S. S., Behera, B., Babu, N., Bhattacharyya, M. K., Pal, K., and Banerjee, I. 2016. Natural gum modified emulsion gel as single carrier for the oral delivery of probiotic-drug combination. *Int J Biol Macromol* 92:504–514.

Park, S., and Kim, D. S. H. L. 2002. Discovery of natural products from *Curcuma longa* that protect cells from beta-amyloid insult: A drug discovery effort against Alzheimer's disease. *J Nat Prod* 65:1227–1231.

Passariello, A., Agricole, P., and Malfertheiner, P. 2014. A critical appraisal of probiotics (as drugs or food supplements) in gastrointestinal diseases. *Curr Med Res Opin* 30:1055–1064.

Prasad, S., Tyagi, A. K., and Aggarwal, B. B. 2014. Recent developments in delivery, bioavailability, absorption and metabolism of curcumin: The golden pigment from golden spice. *Cancer Res Treat* 46:2–18.

Presant, C. A., Blayney, D., Proffitt, R. T., Turner, A. F., Williams, L. E., Nadel, H. I., Kennedy, P., Wiseman, C., Gala, K., Crossley, R. J. et al. 1990. Preliminary report: Imaging of kaposi sarcoma and lymphoma in aids with indium-111-labelled liposomes. *Lancet* 335:1307–1309.

Presant, C. A., Proffitt, R. T., Turner, A. F., Williams, L. E., Winsor, D., Werner, J. L., Kennedy, P., Wiseman, C., Gala, K., McKenna, R. J. et al. 1988. Successful imaging of human cancer with indium-111-labeled phospholipid vesicles. *Cancer* 62:905–911.

Qu, L., Peng, X. 2002. Control of photoluminescence properties of cdse nanocrystals in growth. *J Am Chem Soc* 124:2049–2055.

Rabanel, J. M., Faivre, J., Paka, G. D., Ramassamy, C., Hildgen, P., and Banquy, X. 2015. Effect of polymer architecture on curcumin encapsulation and release from pegylated polymer nanoparticles: Toward a drug delivery nano-platform to the cns. *Eur J Pharm Biopharm* 96:409–420.

Rajam, R., and Anandharamakrishnan, C. 2015. Microencapsulation of lactobacillus plantarum (mtcc 5422) with fructooligosaccharide as wall material by spray drying. *LWT-Food Sci Technol* 60:773–780.

Reddy, L. H., Arias, J. L., Nicolas, J., and Couvreur, P. 2012. Magnetic nanoparticles: Design and characterization, toxicity and biocompatibility, pharmaceutical and biomedical applications. *Chem Rev* 112:5818–5878.

Renukaradhya, G. J., Narasimhan, B., and Mallapragada, S. K. 2015. Respiratory nanoparticle-based vaccines and challenges associated with animal models and translation. *J Control Release* 219:622–631.

Roch, A., Muller, R. N., and Gillis, P. 1999. Theory of proton relaxation induced by superparamagnetic particles. *J Chem Phys* 110:5403.

Roney, C., Kulkarni, P., Arora, V., Antich, P., Bonte, F., Wu, A., Mallikarjuana, N. N., Manohar, S., Liang, H., Kulkarni, A. R., Sung, H., Sairam, M., and Aminabhavi, T. M. 2005. Targeted nanoparticles for drug delivery through the blood–brain barrier for Alzheimer's disease. *J Control Release* 108:193–214.

Rymer, J. A., Harrison, R. W., Dai, D., Roe, M. T., Messenger, J. C., Anderson, H. V., Peterson, E. D., and Wang, T. Y. 2016. Trends in bare-metal stent use in the United States in patients aged ≥65 years (from the cathpci registry). *Am J Cardiol* 118:959–966.

Saha, K., Agasti, S. S., Kim, C., Li, X., and Rotello, V. M. 2012. Gold nanoparticles in chemical and biological sensing. *Chem Rev* 112:2739–2779.

Sanna, V., Pala, N., and Sechi, M. 2014. Targeted therapy using nanotechnology: Focus on cancer. *Int J Nanomedicine* 9:467–483.

Santra, S. 2010. Fluorescent silica nanoparticles for cancer imaging. *Methods Mol Biol* 624:151–162.

Schiffner, R., Kostev, K., and Gothe, H. 2016. Do patients with lactose intolerance exhibit more frequent comorbidities than patients without lactose intolerance? An analysis of routine data from german medical practices. *Ann Gastroenterol* 29:174–179.

Schwarz, C., Mehnert, W., Lucks, J., and Müller, R. 1994. Solid lipid nanoparticles (sln) for controlled drug delivery. I. production, characterization and sterilization. *J Control Release* 30:83–96.

Seetharamu, N., Kim, E., Hochster, H., Martin, F., and Muggia, F. 2010. Phase ii study of liposomal cisplatin (spi-77) in platinum-sensitive recurrences of ovarian cancer. *Anticancer Res* 30:541–545.

Sémiramoth, N., Di Meo, C., Zouhiri, F., Saïd-Hassane, F., Valetti, S., Gorges, R., Nicolas, V., Poupaert, J.-H., Chollet-Martin, S., Desmaële, D., Gref, R., and Couvreur, P. 2012. Self-assembled squalenoylated penicillin bioconjugates: An original approach for the treatment of intracellular infections. *ACS Nano* 6:3820–3831.

Severino, P., Szymanski, M., Favaro, M., Azzoni, A. R., Chaud, M. V., Santana, M. H. A., Silva, A. M., and Souto, E. B. 2015. Development and characterization of a cationic lipid nanocarrier as non-viral vector for gene therapy. *Eur J Pharm Sci* 66:78–82.

Shibu, E. S., Ono, K., Sugino, S., Nishioka, A., Yasuda, A., Shigeri, Y., Wakida, S., Sawada, M., and Biju, V. 2013. Photouncaging nanoparticles for MRI and fluorescence imaging in vitro and in vivo. *ACS Nano* 7:9851–9859.

Shin, T., Choi, Y., Kim, S., and Cheon, J. 2015. Recent advances in magnetic nanoparticle-based multi-modal imaging. *Chem Soc Rev* 44:4501–4516.

Simovic, S., Ghouchi-Eskandar, N., Sinn, A. M., Losic, D., and Prestidge, C. A. 2011. Silica materials in drug delivery applications. *Curr Drug Discov Technol* 8:269–276.

Simovic, S., Hui, H., Song, Y., Davey, A. K., Rades, T., and Prestidge, C. A. 2010. An oral delivery system for indomethicin engineered from cationic lipid emulsions and silica nanoparticles. *J Control Release* 143:367–373.

Singh, H. 2016. Nanotechnology applications in functional foods: Opportunities and challenges. *Prev Nutr Food Sci* 21:1–8.

Singh, R., and Lillard, J. W. J. 2009. Nanoparticle-based targeted drug delivery. *Exp Mol Pathol* 86:215–223.

Sirelkhatim, A., Mahmud, S., Seeni, A., Kaus, N. H. M., Ann, L. C., Bakhori, S. K. M., Hasan, H., and Mohamad, D. 2015. Review on zinc oxide nanoparticles: Antibacterial activity and toxicity mechanism. *Mater Sci Eng C Mater Biol Appl* 7:219–242.

Skrastina, D., Petrovskis, I., Lieknina, I., Bogans, J., Renhofa, R., Ose, V., Dishlers, A., Dekhtyar, Y., and Pumpens, P. 2014. Silica nanoparticles as the adjuvant for the immunisation of mice using hepatitis b core virus-like particles. *PLoS One* 9:e114006.

Sosnik, A. 2014. Alginate particles as platform for drug delivery by the oral route: State-of-the-art. *ISRN Pharm* 2014:926157.

Sousa-Herves, A., Novoa-Carballal, R., Riguera, R., and Fernandez-Megia, E. 2014. Gatg dendrimers and pegylated block copolymers: From synthesis to bioapplications. *AAPS J* 16:948–961.

Stefani, I., and Cooper-White, J. J. 2016. Development of an in-process uv-crosslinked, electrospun PCL/aPLA-co-TMC composite polymer for tubular tissue engineering applications. *Acta Biomater* 36:231–240.

Sun, J., Bi, C., Chan, H. M., Sun, S., Zhang, Q., and Zheng, Y. 2013. Curcumin-loaded solid lipid nanoparticles have prolonged in vitro antitumour activity, cellular uptake and improved in vivo bioavailability. *Colloids Surf B Biointerfaces* 111:367–375.

Swenson, C. E., Haemmerich, D., Maul, D. H., Knox, B., Ehrhart, N., and Reed, R. A. 2015. Increased duration of heating boosts local drug deposition during radiofrequency ablation in combination with thermally sensitive liposomes (Thermodox) in a porcine model. *PLoS One* 10:e0139752.

Szabó, A., Perri, C., Csató, A., Giordano, G., Vuono, V., and Nagy, J. 2010. Synthesis methods of carbon nanotubes and related materials. *Materials* 3:3092–3140.

Tabatt, K., Sameti, M., Olbrich, C., Müller, R. H., and Lehr, C. 2004. Effect of cationic lipid and matrix lipid composition on solid lipid nanoparticle-mediated gene transfer. *Eur J Pharm Biopharm* 57:155–162.

Tagami, T., Ernsting, M. J., and Li, S. 2011. Efficient tumor regression by a single and low dose treatment with a novel and enhanced formulation of thermosensitive liposomal doxorubicin. *J Control Release* 152:303–309.

Tang, L., and Cheng, J. 2013. Nonporous silica nanoparticles for nanomedicine application. *Nano Today* 8:290–312.

Thao, L. Q., Byeon, H. J., Lee, C., Lee, S., Lee, E. S., Choi, H., Park, E., and Youn, Y. S. 2016. Pharmaceutical potential of tacrolimus-loaded albumin nanoparticles having targetability to rheumatoid arthritis tissues. *Int J Pharm* 497:268–276.

Thaxton, C. S., Daniel, W. L., Giljohann, D. A., Thomas, A. D., and Mirkin, C. A. 2009. Templated spherical high density lipoprotein nanoparticles. *J Am Chem Soc* 131:1384–1385.

Thiesen, B., and Jordan, A. 2008. Clinical applications of magnetic nanoparticles for hyperthermia. *Int J Hyperthermia* 24:467–474.

Thomas, C. R., Ferris, D. P., Lee, J., Choi, E., Cho, M. H., Kim, E. S., Stoddart, J. F., Shin, J., Cheon, J., and Zink, J. I. 2010. Noninvasive remote-controlled release of drug molecules in vitro using magnetic actuation of mechanized nanoparticles. *J Am Chem Soc* 132:10623–10625.

Tomalia, D. 1996. Starburst dendrimers-nanoscopic supermolecules according to dendritic rules and principles. *Macromol Symp* 101:243–255.

Tomalia, D., Baker, H., Dewald, J., Hall, M., Kallos, G., Martin, S., Roeck, J., Ryder, J., and Smith, P. 1985. A new class of polymers: Starburst-dendritic macromolecules. *Polym J* 17:117–132.

Tomalia, D., and Fréchet, J. 2002. Discovery of dendrimers and dendritic polymers: A brief historical perspective. *J Polym Sci Pol Chem* 40:2719–2728.

Tomalia, D. A. 2016. Special issue: "Functional dendrimers." *Molecules* 21:1035.

Tong, S., Hou, S., Zheng, Z., Zhou, J., and Bao, G. 2010. Coating optimization of superparamagnetic iron oxide nanoparticles for high T2 relaxivity. *Nano Lett* 10:4607–4613.

Torres, A. G., Gregory, A. E., Hatcher, C. L., Vinet-Oliphant, H., Morici, L. A., Titball, R. W., and Roy, C. J. 2015. Protection of non-human primates against glanders with a gold nanoparticle glycoconjugate vaccine. *Vaccine* 33:686–692.

Torres Martin de Rosales, R., Tavaré, R., Paul, R. L., Jauregui-Osoro, M., Protti, A., Glaria, A., Varma, G., Szanda, I., and Blower, P. J. 2011. Synthesis of ^{64}cu^{II}-Bis(dithiocarbamatebisp hosphonate) and its conjugation with superparamagnetic iron oxide nanoparticles: In vivo evaluation as dual-modality PET-MRI agent. *Angew Chem Int Ed Engl* 50:5509–5513.

Tsai, M., Huang, Y., Wu, P., Fu, Y., Kao, Y., Fang, J., and Tsai, Y. 2011. Oral apomorphine delivery from solid lipid nanoparticles with different monostearate emulsifiers: Pharmacokinetic and behavioral evaluations. *J Pharm Sci* 100:547–557.

Turkevich, J., Stevenson, P., and Hillier, J. 1951. A study of the nucleation and growth process in the synthesis of colloidal gold: Discuss. *Discuss Faraday Soc* 11:55–75.

Uppal, R., Catana, C., Ay, I., Benner, T., Sorensen, A. G., and Caravan, P. 2011. Bimodal thrombus imaging: Simultaneous PET/MR imaging with a fibrin-targeted dual PET/MR probe-feasibility study in rat model. *Radiology* 258:812–820.

U.S. FDA. 2000. Rapamune® monography. Accessed from http://www.fda.gov/ohrms/dock ets/ac/02/briefing/3832b1_03_FDA-RapamuneLabel.htm.

Van der Valk, F. M., van Wijk, D. F., Lobatto, M. E., Verberne, H. J., Storm, G., Willems, M. C. M., Legemate, D. A., Nederveen, A. J., Calcagno, C., Mani, V., Ramachandran, S., Paridaans, M. P. M., Otten, M. J., Dallinga-Thie, G. M., Fayad, Z. A., Nieuwdorp, M., Schulte, D. M., Metselaar, J. M., Mulder, W. J. M., and Stroes, E. S. 2015. Prednisolone-containing liposomes accumulate in human atherosclerotic macrophages upon intravenous administration. *Nanomedicine* 11:1039–1046.

Van Wijk, J., Heunis, T., Harmzen, E., Dicks, L. M. T., Meuldijk, J., and Klumperman, B. 2014. Compartmentalization of bacteria in microcapsules. *Chem Commun (Camb)* 50:15427–15430.

Vanderhoff, J., El-Aassar, M., and Ugelstad, J. 1979. Polymer emulsification process. *U.S. patent* 4 177 177.

Vela Ramirez, J. E., Tygrett, L. T., Hao, J., Habte, H. H., Cho, M. W., Greenspan, N. S., Waldschmidt, T. J., and Narasimhan, B. 2016. Polyanhydride nanovaccines induce germinal center b cell formation and sustained serum antibody responses. *J Biomed Nanotechnol* 12:1303–1311.

Wang, F., Fang, R., Luk, B., Hu, C., Thamphiwatana, S., Dehaini, D., Angsantikul, P., Kroll, A., Pang, Z., Gao, W., Lu, W., and Zhang, L. 2016. Nanoparticle-based antivirulence vaccine for the management of methicillin-resistant *Staphylococcus aureus* skin infection. *Adv Funct Mater* 26:1628–1635.

Wang, M., Gu, X., Zhang, G., Zhang, D., and Zhu, D. 2009. Continuous colorimetric assay for acetylcholinesterase and inhibitor screening with gold nanoparticles. *Langmuir* 25:2504–2507.

Wang, Y., Zhu, Z., Xu, F., and Wei, X. 2012. One-pot reaction to synthesize superparamagnetic iron oxide nanoparticles by adding phenol as reducing agent and stabilizer. *J Nanoparticle Res* 14:755.

Wang, Y. J. 2015. Current status of superparamagnetic iron oxide contrast agents for liver magnetic resonance imaging. *World J Gastroenterol* 21:13400.

Ward, M. A., and Georgiou, T. K. 2011. Thermoresponsive polymers for biomedical applications. *ACS Appl Mater Interfaces* 3:1215–1242.

Woo, K., Hong, J., Choi, S., Lee, H., Ahn, J., Kim, C. S., and Lee, S. W. 2004. Easy synthesis and magnetic properties of iron oxide nanoparticles. *Chem Mater* 16:2814–2818.

Woting, A., and Blaut, M. 2016. The intestinal microbiota in metabolic disease. *Nutrients* 8:202.

Wu, P., Feldman, A. K., Nugent, A. K., Hawker, C. J., Scheel, A., Voit, B., Pyun, J., Fréchet, J. M. J., Sharpless, K. B., and Fokin, V. V. 2004. Efficiency and fidelity in a click-chemistry route to triazole dendrimers by the copper(I)-catalyzed ligation of azides and alkynes. *Angew Chem Int Ed Engl* 43:3928–3932.

Wu, S., Mou, C., and Lin, H. 2013. Synthesis of mesoporous silica nanoparticles. *Chem Soc Rev* 42:3862–3875.

Wu, Y., Loper, A., Landis, E., Hettrick, L., Novak, L., Lynn, K., Chen, C., Thompson, K., Higgins, R., Batra, U., Shelukar, S., Kwei, G., and Storey, D. 2004. The role of biopharmaceutics in the development of a clinical nanoparticle formulation of MK-0869: A beagle dog model predicts improved bioavailability and diminished food effect on absorption in human. *Int J Pharm* 285:135–146.

Wu, Z., Dong, M., Lu, M., and Li, Z. 2010. Encapsulation of β-galactosidase from aspergillus oryzae based on "fish-in-net" approach with molecular imprinting technique. *J Mol Catal B: Enzym* 63:75–80.

Xia, Y., Xiong, Y., Lim, B., and Skrabalak, S. 2009. Shape-controlled synthesis of metal nanocrystals: Simple chemistry meets complex physics? *Angew Chem Int Ed Engl* 48:60–103.

Xu, X., Li, L., Zhou, Z., Sun, W., and Huang, Y. 2016. Dual-pH responsive micelle platform for co-delivery of axitinib and doxorubicin. *Int J Pharm* 507:50–60.

Xuan, S., Wang, Y., Yu, J., and Leung, K. 2009. Tuning the grain size and particle size of superparamagnetic Fe_3O_4 microparticles. *Chem Mater* 21:5079–5087.

Xue, X., Hall, M. D., Zhang, Q., Wang, P. C., Gottesman, M. M., and Liang, X. 2013. Nanoscale drug delivery platforms overcome platinum-based resistance in cancer cells due to abnormal membrane protein trafficking. *ACS Nano* 7:10452–10464.

Yallapu, M. M., Jaggi, M., and Chauhan, S. C. 2012. Curcumin nanoformulations: A future nanomedicine for cancer. *Drug Discov Today* 17:71–80.

Yallapu, M. M., Othman, S. F., Curtis, E. T., Bauer, N. A., Chauhan, N., Kumar, D., Jaggi, M., and Chauhan, S. C. 2012. Curcumin-loaded magnetic nanoparticles for breast cancer therapeutics and imaging applications. *Int J Nanomedicine* 7:1761–1779.

Yang, F., Lim, G. P., Begum, A. N., Ubeda, O. J., Simmons, M. R., Ambegaokar, S. S., Chen, P. P., Kayed, R., Glabe, C. G., Frautschy, S. A., and Cole, G. M. 2005. Curcumin inhibits formation of amyloid beta oligomers and fibrils, binds plaques, and reduces amyloid in vivo. *J Biol Chem* 280:5892–5901.

Yang, X., Grailer, J. J., Rowland, I. J., Javadi, A., Hurley, S. A., Matson, V. Z., Steeber, D. A., and Gong, S. 2010. Multifunctional stable and pH-responsive polymer vesicles formed by heterofunctional triblock copolymer for targeted anticancer drug delivery and ultrasensitive MR imaging. *ACS Nano* 4:6805–6817.

Yang, X., Hong, H., Grailer, J. J., Rowland, I. J., Javadi, A., Hurley, S. A., Xiao, Y., Yang, Y., Zhang, Y., Nickles, R. J., Cai, W., Steeber, D. A., and Gong, S. 2011. cRGD-functionalized, dox-conjugated, and [64]cu-labeled superparamagnetic iron oxide nanoparticles for targeted anticancer drug delivery and PET/MR imaging. *Biomaterials* 32:4151–4160.

Yang, X. X., Li, C. M., and Huang, C. Z. 2016. Curcumin modified silver nanoparticles for highly efficient inhibition of respiratory syncytial virus infection. *Nanoscale* 8:3040–3048.

Yu, Y., Chang, S., Lee, C., and Wang, C. 1997. Gold nanorods: Electrochemical synthesis and optical properties. *J Phys Chem B* 101:6661–6664.

Zhang, Z., Wang, L., Wang, J., Jiang, X., Li, X., Hu, Z., Ji, Y., Wu, X., and Chen, C. 2012. Mesoporous silica-coated gold nanorods as a light-mediated multifunctional theranostic platform for cancer treatment. *Adv Mater* 24:1418–1423.

Zhang, Z., Zhang, R., Chen, L., and McClements, D. J. 2016. Encapsulation of lactase (β-galactosidase) into κ-carrageenan-based hydrogel beads: Impact of environmental conditions on enzyme activity. *Food Chem* 200:69–75.

Zhou, P., Xia, Y., Cheng, X., Wang, P., Xie, Y., and Xu, S. 2014. Enhanced bone tissue regeneration by antibacterial and osteoinductive silica-HACC-zein composite scaffolds loaded with rhBMP-2. *Biomaterials* 35:10033–10045.

4 Green Synthesis and Characterization of Semiconductor and Metal Nanoparticles

Sneha Bhagyaraj and
Oluwatobi Samuel Oluwafemi

CONTENTS

4.1   INTRODUCTION

Nanotechnology, which comprehends the understanding of the fundamental physics, chemistry, biology, and technology of nanometre-scale (10^{-9} meters) objects, has become one of the most exploited research area during last three decades (Murray et al., 1993; Chreigton et al., 1979). Most benefits of nanotechnology depend on the fact that it is possible to tailor the essential structures of materials at the nanoscale to achieve specific properties, thus greatly extending the well-used toolkits of materials science. Using nanotechnology, materials can effectively be made stronger, lighter, more durable, more reactive, more sieve-like, or to be better electrical conductors, among many other traits.

Research on inorganic nanoparticles has been developing rapidly due to their exceptional physical and chemical properties, which are quite different from their respective macroparticles. In nanoscale regime, chemical and physical properties of inorganic crystals are highly dependent on factors such as sizes and shapes (Schmidt and Eberl, 2001). Precise controls of such factors allow us not only to observe unique properties of nanocrystals, but also to tune their chemical and physical properties as desired. These nanoparticles can be synthesized by physical, chemical, and biological methods. The chemical approaches are popular methods for the production of nanoparticles. However, a few chemical methods cannot avoid the use of toxic chemicals in the synthesis procedure (Ouyang et al., 2008). Since noble metal nanoparticles such as gold, silver, and platinum are widely applied to human contacting areas, there is a growing need to develop environmentally benign processes of nanoparticle synthesis that do not use toxic chemicals. Biological methods for nanoparticle synthesis using microorganisms, enzymes, and plants or plant extracts have been suggested as possible eco-friendly alternatives to chemical and physical methods (Talekar et al., 2016). The emphasis of science and technology now shifts towards environmentally friendly and sustainable resources and processes.

4.2   SEMICONDUCTOR NANOPARTICLES

Semiconductor nanocrystals are tiny crystalline particles that exhibit size-dependent optical and electronic properties. With typical dimensions in the range of 1–10 nm, these nanocrystals bridge the gap between small molecules and large crystals, displaying discrete electronic transitions reminiscent of isolated atoms and molecules (Bruchez et al., 1998). A famous demonstration of the size-dependent properties of semiconductor nanoparticles is the drastic color change of their colloidal solutions with decreasing particle size.

Colloidal synthesis of nanoparticles in a suitable solvent medium is often referred to as a "bottom-up" way to obtain nanostructured systems. Using the chemical bottom-up approach, different high-quality semiconductor nanocrystals with desired particle sizes over the largest possible range and with narrow size distributions, good crystallinity, controllable surface functionalization, and high luminescent quantum yields can now be obtained (Peng et al., 2005).

4.3 METAL NANOPARTICLES

Metallic nanoparticles have fascinated scientists for more than a century, and are now heavily utilized in biomedical sciences and engineering (Hermanson et al., 2001). They are a focus of interest because of their huge potential in nanotechnology. Noble metal nanostructures have attracted extensive attention due to their fascinating physical and chemical properties and their relevant applications in optics, catalysis, conducting paste, surface-enhanced Raman scattering (SERS) and sensing. All of these applications are influenced by the size, shape, and morphology of metal nanostructures. Many metals can now be processed into monodisperse particles with controllable composition and structure and can be produced in large quantities at low cost through solution–phase methods. Today, these materials can be synthesized and modified with various chemical functional groups which allow them to be conjugated with antibodies, ligands, and drugs of interest. This opens a wide range of potential applications in biotechnology; magnetic separation; and preconcentration of target analytes, targeted drug delivery, vehicles for gene and drug delivery and more importantly, diagnostic imaging (Mody et al., 2010).

4.4 GREEN SYNTHESIS OF NANOMATERIALS

Over the past decade, the increased emphasis on developing green and sustainable chemical processes has led to numerous efforts toward the elimination or at least minimization of waste. The chemical synthesis of nanoparticles has several occupational exposure hazards like carcinogenicity, genotoxicity, cytotoxicity, and general toxicity (Magaye et al., 2012). So there is a pressing need to develop clean, non-toxic and ecofriendly procedures for synthesis and assembly of nanoparticles. Implementing sustainable methodologies in almost all areas of chemistry, including nanomaterial synthesis entails eliminating toxic reagents and solvents. The choice of an environmentally benign solvent, and the use of a multipurpose agent that serves in reducing, capping, and dispersing agents are some of the key issues that may be addressed in green synthesis of nanomaterials.

To eliminate the use of toxic reducing agents, the use of amino acids, sugars, vitamins, and other eco-friendly biological agents in the synthesis of metal nanoparticles have been reported (Ahmed et al., 2016). Microwave irradiation (MW) is emerging as a rapid and environmentally friendly mode of heating for the generation of nanomaterials. It offers a rapid and volumetric heating of solvents, reagents, and intermediates that provide uniform nucleation and growth conditions for nanomaterial synthesis. Some common reagents used for the green synthesis of nanomaterials are given in Table 4.1.

TABLE 4.1

Common Materials Used for Green Synthesis of Nanomaterials

Material	Example
Biopolymers	PVA, PLGA, PEG
Enzymes	*L*-cysteine
Plants	*Alternanthera dentata*
	Cocos nucifera
Microorganisms	Bacteria: *Pseudomonas strutzeri*
	Fungi: *Fusarium oxysporum*
Polysaccharides	Glucose, dextrose, maltose
Irradiation	Microwave
	Gamma radiation

4.5 CHARACTERIZATION TECHNIQUES FOR NANOPARTICLES

In order to understand the nature and potential of nanoparticle forms, detailed characterization of the particle needs to be done. Various characterization techniques are available for the detailed analysis of optical, morphological, and conducting properties of nanomaterials. The first phase of the analysis will therefore focus on characterization of the material's physical properties. Some of the main parameters for nanomaterial characterization include shape and size of interactive surface, surface area and porosity, particle size distribution, aggregation, solubility, hydrated surface analysis, zeta potential, wettability, adsorption potential, purity, sterility, stability, and so on. Based on the application, various other parameters such as stability in various solvents, toxicity, and compatibility, also need to be analyzed.

4.5.1 OPTICAL CHARACTERIZATION

The optical properties of metal nanoparticles have long been of interest in physical chemistry, starting with Faraday's investigations of colloidal gold in the mid-1800s. However, there are often complicating factors in understanding nanoparticle optical properties, including the presence of a supporting substrate, a solvent layer on top of the particles, and particles that are close enough together that their electromagnetic coupling changes the spectra. Although extinction, absorption, and scattering are still the primary optical properties of interest, other spectroscopic techniques are also being used to characterize these particles, including surface-enhanced Raman spectroscopy (SERS), a variety of nonlinear scattering measurements and time resolved measurements. Nanoparticles made from certain metals, such as gold and silver, strongly interact with specific wavelengths of light, and the unique optical properties of these materials are the foundation for the field of plasmonics.

4.5.1.1 UV-Vis Spectroscopy

Nanoparticles have optical properties that are sensitive to size, shape, concentration, agglomeration state, and refractive index near the nanoparticle surface. This makes

UV/Vis/IR spectroscopy a valuable tool for identifying, characterizing, and studying these materials. UV-visible spectroscopy records the absorption and transmittance of a substance. The transmittance of a sample (T) is defined as the fraction of photons that pass through the sample over the incident number of photons, for instance, $T = I/I_0$. In a typical UV-Vis spectroscopy measurement, we are measuring those photons that are not absorbed or scattered by the sample. It is common to report the absorbance (A) of the sample, which is related to the transmittance by $A = -\log 10$ (T). In the near IR, where the sample does not absorb strongly, the transmittance is close to 100 percent. In the UV portion of the spectrum, where the sample absorbs strongly, the transmittance drops to around 10 percent or less.

Scattering from a sample is typically very sensitive to the aggregation state of the sample, with the scattering contribution increasing as the particles aggregate to a greater extent. For example, the optical properties of silver nanoparticles change when particles aggregate and the conduction electrons near each particle surface become delocalized and are shared amongst neighboring particles. When this occurs, the surface plasmon resonance shifts to lower energies, causing the absorption and scattering peaks to red-shift to longer wavelengths. UV-Vis spectroscopy can be used as a simple and reliable method for monitoring the stability of nanoparticle solutions.

As the particles destabilize, the original extinction peak will decrease in intensity (due to the depletion of stable nanoparticles), and often the peak will broaden or a secondary peak will form at longer wavelengths due to the formation of aggregates.

4.5.1.2 Photoluminescence Spectroscopy

Photoluminescence occurs when a sample is excited by absorbing photons and then emits them with a decay time that is characteristic of the sample environment. *Fluorescence* is a term used by chemists when the absorbing and emitting species is an atom or molecule. Photoluminescence spectroscopy measures the wavelength at which the sample emits the radiation. Highly luminescent materials like CdSe core–shell quantum dots shows significant PL spectra. The spectrum of the wavelengths emitted can be used to identify atoms and molecules, as well as to determine chemical structures. The intensity of the photons emitted can be used to determine the concentration of chemical species.

4.5.1.3 FT-IR Spectroscopy

Vibrational spectroscopy, including both infrared (IR) and Raman spectroscopy, measures the oscillations of atoms in molecules. IR bands arise from an interaction between light and the oscillating dipole moment of a vibrating molecule. The observation of the vibrational transitions yields information about the molecular vibrational energy levels, which in turn are related to molecular conformation, structure, intermolecular interaction, and chemical bonding. In IR spectroscopy, samples are radiated with IR light (wavelength 2.2 mme1 mm) and the observation of IR absorption relies on the change in the dipole moment with the molecular vibration.

4.5.1.4 Raman Spectroscopy

Raman spectroscopy provides information about molecular vibrations that can be used for sample identification and quantization. The technique involves shining a monochromatic light source (i.e., laser) on a sample and detecting the scattered light. Raman spectroscopy can be used for both qualitative and quantitative applications. The spectra are very specific, and chemical identifications can be performed by using search algorithms against digital databases. As in infrared spectroscopy, band areas are proportional to concentration, making Raman amenable to quantitative analysis. In fact, because Raman bands are inherently sharper than their infrared counterparts, isolated bands are often present in the spectrum for more straightforward quantitative analysis. Raman bands arise from an oscillating induced dipole caused by light waves interacting with the polarizability ellipsoid of a vibrating molecule.

Water has very intense IR absorption bands, but is a weak Raman scatterer and thus Raman spectra exhibit much less interference from water. This provides Raman spectroscopy with an advantage over IR spectroscopy for investigating aqueous biological systems, making it an important technique for biomedical research. Raman spectroscopy is also well known for its minimum requirement for sample handling and preparation. In the collection of Raman spectral data, the required sample volume is determined only by the diameter of the focused laser beam, which is of the order of a micron.

4.5.2 Morphological Characterization

Morphological characterization of nanoparticles reveals the size, shape, and crystallinity of the sample. Various characterization techniques are available for this analysis.

4.5.2.1 X-Ray Diffraction Analysis Studies

As a primary characterization tool for obtaining critical features such as crystal structure, crystallite size and strain, X-ray diffraction patterns have been widely used in nanoparticle research. The randomly oriented crystals in nanocrystalline materials cause broadening of diffraction peaks. This has been attributed to the absence of total constructive and destructive interferences of X-rays in a finite-sized lattice. Moreover, inhomogeneous lattice strain and structural faults lead to broadening of peaks in the diffraction patterns. The size calculated from X-ray diffraction peak broadening is a measure of the smallest unfaulted regions or coherently scattering domains of the material. In fact, this is the size of regions bounded by defects and grain boundaries are separated from surrounding by a small misorientation, typically one or two degrees.

4.5.2.2 Dynamic Light Scattering Technique (DLS)

The most common technology of the particle size distribution of nano- and submicron liquid dispersions typically is photon correlation spectroscopy (PCS) or dynamic light scattering (DLS). PCS is a method that depends on the interaction of light with particles. The light scattered by nanoparticles in suspension will fluctuate over time and can be related to the particle diameter.

4.5.2.3   Surface Area Analysis (BET)

The specific surface area of the particles is the summation of the areas of the exposed surfaces of the particles per unit mass. There is an inverse relationship between particle size and surface area. Nitrogen adsorption can be used to measure the specific surface area of a powder. The method of Brunauer, Emmett, and Teller (BET) is commonly used to determine the total surface area. If the particles are assumed to be spherical and of narrow size distribution, the specific surface area provides an average particle diameter in nanometers using this formula: $dBET = 6000/ñs$ in which s is specific surface area in m^2/g and ñ is the theoretical density in g/cm^3. If particles do not bond too tightly, the gas accesses most of the surface area of the powder and provides a good measure of the actual particle size independent of agglomeration. This is the size of the primary particles of which the agglomerate is made up. Thus, surface area measurement gives a value close to that obtained by electron microscopy.

4.5.2.4   X-Ray Photoelectron Spectroscopy

X-ray photoelectron spectroscopy (XPS), also known as electron spectroscopy for chemical analysis (ESCA), involves detection of electrons with kinetic energies between 10 and 2000 electron volts. The average depth of analysis for an XPS measurement is approximately 5 nm. XPS is typically accomplished by exciting a sample surface with mono-energetic Al kα X-rays, causing photoelectrons to be emitted from the sample surface. An electron energy analyzer is used to measure the energy of the emitted photoelectrons. From the binding energy and intensity of a photoelectron peak, the elemental identity, chemical state, and quantity of a detected element can be determined.

4.5.2.5   Atomic Force Microscope (AFM)

The atomic force microscope (AFM) allows for 3D characterization of nanoparticles with sub-nanometer resolution. Nanoparticle characterization using AFM has a number of advantages over dynamic light scattering, electron microscopy, and optical characterization methods. Some of the unique advantages of nanoparticle characterization with an AFM include characterization of nanoparticles that are 0.5 nm in diameter and larger, nanoparticle mixture distributions below 30 nm, characterization of variable geometry nanoparticles, direct visualization of hydrated nanoparticles/liquid medium, and characterization of nanoparticle physical properties such as magnetic fields.

An outstanding feature of the AFM is that it can directly create images of nanoparticles with dimensions between 0.5 nm and 50+ nm. Nanoparticle size distributions are directly calculated from AFM images. The AFM can easily identify and characterize bimodal distributions of nanoparticles. AFM Workshop's built-in nanoparticle analysis software makes nanoparticle characterization fast and easy. The AFM can evaluate variable nanoparticle geometry from traditional spherical nanoparticles to more exotic fractal geometries of nanoparticle clusters. Many AFM modes may be used to measure nanoparticle physical properties such as magnetic fields, mechanical properties, electrical properties, and thermal conductivity.

4.5.2.6   Scanning Electron Microscope (SEM)

The scanning electron microscope uses electrons instead of light to form an image. The electrons in the beam interact with the sample, producing various signals that can be used to obtain information about the surface topography and composition. The scanning electron microscope has many advantages over traditional microscopes. The SEM has a large depth of field, which allows more of a specimen to be in focus at one time. The SEM also has much higher resolution, so that closely spaced specimens can be magnified at much higher levels. Because the SEM uses electromagnets rather than lenses, the researcher has much more control in the degree of magnification.

4.5.2.7   Transmission Electron Microscope (TEM)

The transmission electron microscope (TEM) permits the structural characterization of a collection or isolated nanoparticles. It gives a clear picture regarding the structure, orientation, crystallinity, defects, and so on. TEM operates on the same basic principles as the light microscope but uses electrons instead of light. TEMs use electrons as a "light source" and their much lower wavelength makes it possible to get a resolution a thousand times better than with a light microscope. We can see objects to the order of a few ångström (10^{-10} m). This makes it possible to study small details in the cell or different materials down to near atomic levels. The possibility for high magnifications has made the TEM a valuable tool among medical, biological, and materials research.

4.5.3   ELEMENTAL ANALYSIS

4.5.3.1   Energy Dispersive X-Ray Spectroscopy (EDX)

Energy dispersive X-ray spectroscopy (EDS or EDX) is a chemical microanalysis technique used in conjunction with scanning electron microscopy (SEM). The EDS technique detects X-rays emitted from the sample during bombardment by an electron beam to characterize the elemental composition of the analyzed volume. Features or phases as small as 1 μm or less can be analyzed. When the sample is bombarded by the SEM electron beam, electrons are ejected from the atoms comprising the sample's surface. The resulting electron vacancies are filled by electrons from a higher state, and an X-ray is emitted to balance the energy difference between the two electrons' states. The X-ray energy is characteristic of the element from which it was emitted.

4.5.3.2   Inductively Coupled Plasma Mass Spectrometry (ICP-MS)

Inductively coupled plasma mass spectrometry or ICP-MS is an analytical technique used for elemental determinations. An ICP-MS combines a high-temperature ICP source with a mass spectrometer. The ICP source converts the atoms of the elements in the sample to ions. These ions are then separated and detected by the mass spectrometer. This technique is very useful to characterize the amount of metal precursors remaining after the reaction during a synthesis protocol.

The percentage conversion of metal ions to metal nanoparticles is obtained by the following equation.

$$Q = \left(\frac{C_0 - C_f}{C_0} \right) \times 100 \tag{4.1}$$

where C_0 and C_f are the initial and final concentrations of metal ion (mg/l), and Q is the percentage conversion of metal ions to metal nanoparticles.

Inductively coupled plasma—atomic emission spectrometry (ICP-AES) is an emission spectrophotometric technique, exploiting the fact that excited electrons emit energy at a given wavelength as they return to ground state after excitation by high temperature argon plasma. The fundamental characteristic of this process is that each element emits energy at specific wavelengths peculiar to its atomic character. The energy transfer for electrons when they fall back to ground state is unique to each element as it depends upon the electronic configuration of the orbital. The energy transfer is inversely proportional to the wavelength of electromagnetic radiation, $E = hc/\lambda$ (where h is Planck's constant, c is the velocity of light, and λ is wavelength), and hence the wavelength of light emitted is also unique.

Although each element emits energy at multiple wavelengths, in the ICP-AES technique it is most common to select a single wavelength (or a very few) for a given element. The intensity of the energy emitted at the chosen wavelength is proportional to the amount (concentration) of that element in the sample being analyzed. Thus, by determining which wavelengths are emitted by a sample and by determining their intensities, the analyst can qualitatively and quantitatively find the elements from the given sample relative to a reference standard.

4.5.4 BIOLOGICAL CHARACTERIZATION

The increased global production of engineered nanoparticles (NPs) and their application in various fields require a detailed understanding of their potential toxicity. *In vitro* and *in vivo* studies demonstrated that NPs may display a higher toxic potential than fine-sized particles of identical composition. Preclinical physicochemical characterization of a nanoparticle includes measurement of size and shape, surface chemistry, and aggregation state. Many properties of nanoparticles are environment and condition dependent. In aqueous biological systems, the nanoparticle surface is dramatically altered by solvation, the adsorption of small molecules, and ionic species. This forms the solid–liquid interface, which is key to understanding the behavior of nanoparticles in biological systems because it determines the colloidal stability of the nanoparticle in aqueous solutions and determines the affinity and selectivity of biomolecules when forming nanoparticle–protein interfaces. Biological characterization of nanoparticles basically includes the *in vitro* and *in vivo* analysis of the sample in various biological conditions.

4.5.4.1 *In Vitro* Analysis

In vitro experiments can provide an initial cost-effective assessment of the toxicity and efficacy of a nanomaterial-based therapeutic and inform the design of animal studies. *In vitro* studies also enable the elucidation of biochemical mechanisms—under controlled conditions not achievable by *in vivo* studies. Nanoparticle's binding, pharmacology, and uptake properties can be monitored by common cell and molecular biology methods, such as ELISA (enzyne-linked immunosorbent assay) and fluorescence microscopy. Scanning electron microscopy (SEM) and transmission electron microscopy (TEM) can also be used as tools to observe the particle's interaction with cellular-level components. Electron microscopy, chromatography, and electrophoresis protocols allow characterization of nanomaterial's blood contact properties, such as opsonization and macrophage phagocytosis, as well as pinocytosis and uptake by nonphagocytic cells.

In vitro characterization also includes a thorough examination of the nanoparticle's therapeutic and diagnostic functionality. For example, particles with imaging modalities will be examined for their signal intensity. Nanotechnology strategies that incorporate therapeutic or preventative agents will be characterized for their drug-release kinetics and ability to cross biological barriers.

A list of assays and equipment used for the *in vitro* characterization is shown in Table 4.2.

For *in vitro* drug release studies, sample and separate methods (SS) is the most widely used technique. Briefly, drug-loaded micro-/nanoparticles are introduced into

TABLE 4.2
***In Vitro* Analysis Parameters and Their Assays and Instruments**

Property	Assay	Instrumentation
Binding and pharmocology	Enzyme-linked immunosorbent Assay	Flow cytometry, fluorescent microscopy, liquid scintillation counter
Blood contact	Lumilus amebocyte lysate (LAL) Rabbit pyrogen	Chromatography, HPLC, gel electrophoresis
Cellular uptake	Caco-2 cell line	Fluorescence microscopy, electrophoresis, SEM
Toxicity, *in vitro* absorption, distribution, metabolism, and excretion	MTT (3-(4,5-Dimethylthiazol-2-yl)-2,5-diphenyltetrazoliumbromide) Human lung fibroblast cells (IMR-90)	Microscopy, spectroscopy, high performance liquid chromatography, liquid scintillation, electrophoresis
Oxidative stress	DCF 2',7'-Dichlorofluorescein	Fluorescence microscopy
Cell viability	MTT (3-(4,5-Dimethylthiazol-2-yl)-2,5-diphenyltetrazoliumbromide)	Absorption spectroscopy
Cell death	LDH	Absorption spectroscopy
Cytokine production	IL-8 ELISA	Absorption spectroscopy

a vessel containing media and release is assessed over time. Media selection is based on drug solubility and stability over the duration of the release study. Modifications of the basic technique to study drug release include size of container, use of agitation, and sampling methods.

4.5.4.2 *In Vivo* Analysis

After the *in vitro* analysis, the nanomaterials are intended for *in vivo* diagnostic and therapeutic purposes. The primary goal of the *in vivo* characterization is to elucidate the nanomaterial's safety, efficacy, and toxicokinetic properties in animal models. *In vivo* assays can supply essential information regarding what may happen when the NPs are inside the body. Some *in vivo* tests which are important in nanoparticle analysis include dose-response; biodistribution; acute and multi-dose safety and efficacy; administration route determination; and absorption, distribution, metabolism, and excretion (ADME).

As is the case with any new chemical entity (NCE), these properties and other ADME data must be obtained prior to transitioning the nanoparticles to clinical applications. This phase will leverage the plethora of knowledge and protocols used to characterize drugs and devices *in vivo*.

Animal studies conducted under the *in vivo* phase for the study of nanoparticles will be in support of the FDA's Guidance for Industry, Single Dose Acute Toxicity Testing for Pharmaceuticals. The nanoparticle will be administered to animals to identify (1) doses causing no adverse effect and (2) doses causing life-threatening toxicity. The information obtained from these tests will provide preliminary identification of target organs of acute toxicity, and may aid in the selection of starting doses for Phase I human trials. Preliminary data on the nanoparticle ADME profile will also be obtained in this phase. *In vivo* studies will characterize the nanoparticle absorption, pharmacokinetics, serum half-life, protein binding, tissue distribution/accumulation, enzyme induction or inhibition, metabolism characteristics and metabolites, and excretion pattern.

Given the multifunctional potential of nanoparticles, the *in vivo* characterization phase will also include an assessment of the strategy's targeting and imaging capabilities. Targeting will be assessed, for example, by comparing a nanoparticle distribution profile with a non-targeting nanoparticle from the same class. For those particles used with imaging modalities, the signal enhancement will be monitored using the appropriate magnetic resonance, ultrasound, optical, or positron emission tomography imaging instrumentation.

4.6 NANOPARTICLES IN VARIOUS APPLICATIONS

Improved production methods have led to more widespread employment of nanomaterials in commercially available products. The noble metallic nanoparticle such as gold, silver, and platinum play an important role in the field of organic chemistry, bioelectronics, and pharmaceuticals. Among these nanomaterials, silver nanoparticles are being used increasingly as a broad-spectrum antimicrobial agent in clothing, food storage containers, pharmaceuticals, cosmetics, electronics, and optical devices. Ag nanoparticles have been used as a class of broad-spectrum antimicrobial reagents in medical and consumer products such as household antiseptic sprays and antimicrobial coating for medical devices. Water filters incorporating Ag nanowires have been demonstrated to be very efficient for cleaning water that is polluted with bacteria. Due to the large surface-to-volume ratios of the Ag nanoparticles in comparison with their bulk counterparts, Ag nanoparticles have been used as classic catalysts for important industrial reactions. The high electrical and thermal conductivities of Ag cause Ag nanoparticles to be used widely in the electronics industry as conductive fillers in conductive adhesives and thermal interfacial materials. Most recently, two-dimensional (2D) random networks of Ag nanowires have been exploited to serve as transparent conductive films due to the fact that the low percolation threshold for Ag nanowires assures a high percentage of open areas in the conductive networks (Sun, 2010). In combination with the thin diameters of Ag nanowires that are responsible for the mechanical flexibility of the nanowires, such 2D networks are very promising replacements for the traditional rigid doped metal oxide conductive films, such as the most commonly used tin-doped indium oxide (ITO).

Gold nanoparticles (AuNPs) are found to be highly active and selective in a variety of important catalytic reactions. Some of the important applications of AuNPs include the following:

1. *In vivo* cell-tracking in cell-based therapy applications (Dykman and Khlebtsov, 2011).
2. Conductors from printable inks to electronic chips.
3. Photodynamic therapy–near-IR absorbing gold nanoparticles (including gold nanoshells and nanorods) produce heat when excited by light at wavelengths from 700 to 800 nm. This enables these nanoparticles to eradicate targeted tumors (Cai et al., 2008).
4. Sensors. For example, a colorimetric sensor based on gold nanoparticles can identify if foods are suitable for consumption.
5. Detection of biomarkers in the diagnosis of heart diseases, cancers, and infectious agents.

Nanoscale additives in polymer composite materials such as baseball bats, tennis rackets, motorcycle helmets, automobile bumpers, luggage, and power tool housings can make them simultaneously lightweight, stiff, durable and resilient. Surface treatments or additives of nanomaterials to fabrics help them resist wrinkling, staining, bacterial growth, and provide lightweight ballistic energy deflection in personal body armor. Nanoscale thin films on eyeglasses, computers, camera displays, windows, and other surfaces can make them water-repellent, antireflective, self-cleaning, resistant to ultraviolet or infrared light, antifog, antimicrobial, scratch-resistant, or electrically conductive. Addition of nanoscale materials in cosmetic products provide greater transparency, cleansing, absorption, antioxidant, antimicrobial, and add other health properties in sunscreens, cleansers, complexion treatments, creams and lotions, shampoos, and specialized makeup. Application of nanomaterials in the food industry includes nanocomposites in food containers to minimize carbon dioxide leakage out of carbonated beverages, and to reduce oxygen inflow, moisture outflow, or the growth of bacteria in order to keep food fresher and safer for longer.

Nanosensors built into plastic packaging can warn against spoiled food. Nanosensors are being developed to detect salmonella, pesticides, and other contaminates on food before packaging and distribution. Application in automotive products include high-power rechargeable battery systems; thermoelectric materials for temperature control; lower-rolling resistance tires; high-efficiency/low-cost sensors and electronics; thin-film smart solar panels; and fuel additives and improved catalytic converters for cleaner exhaust and extended range.

4.7 CONCLUSIONS

The development of efficient green chemistry methods for the synthesis of metal nanoparticles has become a recent major focus of researchers. Nanomaterials synthesis have evolved from chemical reduction, which uses toxic reagents, to green synthesis, which uses bio-organisms and plant extracts. Detailed chemical, physical, and biological characterizations of synthesized materials are now possible. Applications of nanotechnology are delivering in both expected and unexpected ways to benefit society.

REFERENCES

Ahmed, S., Ahmad, M., Swami, B., and Ikram, S. 2016. A review on plants extract mediated synthesis of silver nanoparticles for antimicrobial applications: A green expertise. *J. Adv. Res.* 7:17–28.

Bruchez, M. J., Moronne, M., Gin, P., Weiss, S., and Alivisatos, A. P. 1998. Semiconductor nanocrystals as fluorescent biological labels. *Science* 281:2013.

Cai, W., Gao, T., Hong, H., and Sun, J. 2008. Applications of gold nanoparticles in cancer nanotechnology. *Nanotechnol. Sci. Appl.* 2008(1):10.2147/NSA.S3788.

Chreigton, J. A., Blatchford, C. G., and Albrecht, M. G. 1979. Plasma resonance enhancement of Raman scattering by pyridine adsorbed on silver or gold sol particles of size comparable to the excitation wavelength. *J. Chem. Soc. Faraday Transactions* 75:790–798.

Dykman, L. A., and Khlebtsov, N. G. 2011. Gold nanoparticles in biology and medicine: Recent advances and prospects. *Acta Naturae* 3(2):34–55.

Hermanson, K. D., Lumsdon, S. O., Williams, J., Kaler, P., and Velev, E. W. O. D. 2001. Dielectrophoretic assembly of electrically functional microwires from nanoparticle suspensions. *Science* 294:1082–1086.

Magaye, R., Zhao, J., Bowman, L., and Ding, M. 2012. Genotoxicity and carcinogenicity of cobalt-, nickel- and copper-based nanoparticles. *Exp. Ther. Med.* 4(4):551–561.

Mody, V. V., Siwale, R., Singh, A., and Mody, H. R. 2010. Introduction to metallic nanoparticles. *J. Pharm. Bioall. Sci* 2:282–289.

Murray, C. B., Norris, D. J., and Bawendi, M. G. 1993. Synthesis and characterization of nearly monodisperse CdE (E = sulfur, selenium, tellurium) semiconductor nanocrystallites. *J. Am. Chem. Soc.* 115:8706–8715.

Ouyang, J. Y., Zaman, M. B., Yan, F. J., Johnston, D., Li, G., Wu, X. H., Leek, D., Ratcliffe, C. I., Ripmeester, J. A., and Yu, K. 2008. Multiple families of magic-sized CdSe nanocrystals with strong bandgap photoluminescence via noninjection one-pot syntheses. *J. Phys. Chem. C* 112:13805–13811.

Peng, P., Milliron, D. J., Hughes, S. M., Johnson, J. C., Alivisatos, A. P., and Saykally, R. J. 2005. Femtosecond spectroscopy of carrier relaxation dynamics in type II CdSe/CdTe tetrapod heteronanostructures. *Nano Lett.* 5:1809–1813.

Schmidt, O. G., and Eberl, K. 2001. Nanotechnology: Thin solid films roll up into nanotubes. *Nature* 410:168.

Sun, Y. 2010. Silver nanowires: Unique templates for functional nanostructures. *Nanoscale* 2:1626–1642.

Talekar, S., Joshi, A., Chougle, R., Nakhe, A., and Bhojwani, R. 2016. Immobilized enzyme mediated synthesis of silver nanoparticles using cross-linked enzyme aggregates (CLEAs) of NADH-dependent nitrate reductase. *Nano-Structures & Nano-Objects* 6:23–33.

Section II

Interaction with
Biological Systems

5 The Nanoparticle "Coronome" Is Mainly Explained by InterPro Domains of Proteins

Olivier Joubert, Phèdre Rihn,
and Bertrand Henri Rihn

CONTENTS

There is a considerable interest in changes of the physicochemical properties of nanoparticles (NP) once they are surrounded by biological media. To target cells efficiently and to avoid being cleared by scavenger cells like macrophages, many researchers in nanomedicine are looking for their "stealth" property in biological fluids. However, even in the presence of polyethylene glycol (PEG), a crown of plasma proteins is shown around them that seems to influence nanoparticle determinism. That crown was named *corona* after a Latin term analogous to the ancient Greek "κορώνη," meaning crown, *couronne* in French, and *krone* in German. As far as is our knowledge, the first occurrence, of "corona" appeared in the year 2000 (Gref et al., 2000). Using various cores of nanoparticles, for example, poly(lactic-co-glycolic) acid (PLGA) or PEG, albumin, fibrinogen, IgG, Ig light chains, apoA-I, and apoE were identified in nanoparticle corona: Their distribution did not vary as a function of corona thickness and density (Gref et al., 2000). The "corona" term was reused in 2007 by Cedervall et al., who defined the parameters of kinetics of acrylamide-based polymeric NP interactions with albumin and fibrinogen.

The notion of "biological identity" or protein fingerprinting of NP, driven by the discovery of adhesion forces between specific proteins of biological fluids and NP, emerged in studies published recently (Walkey et al., 2011; Pearson et al., 2014). Those proteins are supposed to alter the synthetic identity of NP and change it into

113

biological identity that may modify the initial determinism of NPs as was shown recently (Hussien et al., 2013; Walter, 2014). As a matter of fact, whatever the synthetic identity of NP, various proteins are eluted and characterized, once they are incubated in plasma, by increasing or diminishing ionic strength, heating, denaturing or adding chaotropic substances. Moreover, by modeling protein/NP interactions, size (Shannahan et al., 2013) and charge (Lundqvist et al., 2008; Sakulkhu et al., 2014) have been shown to play a role in selecting proteins from plasma.

In the present study, we reanalyze data from a panel of nine published studies and suggest that (1) hydrophobicity of proteins is an important parameter for their adhesive properties, (2) subsets of proteins identified in corona should be considered as interactomes, namely, proteins linked by explainable biological interplays that were recently called *coronome* (Rihn and Joubert, 2015), a contraction of *cor*ona prote*ome*, and (3) InterPro Domains (IPD) of proteins reflect protein–protein or protein–NP interactions well and should be extensively determined by protein identification using MS tools.

5.1 EXPERIMENTAL DESIGN: NANOPARTICLE, PLASMA INCUBATION, AND ELUTION METHOD VARY HIGHLY

Chemical compositions of NP analyzed in our study were highly heterogeneous. Four were entirely polymeric (Lundqvist et al., 2008; Hussien et al., 2013; Sempf et al., 2013; Pozzi et al., 2015); five were modified metals: iron (Hirsch et al., 2013; Sakulkhu et al., 2014) and either silver (Shannahan et al., 2014) or gold (Walkey et al., 2011; Kreyling et al., 2014). Mean diameters varied from 15 to 227 nm and ζ-potential from −46.6 to +65 mV (Table 5.1).

If those physical and chemical characteristics were highly different, one should note that the chemical surface modifications generate a high number of hydroxyl radicals or oxygen atoms at NP surface as found in polyvinyl alcohol (PVA), PEG, Eudragit™, PLGA nanoparticles, and polystyrene amine and AuNP bis (p-sulfonatophenyl) phenylphosphine modified NP. Remarkably, all types of surface modifications of nanoparticles may be involved in hydrogen bonding or in hydrophobic and aromatic interactions as happens when derivatives of phenylphosphine, styrene, and bioethers are used to modify NP.

5.2 PROTEINS RETRIEVED FROM CORONA ARE FREQUENTLY LINKED IN INTERACTOMES

Proteins were eluted from nanoparticles in the presence of: (1) ionic detergents (SDS or LDS), (2) reducing or denaturing conditions, (3) buffer with various ionic strength (0 to 2 M NaCl or equivalent cation), and (4) chaotropic substances (Table 5.1). In a previous work we identified 178 proteins having molecular weight (MM) ranging from 8,765 to 3,715,733 Da and pH$_i$ varying from 4.2 to 10.5 by nano-electrospray ion trap MS (Hussien et al., 2013). Their interactome was analyzed using the String-developed software (http://string-db.org/): 70 percent of proteins showed interaction at the evidence level and 42 percent of them interact at the action level demonstrating

TABLE 5.1

Summary of the Nine Analyzed Experiments

Composition of Nanoparticles	Diameter (nm)	ζ-Potential (mV)	Origin and Elution Method of Proteins	Authors and Year of the Study
Polystyrene amine modified	50	+23	H; SDS @ 95°C	2008 Lundqvist et al.
Au grafted with PEG (0.32–0.96 nm²)	15	ND	H; LDS + DTT @ 70°C, 1 h	2011 Walkey et al.
Carboxylated PVA-SPION	38.1	−5.9	B; 50 and 100 mM KCl	2013 Hirsch et al.
Eudragit® RS NP	65	+51.0	B; 6 M guanidine thiocyanate	2013 Hussien et al.
PLGA	227	−18.7	H; H₂O DTT and trypsin	2013 Sempf et al.
Au bis (p-sulfonatophenyl) phenylphosphine modified	15	−51	M; LDS	2014 Kreyling et al.
Neutral PVA-SPION	95	+5	R; 2 M NaCl and magnet	2014 Sakulkhu et al.
Ag citrate modified	24.4	−46.6	B; 8 M urea; 10 mM DTT	2014 Shannahan et al.
PEGylated cationic liposome	65	+65	H; ND	2015 Pozzi et al.

Note: B: *Bos taurus*; DTT: Dithiothreitol; H: Homo sapiens; L/SDS: Lithium/sodium dodecylsufate; M: *Mus musculus*; ND: Nondetermined; PEG: Polyethylene glycol; PLGA: Poly(lactic-co-glycolic) acid; PVA-SPION: Polyvinyl alcohol supramagnetic iron oxide nanoparticle; R: *Rattus norvegicus* plasma and protein database.

that protein are not randomly distributed in the corona despite their high dispersity of pH_i and MM. Thus we determined interactomes in the eight other studies that are presented in Table 5.1. Indeed, in those studies interactomes were not determined: Lundqvist et al., 2008; Walkey et al., 2011; Hirsch et al., 2013; Shannahan et al., 2013; Sempf et al., 2013; Kreyling et al., 2014; Pozzi et al., 2014; and Sakulkhu et al., 2014. The nine schemes obtained by the String database show all relationships existing at the action level represented in colored bold lines. Relationships existing at the evidence level, for example, co-citation of both involved proteins in Medline, was drawn by faint gray lines (Figure 5.1).

This is in favor of non-random adhesion of proteins, namely if a given protein X is present in the corona, a given protein Y that displays interaction with X has more probability to be in the corona than another protein Z that displays no interaction with X. Noteworthy proteins that do not display any interaction with each other at the evidence level were rarely noted in coronomes presented in our study. On average, 65 ± 22% of all proteins identified in the nine studies interact at the most documented action level that is drawn by bold lines in Figure 5.1a to 5.1i. This fact confirms our study and previous hypothesis (Hussien et al., 2013; Brooks et al., 2015).

Moreover, we retrieved all proteins that were eluted from nanoparticles in at least four of nine analyzed coronomes; they were encoded by the twenty-three following human genes as assessed by Genecards (http://www.genecards.org/): *A2M, AHSG, ALB, APOA1, APOA2, APOA4, APOB, APOC3, APOE, C3, CD5L, CFH, CLU, FGA, FGB, FGB, HBB, HPR, IGKC, KNG1, SERPINA1, SERPING1, VTN*. All but *CD5L* encoded proteins displayed multiples interactions at the evidence level (data not shown) and, more importantly, all but *AHSG-, CD5L-, HBB-* and *VTN*-encoded proteins showed interactions with the highest confidence (>90 percent) at the action level demonstrating that they were not randomly present in the corona but rather associated due to their biological action and molecular affinity (Figure 5.2).

As those proteins were identified in nine totally different experimental conditions, their presence in the NP corona is not dependent on the NP type but rather on the ability of a certain subset of proteins to fix by adhesion to every foreign

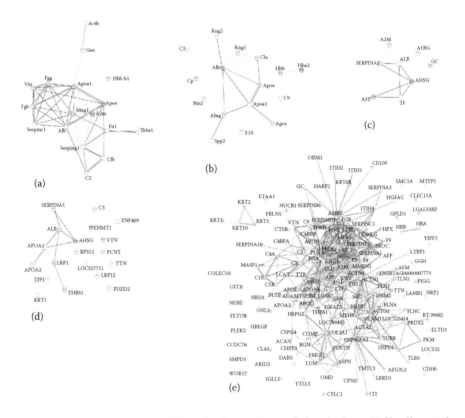

FIGURE 5.1 Interactomes at evidence level according to String database. (a) Kreyling et al. (2014), 17 items as retrieved from *Mus musculus* database; (b) Sakulkhu et al. (2014), 15 items as retrieved from *Rattus norvegicus* database; (c) Hirsch et al. (2013), 8 items as retrieved from *Bos taurus* database; (d) Shannahan et al. (2013), 16 items as retrieved from *Bos taurus* database; (e) Hussien et al. (2013), 158 items as retrieved from *Bos taurus* database.   (*Continued*)

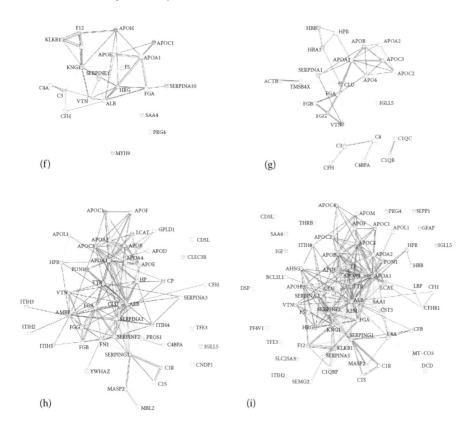

FIGURE 5.1 (CONTINUED) Interactomes at evidence level according to String database. (f) Sempf et al. (2013), 24 items as retrieved from Homo sapiens database; (g) Pozzi et al. (2014), 29 items as retrieved from Homo sapiens database; (h) Lundqvist et al. (2008), 47 items as retrieved from Homo sapiens database. (i) Walkey et al. (2011), 65 items as retrieved from Homo sapiens database. Relationships existing at the evidence level, for example, co-citation of both involved proteins in Medline, was drawn by faint gray lines; relationships existing at the action level are drawn in bold colored lines. Interactome were calculated at medium confidence level (>0.7).

material. By the way, our reanalysis of those nine independent experiments showed that certain proteins have a high probability to be present in corona as they are associated with each other in clusters or interactomes. Interestingly, Shannahan et al. (2013) also identified a subset of eleven corona proteins that were equally eluted from four types of silver NP behaving in various charges and ζ-potentials. It is not surprising that gene ontology (GO) pathways associated with those proteins were mainly described as binding activity for anion, antioxidant, apolipoprotein receptor, chaperone, hemoglobin, heparin, lipid, lipoprotein particle, protein, or receptor (false discovery rate < 0.0008). String analysis reveals that the most relevant KEGG pathway associated with those protein subsets is #4610 or "complement and coagulation cascades." As a matter of fact, NP interaction with complement components was largely described with various kind of modified or unmodified NP (Camacho

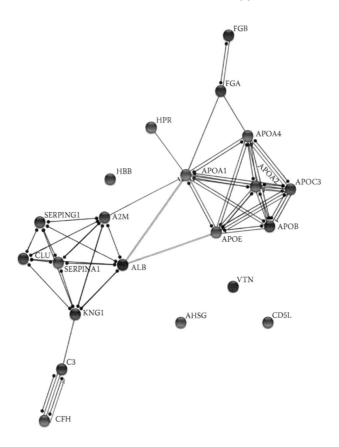

FIGURE 5.2 Action levels of shared proteins that were identified in at least four different studies. Action levels were calculated at the highest confidence score (>0.9) in the String database. Line shapes indicate the predicted mode of action: Activation, binding, catalysis, inhibition, reaction. Only four proteins do not display any interaction at that level of confidence score (AHSG, CD5L, HBB, and VTN). However, AHSG and VTN display interaction at the evidence level (data not shown, confidence score >0.4).

et al., 2011). As for pathway functions, nearly all proteins retrieved in at least four experiments display binding activity for anion, apolipoprotein receptor, chaperone, cholesterol, hemoglobin, heparin, high-density lipoprotein particle, lipid, lipoprotein particle, lipoprotein particle receptor, phosphatidylcholine, phospholipid, protein, and receptor (false discovery rate in String database < 0.0033). This is in favor of corona formation whatever the nature and surface of NP. Pathway process analysis of shared corona proteins are partially presented in Table 5.2. Gene Ontology "transport," "vesicle-mediated transport," and "single-organism transport" are frequently cited and retrieved at a very low false discovery rate indicating that proteins involved in transport have a strong ability to affix to NP corona. "Response to stress," "inflammatory response," and "regulation of inflammatory response" are

TABLE 5.2

Main Pathway Processes of Coronomes Retrieved in the Meta-Analysis

Pathway #	Pathway ID	Observed Protein Count
GO.0050896	Response to stimulus	20
GO.0050789	Regulation of biological process	20
GO.0006810	Transport	19
GO.0050794	Regulation of cellular process	19
GO.0006950	Response to stress	18
GO.0019222	Regulation of metabolic process	18
GO.0016192	Vesicle-mediated transport	16
GO.0048523	Negative regulation of cellular process	16
GO.0044710	Single-organism metabolic process	16
GO.0048518	Positive regulation of biological process	16
GO.0080090	Regulation of primary metabolic process	16
GO.0031323	Regulation of cellular metabolic process	16
GO.0044765	Single-organism transport	15
GO.0065008	Regulation of biological quality	15
GO.0048583	Regulation of response to stimulus	15
GO.0060255	Regulation of macromolecule metabolic process	15
GO.0044707	Single-multicellular organism process	15

Note: Process pathway IDs with the highest count of common proteins (≥ 15) all behave at a false discovery rate <0.0003.

also associated processes in protein corona of NP that are known to induce oxidative stress in cellular systems (Ronzani et al., 2013).

5.3   CERTAIN INTERPRO DOMAINS (IPD) ARE MORE FREQUENTLY RETRIEVED

In order to try to explain the high variability of the isolated proteins, we chose to collect all their IPD as performed previously (Hussien et al., 2013). We remarked that highly different proteins at the structural or functional level present in the corona may have similar IPD. For every IPD, we calculated its frequency by calculating the ratio of the number of a given domain on the number of all IPD in all eight reanalyzed studies (Lundqvist et al., 2008; Walkey et al., 2011; Hirsch et al., 2013; Shannahan et al., 2013; Sempf et al., 2013; Kreyling et al., 2014; Pozzi et al., 2014; Sakulkhu et al., 2014), and one experiment for which analysis was already done (Hussien et al., 2013). IPD were ranked together if they were identified in at least two experiments (see Table 5.3). Thus, all frequencies were listed in seven subsets corresponding to different experiments, namely, IPD shared in 8, 7, 6, 5, 4, 3, 2 studies.

We calculated the mean and the standard deviation of IPD occurrence and finally evidenced three groups of IPD as assessed by one-way ANOVA post-hoc Tukey Kramer (Figure 5.3).

TABLE 5.3

Frequency Mean and SD of InterPro Domains (IPD) Retrieved in at Least Two Experiments

InterPro Domain Name	N	F Mean	F SD
IPR000074 ApoA1_A4_E	8	0.0219	0.0089
IPR000264 ALB/AFP/VDB	8	0.0232	0.0294
IPR001314 Peptidase_S1A	8	0.0295	0.0150
IPR001599 Macroglobln_a2	8	0.0223	0.0120
IPR002890 A2M_N	8	0.0223	0.0120
IPR008930 Terpenoid_cyclase/PrenylTrfase	8	0.0217	0.0126
IPR009048 A-macroglobulin_rcpt-bd	8	0.0223	0.0120
IPR011625 6_N_2	8	0.0223	0.0120
IPR011626 A2M_comp	8	0.0223	0.0120
IPR014760 Serum_albumin_N	8	0.0214	0.0294
IPR019742 MacrogloblnA2_CS	8	0.0220	0.0123
IPR020858 Serum_albumin-like	8	0.0214	0.0294
IPR021177 Serum_albumin/AFP	8	0.0172	0.0186
IPR023795 Serpin_CS	8	0.0229	0.0092
IPR023796 Sepin_dom	8	0.0251	0.0086
IPR000020 Anaphylatoxin/fibulin	7	0.0156	0.0086
IPR000215 Serpin_fam	7	0.0246	0.0092
IPR000585 Hemopexin/matrixin	7	0.0131	0.0072
IPR000742 EGF_3	7	0.0166	0.0103
IPR001134 Netrin_domain	7	0.0153	0.0089
IPR001212 Somatomedin_B_dom	7	0.0128	0.0076
IPR001254 Peptidase_S1_S6	7	0.0274	0.0148
IPR001840 Anaphylatoxn	7	0.0153	0.0089
IPR007110 Ig-like_dom	7	0.0353	0.0233
IPR008993 TIMP-like_OB-fold	7	0.0153	0.0089
IPR009003 Pept_cys/ser_Trypsin-like	7	0.0267	0.0153
IPR013032 EGF-like_reg_CS	7	0.0230	0.0086
IPR013783 Ig-like_fold	7	0.0378	0.0220
IPR018081 Anaphylatoxin_comp_syst	7	0.0153	0.0089
IPR018486 Hemopexin_CS	7	0.0131	0.0072
IPR018487 Hemopexin-like_repeat	7	0.0131	0.0072
IPR018933 Netrin_module_non-TIMP	7	0.0153	0.0089
IPR019565 MacrogloblnA2_thiol-ester-bond	7	0.0230	0.0131
IPR020436 Somatomedin_B_chordata	7	0.0128	0.0076
IPR020857 Serum_albumin_CS	7	0.0223	0.0316
IPR000010 Prot_inh_cystat	6	0.0240	0.0136
IPR000436 Sushi_SCR_CCP	6	0.0331	0.0207
IPR001881 EGF-like_Ca-bd	6	0.0233	0.0095
IPR002181 Fibrinogen_a/b/g_C	6	0.0205	0.0140
IPR012290 Fibrinogen_a/b/g_coil_dom	6	0.0205	0.0140
IPR014715 Fibrinogen_a/b/g_C_2	6	0.0205	0.0140

(Continued)

TABLE 5.3 (CONTINUED)

Frequency Mean and SD of InterPro Domains (IPD) Retrieved in at Least Two Experiments

InterPro Domain Name	N	F Mean	F SD
IPR014716 Fibrinogen_a/b/g_C_1	6	0.0205	0.0140
IPR018114 Peptidase_S1_AS	6	0.0257	0.0115
IPR020837 Fibrinogen_CS	6	0.0229	0.0167
IPR000083 Fibronectin_type1	5	0.0095	0.0045
IPR000152 EGF-type_Asp/Asn_hydroxyl_site	5	0.0207	0.0097
IPR000562 FN_type2_col-bd	5	0.0095	0.0045
IPR000753 Clusterin-like	5	0.0091	0.0051
IPR000971 Globin_subset	5	0.0163	0.0115
IPR001363 Prot_inh_fetuin_CS	5	0.0134	0.0107
IPR001751 S100/CaBP-9k_CS	5	0.0066	0.0049
IPR002337 Haemoglobin_b	5	0.0102	0.0057
IPR002355 Cu_oxidase_Cu_BS	5	0.0095	0.0045
IPR003006 Ig/MHC_CS	5	0.0361	0.0226
IPR003597 Ig_C1-set	5	0.0356	0.0233
IPR006801 ApoA-II	5	0.0083	0.0044
IPR008972 Cupredoxin	5	0.0095	0.0045
IPR008985 ConA-like_lec_gl	5	0.0132	0.0035
IPR009050 Globin-like	5	0.0163	0.0115
IPR011707 Cu-oxidase_3	5	0.0095	0.0045
IPR012292 Globin_dom	5	0.0192	0.0127
IPR013806 Kringle-like	5	0.0138	0.0089
IPR016014 Clusterin_N	5	0.0091	0.0051
IPR016015 Clusterin_C	5	0.0091	0.0051
IPR016016 Clusterin	5	0.0091	0.0051
IPR018097 EGF_Ca-bd_CS	5	0.0216	0.0103
IPR021996 Fibrinogen_aC	5	0.0089	0.0049
IPR000859 CUB	4	0.0167	0.0076
IPR000884 Thrombospondin_1_rpt	4	0.0115	0.0038
IPR001791 Laminin_G	4	0.0107	0.0027
IPR002035 VWF_A	4	0.0189	0.0110
IPR002338 Haemoglobin_a	4	0.0082	0.0069
IPR002395 Kininogen	4	0.0092	0.0059
IPR003961 Fibronectin_type3	4	0.0112	0.0024
IPR009454 Lipid_transpt_open_b-sht	4	0.0078	0.0048
IPR011030 Vitellinogen_superhlx	4	0.0078	0.0048
IPR013320 ConA-like_subgrp	4	0.0129	0.0040
IPR014756 Ig_E-set	4	0.0177	0.0144
IPR015255 Vitellinogen_open_b-sht	4	0.0078	0.0048
IPR015553 C1-inh	4	0.0079	0.0051
IPR015816 Vitellinogen_b-sht_N	4	0.0078	0.0048
IPR015817 Vitellinogen_open_b-sht_sub1	4	0.0078	0.0048

(Continued)

TABLE 5.3 (CONTINUED)
Frequency Mean and SD of InterPro Domains (IPD) Retrieved in at Least Two Experiments

InterPro Domain Name	N	F Mean	F SD
IPR015818 Vitellinogen_open_b-sht_sub2	4	0.0078	0.0048
IPR015819 Lipid_transp_b-sht_shell	4	0.0078	0.0048
IPR022176 ApoB100_C	4	0.0078	0.0048
IPR025760 Cystatin_Fetuin_A	4	0.0156	0.0109
IPR000001 Kringle	3	0.0096	0.0038
IPR000421 Coagulation_fac_5/8-C_type_dom	3	0.0089	0.0042
IPR000895 Transthyretin/HIU_hydrolase	3	0.0058	0.0033
IPR001007 VWF_C	3	0.0105	0.0039
IPR001117 Cu-oxidase	3	0.0085	0.0061
IPR001156 Peptidase_S60	3	0.0140	0.0150
IPR001190 Srcr_rcpt	3	0.0058	0.0033
IPR001664 IF	3	0.0107	0.0046
IPR002172 LDrepeatLR_classA_rpt	3	0.0133	0.0084
IPR002339 Haemoglobin_pi	3	0.0101	0.0069
IPR003014 PAN-1_domain	3	0.0120	0.0135
IPR003367 Thrombospondin_3-like_rpt	3	0.0105	0.0039
IPR003386 LACT/PDAT_acylTrfase	3	0.0058	0.0033
IPR003598 Ig_sub2	3	0.0176	0.0118
IPR003609 Pan_app	3	0.0120	0.0135
IPR004000 Actin-relat	3	0.0123	0.0031
IPR004001 Actin_CS	3	0.0123	0.0031
IPR006781 ApoC-I	3	0.0096	0.0038
IPR008160 Collagen	3	0.0158	0.0101
IPR008292 Haptoglobin	3	0.0096	0.0038
IPR008403 Apo-CIII	3	0.0096	0.0038
IPR008859 Thrombospondin_C	3	0.0105	0.0039
IPR008979 Galactose-bd-like	3	0.0089	0.0042
IPR009030 Growth_fac_rcpt_N_dom	3	0.0113	0.0029
IPR010600 ITI_HC_C	3	0.0168	0.0161
IPR010916 TonB_box_CS	3	0.0173	0.0127
IPR011038 Calycin-like	3	0.0102	0.0065
IPR011042 6-blade_b-propeller_TolB-like	3	0.0115	0.0058
IPR011706 Cu-oxidase_2	3	0.0085	0.0061
IPR013694 VIT	3	0.0168	0.0161
IPR014394 Coagulation_fac_XIIa/HGFA	3	0.0074	0.0058
IPR015104 Sushi_2	3	0.0074	0.0058
IPR016024 ARM-type_fold	3	0.0096	0.0038
IPR016357 Transferrin	3	0.0140	0.0150
IPR017448 Srcr_rcpt-rel	3	0.0058	0.0033
IPR017857 Coagulation_fac_subgr_Gla_dom	3	0.0107	0.0033
IPR017897 Thrombospondin_3_rpt	3	0.0105	0.0039

(Continued)

TABLE 5.3 (CONTINUED)
Frequency Mean and SD of InterPro Domains (IPD) Retrieved in at Least Two Experiments

InterPro Domain Name	N	F Mean	F SD
IPR018039 Intermediate_filament_CS	3	0.0107	0.0046
IPR018073 Prot_inh_cystat_CS	3	0.0150	0.0134
IPR018159 Spectrin/alpha-actinin	3	0.0071	0.0031
IPR018195 Transferrin_Fe_BS	3	0.0140	0.0150
IPR018331Haemoglobin_alpha_chain	3	0.0101	0.0069
IPR020902 Actin/actin-like_CS	3	0.0123	0.0031
IPR023415 LDLR_class-A_CS	3	0.0133	0.0084
IPR023416 Transthyretin/HIU_hydrolase_SF	3	0.0058	0.0033
IPR023418 Thyroxine_BS	3	0.0058	0.0033
IPR023419 Transthyretin_CS	3	0.0058	0.0033
IPR024715 Factor_5/8	3	0.0081	0.0049
IPR027358 Kininogen-type_cystatin_dom	3	0.0163	0.0116
IPR000048 IQ_motif_EF-hand-BS	2	0.0080	0.0081
IPR000096 Serum_amyloid_A	2	0.0131	0.0008
IPR000177 Apple	2	0.0168	0.0150
IPR000213 VitD-bd	2	0.0167	0.0205
IPR000294 GLA_domain	2	0.0088	0.0000
IPR000566 Lipocln_cytosolic_FA-bd_dom	2	0.0122	0.0078
IPR000719 Prot_kinase_cat_dom	2	0.0097	0.0012
IPR001028 Gprt_PLipase_D	2	0.0055	0.0047
IPR001073 C1q	2	0.0159	0.0163
IPR001124 Lipid-bd_serum_glycop_C	2	0.0042	0.0029
IPR001304 C-type_lectin	2	0.0122	0.0078
IPR001452 SH3_domain	2	0.0075	0.0043
IPR001589 Actinin_actin-bd_CS	2	0.0097	0.0012
IPR001609 Myosin_head_motor_dom	2	0.0080	0.0081
IPR001703 Alpha-fetoprotein	2	0.0178	0.0190
IPR001715 CH-domain	2	0.0097	0.0012
IPR001862 MAC_perforin	2	0.0084	0.0087
IPR002017 Spectrin_repeat	2	0.0075	0.0043
IPR002110 Ankyrin_rpt	2	0.0064	0.0059
IPR002223 Prot_inh_Kunz-m	2	0.0077	0.0016
IPR002290 Ser/Thr_kinase_dom	2	0.0075	0.0043
IPR002345 Lipocalin	2	0.0111	0.0094
IPR002640 Arylesterase	2	0.0120	0.0081
IPR002928 Myosin_tail	2	0.0080	0.0081
IPR002968 A1-microglobln	2	0.0055	0.0047
IPR002969 ApolipopD	2	0.0055	0.0047
IPR003599 Ig_sub	2	0.0097	0.0012
IPR004009 Myosin_N	2	0.0080	0.0081
IPR004168 PPAK_motif	2	0.0064	0.0059

(Continued)

TABLE 5.3 (CONTINUED)

Frequency Mean and SD of InterPro Domains (IPD) Retrieved in at Least Two Experiments

InterPro Domain Name	N	F Mean	F SD
IPR007087 Znf_C2H2	2	0.0075	0.0043
IPR007122 Villin/Gelsolin	2	0.0084	0.0087
IPR007123 Gelsolin_dom	2	0.0084	0.0087
IPR008019 Apo-CII	2	0.0100	0.0053
IPR008266 Tyr_kinase_AS	2	0.0086	0.0028
IPR008363 Paraoxonase1	2	0.0075	0.0018
IPR008983 Tumour_necrosis_fac-like	2	0.0170	0.0147
IPR011360 Compl_C2_B	2	0.0104	0.0058
IPR012224 Pept_S1A_FX	2	0.0095	0.0071
IPR012674 Calycin	2	0.0122	0.0078
IPR013098 Ig_I-set	2	0.0108	0.0004
IPR013106 Ig_V-set	2	0.0080	0.0081
IPR015129 Titin_Z	2	0.0064	0.0059
IPR015247 VitD-bind_III	2	0.0167	0.0205
IPR015555 AT-III	2	0.0084	0.0087
IPR015880 Znf_C2H2-like	2	0.0075	0.0043
IPR016137 Regulat_G_prot_signal_superfam	2	0.0080	0.0081
IPR016186 C-type_lectin-like	2	0.0122	0.0078
IPR016187 C-type_lectin_fold	2	0.0133	0.0063
IPR017942 Lipid-bd_serum_glycop_N	2	0.0042	0.0029
IPR017943 Bactericidal_perm-incr_a/b_dom	2	0.0042	0.0029
IPR017954 Lipid-bd_serum_glycop_CS	2	0.0042	0.0029
IPR018378 C-type_lectin_CS	2	0.0133	0.0063
IPR020683 Ankyrin_rpt-contain_dom	2	0.0064	0.0059
IPR020863 MACPF_CS	2	0.0084	0.0087
IPR020864 MACPF	2	0.0084	0.0087
IPR020901 Prtase_inh_Kunz-CS	2	0.0077	0.0016
IPR022271 Lipocalin	2	0.0055	0.0047
IPR022272 Lipocalin_CS	2	0.0111	0.0094
IPR023121 ApoC-II_domain	2	0.0100	0.0053
IPR024175 Pept_S1A_C1r/C1S/mannan-bd	2	0.0271	0.0118
IPR026114 APOF	2	0.0075	0.0018
IPR027150 CP	2	0.0117	0.0040
IPR027417 P-loop_NTPase	2	0.0121	0.0022
IPR028499 Thrombospondin-1	2	0.0125	0.0028

Note: **N** is the number of experiments in which a given common InterPro domain, listed by increasing ID number, was retrieved (N is varying from 8 to 2). Only InterPro domains (IPD) found by more than 2 studies were noted. **N**, **F Mean** and **F SD** are respectively the mean and the standard deviation of the means of all domains found in 8, 7, 6, 5 4, 3, and 2 experiments. All the experiments were analyzed but the study of Hussien et al. (2013). For consulting extensive analysis of the last experiment, refer to U.S. patent N° WO2015026947 (Brooks et al., 2015).

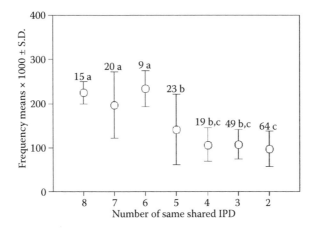

FIGURE 5.3 Single classification ANOVA of the seven InterPro domain groups. Groups not sharing the same letter are different on the 95 percent level (Tukey–Kramer method). ANOVA source of variation analysis (p < 0.0001). IPD: InterPro domain.

Thus, three groups of IPD were defined: series "8-7-6," "5-4-3," and "2," which were different at the 95 percent level by the Tukey Kramer method, indicating that IPD shared in 8, 7, 6 experiments has a statistically significant higher occurrence than the ones shared in 5, 4, or 3 experiments and the ones displayed in only 2 different experiments. For example, an IPD shared in different studies which occurred in 6 experimental designs has a same probability to occur at the same frequency in 7 or 8 experiments. The more numerous the corona analysis, the higher the occurrence frequency of a given IPD.

Moreover, we compared the 199 most frequent IPD retrieved from the eight reanalyzed studies (Lundqvist et al., 2008; Walkey et al., 2011; Hirsch et al., 2013; Shannahan et al., 2013; Sempf et al., 2013; Kreyling et al., 2014; Pozzi et al., 2014; Sakulkhu et al., 2014) to the 199 most frequent ones that were identified by Hussien et al. (2013). Surprisingly, 271 of them were common (68 percent) and only 63 (~16 percent) and 64 (~16 percent) were described in the Hussien et al. (2013) coronome and in the pooled eight other coronomes, respectively. Percentage of shared IPD are much higher than percentage of shared proteins. As mentioned previously, experimental conditions, type of NP, coronome extraction, and protein identification are highly different in all experiments, indicating that apparent discrepancy at the protein level is largely smoothed at the IPD level. If careful MS analysis is done, one can consider that the specificity of IPD is limited to only 16 percent of all IPD retrieved in coronomes.

Moreover, the 33 most frequent domains determined in the study of Hussien et al. (2013) were compared to the 33 most frequent domains retrieved from the other eight reanalyzed studies. Table 5.4 showed that 30 percent of the most frequent domains are shared in all nine studies, 36 percent were specific of Hussien's study (2013), and 34 percent of all other eight studies taken together.

TABLE 5.4

Most Common InterPro Domains (IPD)

IPR#	Description
IPR000010	Prot_inh_cystat
IPR000215	Serpin_fam
IPR000264	ALB/AFP/VDB
IPR000436	Sushi_SCR_CCP
IPR001254	Peptidase_S1_S6
IPR001599	Macroglobln_a2
IPR007110	Ig-like_dom
IPR009003	Pept_cys/ser_Trypsin-like
IPR013783	Ig-like_fold
IPR020837	Fibrinogen_CS

Interestingly, among those most frequently identified IPD, IPD related to proteases inhibitors, namely IPR000010 (Prot_inh_cystat), IPR000215 (Serpin_fam), IPR001599 (Macroglobln_a2), and proteases, for example, IPR001254 (Peptidase_S1_S6) and IPR009003 (Pept_cys/ser_Trypsin-like), are overrepresented. The recognition process is also in the most frequently shared IPD, for example, by IPR000436 Sushi_SCR_CCP and two others involved in a variety of functions, including cell–cell recognition, cell–surface receptors, and immune system (IPR007110 Ig-like_dom; IPR013783 Ig-like_fold). The last one, IPR020837 Fibrinogen_CS, may be involved in NP aggregation as it is known to play a key role in blood clotting.

5.4   DETERMINATION OF IPD FACILITATES BETTER KNOWLEDGE OF NP "BIOLOGICAL IDENTITY"

The action level of the eight reanalyzed studies, illustrated by full-color lines in Figure 5.1, was further defined with IPD-associated GO terms of shared proteins as was previously performed using Uniprot (http://www.uniprot.org/) databases (Hussien et al., 2013). As for the IPD biological process: "Lipid transport," "proteolysis," "cell adhesion," "immune response," "oxidation-reduction process," "iron binding," "oxygen transport," "lipoprotein metabolism," "regulation of blood coagulation," and "platelet activation" were frequently described (an extractum of GO terms is shown in Table 5.5). Thus, IPD involved in such biological functions display a higher affinity for NP, whatever their structure.

IPD molecular functions were mainly represented by (1) catalytic activities like serine-type endopeptidase activity (four times) and serine- and cysteine-type endopeptidase inhibitor activity (six times); and (2) binding activity protein (nine times), iron (eight times), heme (seven times), dioxygen (five times), calcium (five times), copper (four times), lipid (three times), and polysaccharide (two times). Not surprisingly, cellular components were mainly represented by "extracellular region"

TABLE 5.5

GO Terms of a Selection of 19/299 IPRO Domains (IPD) Describing Their Biological Process, Molecular Function, Cellular Component, and Related IPD

IPD #	Biological Process	Molecular Function	Cellular Component	Related IPD	Related IPD
IPR000074 ApoA1_A4_E	GO 0006869 lipid transport; GO 0042157 lipoprotein metabolic process	GO 0008289 lipid binding	GO 0005576 extracellular region		Vitamin D-binding protein (IPR000213)
IPR000264 ALB/AFP/VDB	GO 0006810 transport		GO 0005615 extracellular space	Serum albumin/Alpha-fetoprotein (IPR021177)	
IPR001314 Peptidase_S1A	GO 0006508 proteolysis	GO 0004252 serine-type endopeptidase activity		Coagulation factor XIIa/hepatocyte growth factor activator (IPR014394); Complement B/C2 (IPR011360)	Peptidase S1A, complement C1r/C1S/mannan-binding (IPR024175); Haptoglobin (IPR008292)
IPR001599 Macroglobln_a2		GO 0004866 endopeptidase inhibitor activity			
IPR002890 A2M_N		GO 0004866 endopeptidase inhibitor activity			
IPR008930 Terpenoid_cyclase/PrenylTrfase				Alpha-macroglobulin complement component (IPR011626)	
IPR009048 A-macroglobulin_rcpt-bd					
IPR011625 A2M_N			GO 0005576 extracellular region		

(Continued)

TABLE 5.5 (CONTINUED)

GO Terms of a Selection of 19/299 IPRO Domains (IPD) Describing Their Biological Process, Molecular Function, Cellular Component, and Related IPD

IPD #	Biological Process	Molecular Function	Cellular Component	Related IPD	Related IPD
IPR011626 A2M_comp			GO 0005615 extracellular space	Terpenoid cyclases/protein prenyltransferase alpha-alpha toroid (IPR008930)	
IPR014760 Serum_albumin_N IPR019742 MacroglobinA2_CS			GO 0005615 extracellular space	Serum albumin-like (IPR020858)	
IPR020858 Serum_albumin-like			GO 0005615 extracellular space	Serum albumin, N-terminal (IPR014760)	Vitamin D binding protein, domain III (IPR015247) ALB/AFP/VDB (IPR000264)
IPR021177 Serum_albumin/AFP IPR023795 Serpin_CS IPR023796 Sepin_dom			GO 0005615 extracellular space	Alpha-fetoprotein (IPR001703)	
IPR000020 Anaphylatoxin/fibulin			GO 0005576 extracellular region	Anaphylatoxin, complement system (IPR018081)	
IPR000215 Serpin_fam			GO 0005615 extracellular space	Antithrombin-III (IPR015555)	Plasma protease C1 inhibitor (IPR015553)
IPR000585 Hemopexin-like_dom IPR000742 EG-like_dom		GO 0005515 protein binding			

(eleven) and "extracellular space" (eight) and more scarcely by "hemoglobin-" or "fibrinogen-complex."

Last but not least on the 199 IPD of the eight reanalyzed studies, 28.5 percent of them are related to each other, for example, of "IPR001314 Peptidase_S1A" that was related to "coagulation factor XIIa/hepatocyte growth factor activator (IPR014394)," "Peptidase S1A, complement C1r/C1S/mannan-binding (IPR024175)," "Complement B/C2 (IPR011360)," and also "Haptoglobin (IPR008292)" (Table 5.5). Remarkably, all of them were retrieved in our previous experiment (Hussien et al., 2013). Thus, despite the heterogeneity of nanoparticles, protein source, and elution as well as protein identification methods, it is likely that a high subset of IPD (84 percent) and consequently a high subset of proteins—roughly estimated to two-thirds of the proteins identified in our study—are on average involved in the corona formation, whatever the nature of nanoparticle. Involvement of IPD that are specific to a given type of nanoparticle remains incidental, even if one cannot completely exclude a certain degree of fingerprinting or protein signature. Indeed, when one considers the chemical nature of the modifying agents used in NP preparation, 89 percent of them behave as hydroxyl groups and oxygen moieties that may be involved in hydrogen bonds. Thus, a certain degree of selection bias may not be excluded.

However, we hypothesize that specific IPD, namely no more than 16 percent of all retrieved IPD, may confer the "protein signature" together with the biological determinism of cells exposed to NP that induce their binding. Some of those biological fates were recently described: (1) epithelium differentiation of Human Mammary Epithelial Cells provoked by polymeric nanoparticles due to their specific protein cargo or coronome (Hussien et al., 2013), (2) autophagy program in macrophages (Eidi et al., 2012), or (3) the opposite, lack of cytotoxicity in macrophages exposed to NP (Lee et al., 2014; Ronzani et al., 2014). Sisco et al. (2014) suggested as we did previously (Hussien et al., 2013) that proteins adsorbed to nanorods mediate cell–cell interaction and fibroblast-mediated matrix remodeling. Nevertheless, corona formation seems more to depend on the given properties of IPD that allow their interactions as well as their adhesion on a given nanoparticle surface, mainly by hydrogen bonding and hydrophobic interaction (Cedervall et al., 2007; Pearson et al., 2014).

Thus, we propose that the subset of corona proteins has to be analyzed by mass spectrometry following incubation with nanoparticles and their list should be determined as well as other physicochemical characteristics following their elution with high stringency solution as was performed in three previous studies: Lundqvist et al. (2008), Hussien et al. (2013), and Shannahan et al. (2014). Therefore, the exact determination of coronome, namely, the protein cargo of corona, is necessary but not sufficient, as IPD reflect more precisely biological activity of attached proteins and seem critical for determining the fate of NP and cells after their complex interplay. Characterizing coronomes is a new research field that will allow researchers to better understand interactions with plasma proteins of living or inert nanoparticles, like carbone nanotubes, metal NP, and viruses, even if they interact specifically with receptor proteins but are also able to induce autophagy in infected immune cells. The knowledge of specific interaction may also be beneficial for diagnosis purposes, for example, AuNP for protein characterization in broncho-alveolar lavage (Kreyling et al., 2014) or in other biological fluids as it was claimed in a recent U.S. patent

(Brooks et al., 2015). Last but not least, liposome NP, for example, will further be powerful paradigms of protein–biological membranes interaction studies.

ACKNOWLEDGMENTS

B. H. R. was supported by National Academy of Medicine (France). B. H. R. and P.R. are debt in GA Brooks (Department of Integrative Biology, University of California, Berkeley, California, 94720-3140) to allow them to work on this project in his laboratory.

REFERENCES

Brooks, G. A., Hussien, R., and Rihn, B. 2015. Composition and methods for culturing cells. U.S. patent N° WO2015026947.

Camacho, A. I., Da Costa Martins, R., Tamayo, I., de Souza, J., Lasarte, J. J., Mansilla, C., Esparza, I., Irache, J. M., and Gamazo, C. 2011. Poly(methyl vinyl ether-co-maleic anhydride) nanoparticles as innate immune system activators. *Vaccine* 29(41):7130–7135.

Cedervall, T., Lynch, I., Lindman, S., Berggård, T., Thulin, E., Nilsson, H., Dawson, K. A., and Linse, S. 2007. Understanding the nanoparticle-protein corona using methods to quantify exchange rates and affinities of proteins for nanoparticles. *Proc Natl Acad Sci USA* 104(7):2050–2055.

Eidi, H., Joubert, O., Némos, C., Grandemange, S., Mograbi, B., Foliguet, B., Tournebize, J., Maincent, P., Le Faou, A., Aboukhamis, I., and Rihn, B. H. 2012. Drug delivery by polymeric nanoparticles induces autophagy in macrophages. *Int J Pharm* 422(1–2):495–503.

Gref, R., Lück, M., Quellec, P., Marchand, M., Dellacherie, E., Harnisch, S., Blunk, T., and Müller, R. H. 2008. 'Stealth' corona-core nanoparticles surface modified by polyethylene glycol (PEG): Influences of the corona (PEG chain length and surface density) and of the core composition on phagocytic uptake and plasma protein adsorption. *Colloids Surf B Biointerfaces* 18(3–4):301–313.

Hirsch, V., Kinnear, C., Moniatte, M., Rothen-Rutishauser, B., Clift, M. J., and Fink, A. 2013. Surface charge of polymer coated SPIONs influences the serum protein adsorption, colloidal stability and subsequent cell interaction in vitro. *Nanoscale* 7;5(9):3723–3732.

Hussien, R., Rihn, B. H., Eidi, H., Ronzani, C., Joubert, O., Ferrari, L., Vazquez, O., Kaufer, D., and Brooks, G. A. 2013. Unique growth pattern of human mammary epithelial cells induced by polymeric nanoparticles. *Physiol Rep* 1(4):e00027.

Kreyling, W. G., Fertsch-Gapp, S., Schäffler, M., Johnston, B. D., Haberl, N., Pfeiffer, C., Diendorf, J., Schleh, C., Hirn, S., Semmler-Behnke, M., Epple, M., and Parak, W. J. 2014. In vitro and in vivo interactions of selected nanoparticles with rodent serum proteins and their consequences in biokinetics. *Beilstein J Nanotechnol* 5:1699–1711.

Lee, Y. K., Choi, E. J., Webster, T. J., Kim, S. H., and Khang, D. 2014. Effect of the protein corona on nanoparticles for modulating cytotoxicity and immunotoxicity. *Int J Nanomedicine* 10:97–113.

Lundqvist, M., Stigler, J., Elia, G., Lynch, I., Cedervall, T., and Dawson, K. A. 2008. Nanoparticle size and surface properties determine the protein corona with possible implications for biological impacts. *Proc Natl Acad Sci USA* 105(38):14265–14270.

Pearson, R. M., Juettner, V. V., and Hong, S. 2014. Biomolecular corona on nanoparticles: A survey of recent literature and its implications in targeted drug delivery. *Front Chem* 2:108.

Pozzi, D., Caracciolo, G., Capriotti, A. L., Cavaliere, C., Piovesana, S., Colapicchioni, V., Palchetti, S., Riccioli, A., and Laganà, A. 2014. A proteomics-based methodology to investigate the protein corona effect for targeted drug delivery. *Mol Biosyst* 10(11):2815–2819.

Rihn, B. H., and Joubert, O. 2015. Comment on "Protein Corona Fingerprinting Predicts the Cellular Interaction of Gold and Silver Nanoparticles." *ACS Nano* 9(6):5634–5635.

Ronzani, C., Safar, R., Diab, R., Chevrier, J., Paoli, J., Abdel-Wahhab, M. A., Le Faou, A., Rihn, B. H., and Joubert, O. 2014. Viability and gene expression responses to polymeric nanoparticles in human and rat cells. *Cell Biol Toxicol* 30(3):137–146.

Sakulkhu, U., Maurizi, L., Mahmoudi, M., Motazacker, M., Vries, M., Gramoun, A., Ollivier Beuzelin, M. G., Vallée, J. P., Rezaee, F., and Hofmann, H. 2014. Ex situ evaluation of the composition of protein corona of intravenously injected superparamagnetic nanoparticles in rats. *Nanoscale* 6(19):11439–11450.

Sempf, K., Arrey, T., Gelperina, S., Schorge, T., Meyer, B., Karas, M., and Kreuter, J. 2013. Adsorption of plasma proteins on uncoated PLGA nanoparticles. *Eur J Pharm Biopharm* 85(1):53–60.

Shannahan, J. H., Lai, X., Ke, P. C., Podila, R., Brown, J. M., and Witzmann, F. A. 2013. Silver nanoparticle protein corona composition in cell culture media. *PLoS ONE* 8(9):e74001.

Sisco, P. N., Wilson, C. G., Chernak, D., Clark, J. C., Grzincic, E. M., Ako-Asare, K., Goldsmith, E. C., and Murphy, C. J. 2014. Adsorption of cellular proteins to polyelectrolyte-functionalized gold nanorods: A mechanism for nanoparticle regulation of cell phenotype? *PLoS ONE* 9(2):e86670.

Walkey, C. D. 2014. The Biological Identity of Nanoparticles. Doctor of Philosophy Thesis. Toronto: University of Toronto, 263 pp.

Walkey, C. D., Olsen, J. B., Guo, H., Emili, A., and Chan, W. C. 2012. Nanoparticle size and surface chemistry determine serum protein adsorption and macrophage uptake. *J Am Chem Soc* 1;134(4):2139–2147.

6 Nanoparticles and Viruses as Mitophagy Inducers in Immune Cells

Housam Eidi, Zahra Doumandji,
Lucija Tomljenovic, and Bertrand Henri Rihn

CONTENTS

6.1 WELCOME TO THE SYNTHETIC AND NATURAL "NANOWORLD"

Nowadays, nanobodies are used every day and everywhere. Everybody has been exposed to a foreign particle measuring a few nanometers. We inhale them with each of our breaths, we intake them with each mouthful of consumption, and we spread them on our skin.

Many studies show that nanoorganisms such as viruses provoke chronic disease. Diseases caused by persistent virus infections include liver cancer (hepatitis virus; Levrero 2006), subacute sclerosing panencephalitis (measles virus; Wild 1981), progressive multifocal leukoencephalopathy (papovavirus; Padgett et al. 1976), and spongiform encephalopathies (proteins prions; Budka et al. 1995). Further, γ-herpesviruses, Epstein–Barr virus, and Kaposi's sarcoma–associated herpesvirus induce neoplasia (Shelby et al. 2005). The pathogenic mechanisms by which these viruses cause disease include disorders of biochemical, cellular, immune, and physiologic processes (Boldogh et al. 1996).

One might think that nanoparticles (NPs) induce the same damage as the one of these viruses, knowing that they are similar in size. One might also think that NPs are less harmful, because unlike viruses, they are unable to replicate. However, it has long been recognized that workers in the silicon alloy industry develop a progressive form of silicosis rapidly (Bruce 1937). Furthermore, the previously unknown causes of certain diseases have been recently correlated with NPs exposure. Crohn's and Parkinson's diseases, for example, are both due to exposure to titanium dioxide NPs (Ruiz et al. 2016, Wu and Xie 2014). Despite the potential hazard of NPs, this does not impede the constant evolution of nanotechnology in different fields, ranging from medicine and scientific equipment to electronics. The use of nanoparticles seems to make life easier. In medicine, for instance, nanoparticles are used for targeted treatments, either by surface targeting or by magnetic guidance. This is done by manipulating the size and characteristics of the particles while choosing the matrix constituents. The system can be used for various routes of administration including oral, nasal, parenteral, intra-ocular, and so on (Mohanraj and Chen 2006). The objective is to make a faster development of new safe medicines. Unfortunately, technological advancements progress faster than safety evaluations.

Due to their small size, NPs, even with reduced mass, are deprived of large values in terms of number, surface area, and concentrations. NPs are classified according to their morphology, composition, and ability to disperse. NP production around the world exceeds 11×103 tons per year, with SiO_2 and TiO_2 at the top of the list (Piccinno et al. 2012, Hendren et al. 2011, Huang et al. 2016). NPs are produced for cosmetics (Comiskey et al. 1998), paints (Zuccheri et al. 2013), plastics (Koivisto et al. 2012), fuel (Wang and Feng 2003), textiles (Dubas et al. 2006), and so on. All living creatures in the environment are permanently exposed to NPs. Humans are exposed to various nanoscale materials since childhood through their skin, lungs, and digestive tract, and the new emerging field of nanotechnology has become another threat to human life (Oberdorster et al. 2005). There are three principal mechanisms that lead to pulmonary deposition: inertial impaction, gravitational sedimentation, and Brownian diffusion (Byron 1986, Courrier et al. 2002).

Given the application increase of NPs and our exposure to them, their toxicity assessment has become imperative. The potential toxicity of NPs changes from one NP to another, depending on their substance, size, and shape. Almost all NP disturb the cell viability, increase cellular oxidation, alter mitochondrial potential, and cause DNA damage (Chen et al. 2008, De Matteis et al. 2016).

6.2 AUTOPHAGY

Macroautophagy (autophagy) was described for the first time by Christian De Duve in 1963 (De Duve 1963). *Autophagy* (self-eating) means the sequestration of intracellular cargo such as cellular organelles, proteins, and pathogens inside autophagosome, a double-membrane structure (Xie and Klionsky 2007, Klionsky 2007, Klionsky et al. 2008; see Figure 6.1). Autophagosome/lysosome fusion forms

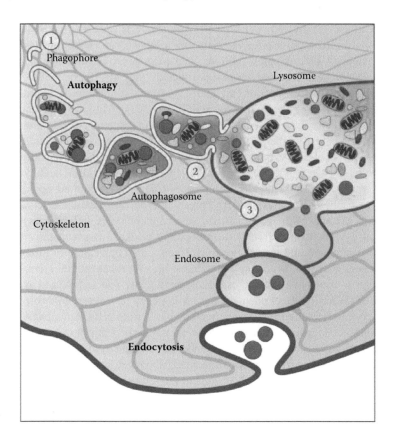

FIGURE 6.1 Autophagy: (1) The autophagosome, a double membrane structure, is formed that surrounds the damaged organelles resulting in their degradation; (2) the autophagosome and lysosome fusion where autophagosome contents will be dismantled by lysosome enzymes; (3) the autophagy is linked to endocytosis pathways, with most endosomes eventually merging with the lysosome. (Adapted from Stern, S. T. et al., *Part Fibre Toxicol* 9, 20, 2012.)

autophagolysosome, a multimembrane structure, inducing the breakdown of encapsulated materials to components that could be useful in cell growth and homeostasis processes.

Autophagy can be assessed by electron microscopy to observe the intracellular specific double- and multi-membrane structures of autophagy: Autophagosomes and autophagolysosomes. However, as imaging techniques are generally associated with artifacts, it should be validated by quantitative methods (Brandenberger et al. 2010, Seib et al. 2006, Manunta et al. 2007). Actually, autophagy can be confirmed by different quantitative methods such as evaluation of its biomarker LC3-II using lysosomotropic dyes, and by the use of genetically modified cells and animals such as GFP-LC3 (Barth et al. 2010).

Different stress conditions can induce autophagy activation such as starvation, depletion of growth factors, endoplasmic reticulum stress, oxidative stress, and infections (He and Klionsky 2009). Autophagy is seen as a nonselective cellular response to stress or a homeostatic and selective one in the removal of damaged organelles, ubiquitinated proteins, and pathogens (He and Klionsky 2009). Autophagy can be also selectively compartmentalizing NPs (Stern et al. 2010).

Mitochondrial depolarization can induce lysosomal mitochondria alteration using a process called *mitophagy* (Barbour and Turner 2014). Mitophagy (mitochondrial autophagy; it also can be called autophagy) plays an essential role in mitochondrial homeostasis, regulating their size and quality. Mitophagy eliminates damaged mitochondria, which could be induced under diverse stress conditions including pathogens and biopersistent NPs. In addition to damaged mitochondria, healthy ones are also removed when mitochondrial attenuation function is required upon hypoxia, caloric restriction, and certain developmental processes (Palikaras et al. 2016). Mitophagy declines with age and during several pathologies with progressive mitochondrial dysfunction. Nevertheless, mitophagy blockade is specifically linked to cancer development and mitophagy impairment could contribute to tumorigenesis (Palikaras et al. 2016). Mitophagy is induced in several cancer cell types to adjust themselves to their environment, especially limited nutrient and oxygen availability conditions (Warburg effect phenomenon). Mitophagy has an essential role in mammalian erythrocyte maturation from hematopoietic stem cells. Autophagy dysfunction in these cells induces myeloproliferation and early death in mice, which could be linked to human myelodysplastic syndrome. In *C. elegans*, mitophagy inhibition induces mitochondrial size increase, reactive oxygen species (ROS) production, increase of calcium levels in cytoplasm, and DNA damage (Watson et al. 2011).

Several studies report that internalized NPs induce autophagic sequestration and autophagy dysfunction, which play an essential role in NPs cytotoxicity. NPs have been shown to induce autophagy pathway dysfunction which was considered a link to their toxicity mechanism (Stern et al. 2010).

6.3   NPs AND AUTOPHAGY

Autophagy perturbation can be induced consistently across several classes of NPs and biological models (Stern et al. 2012). NPs were reported to be within the autophagosomes in alveolar macrophages, dendritic cells, lung cancer cells, human mesenchymal stem cells, and human lung adenocarcinoma cells post-treated with carbon NPs, alumina NPs, gold-coated iron oxide NPs, quantum dots, and silica NPs, respectively (Herd et al. 2011, Li et al. 2011, Monick et al. 2010, Seleverstov et al. 2006).

6.3.1   AUTOPHAGY ACTIVATION BY NPS

Autophagy induction by nanomaterials can be explained by several mechanisms, as shown in Figure 6.2. Actually, NPs induce autophagy via the oxidative stress mechanism (Li et al. 2008) or mitochondrial damage (Figure 6.3; He and Klionsky 2009). The role of the oxidative stress mechanism can be explained by the accumulation of damaged proteins and subsequent endoplasmic reticulum stress. Autophagy can be induced by fullerene in HeLa cells and can be inhibited by different antioxidants such as reduced glutathione, N-acetyl-L-cysteine, and L-ascorbic acid (Li et al. 2008).

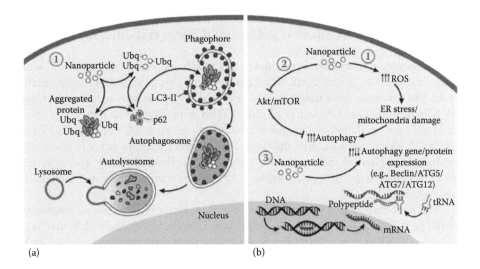

(a)   (b)

FIGURE 6.2 Autophagy induction and dysfunction by NPs: (a) NPs ubiquitination through with protein aggregates, suggesting that cell reaction to NPs is via autophagy through a p62-LC3 II pathway similar to invading pathogens; (b) NPs also could induce autophagy dysfunction via (1) oxidative stress signals, (2) suppression of Akt-mTOR signaling, and (3) involved gene and protein expression. (Adapted from Stern, S. T. et al., *Part Fibre Toxicol* 9, 20, 2012.)

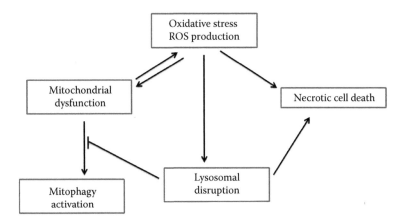

FIGURE 6.3 Oxidative stress induces mitochondrial dysfunction and lysosomal disruption, leading to mitophagy blockade and necrotic cell death.

NPs can affect autophagy by signaling pathways or by gene/protein expression. Autophagy induction by NPs could be considered a degradation process of foreign or aberrant agents for cells, such as bacteria and virus. NPs are often visualized inside autophagosomes, suggesting that autophagy could be the organisms' attempt to sequester and degrade these NPs after their internalization by the cell. Recent evidence suggests that cells could select NPs for autophagy pathway similar to invading pathogens such as virus and bacteria (Calzolai et al. 2010, Wu et al. 2010, Li et al. 2011).

Autophagy activation was reported in HeLa cells following their treatment with gadolinium oxide as rare earth oxide nanocrystals (Yu et al. 2009). Additionally, gold NPs that have been used recently in drug delivery systems induce autophagy in human fibroblasts (Powell et al. 2010). This autophagy induction was associated with up-regulation of the specific autophagy proteins LC3 and ATG7 (Yu et al. 2009). Quantum dots, NPs that emit light of specific frequencies if electricity or light is applied to them and have very large applications, were also reported to induce autophagy in porcine kidney cells and human mesenchymal stem cells (Stern et al. 2008).

The nanoscale size is considered an important factor in autophagy response in cells (Stern et al. 2012). Indeed, autophagy is not affected by quantum dots that have a tendency to aggregate, forming microparticles after their internalization by cells (Seleverstov et al. 2006). Another example of nanoscale size effect on autophagy response was also reported for neodymium oxide NPs as compared to larger particles (Chen et al. 2005).

Autophagosome accumulation was induced in human lung adenocarcinoma cells post-treated with cationic dendrimers and carboxylated carbon nanotubes (Li et al. 2009, Liu et al. 2011). Cytotoxicity associated with these nanomaterials in lung cancer cells can be blocked using the autophagy inhibitor 3-methyladenine (3-MA) or knockdown autophagy gene ATG6, suggesting that the autophagy pathway is an essential factor in NPs cytotoxicity (Stern et al. 2012). Furthermore, autophagy induction by both the cationic dendrimers and carbon nanotubes was the outcome of mTOR signaling blockade.

The *in vitro* findings mentioned above were confirmed in mice treated with cationic dendrimers and carbon nanotubes. Autophagosome accumulations in lung tissue and lung inflammation associated with animal death were observed in mice treated with these NPs. However, these pathologies were prevented in mice co-treated with 3-MA. Moreover, hepatic lesions were observed in mice treated intraperitoneally with cationic dendrimers while a typical lysosomal dysfunction was observed using polycationic drugs such as vacuolization (Schneider et al. 1997, Anderson and Borlak 2006, Roberts et al. 1996).

6.3.2 Autophagy Blockade by NPs

Autophagy activation induced by nanomaterial treatment is generally followed by cell death. However, blockade of autophagy's pro-survival mechanisms could be considered the most expected scenario of NPs cytotoxicity (Stern et al. 2012). Autophagy dysfunction is defined as excessive autophagy activation or blockade of autophagy flux (Stern et al. 2012). Actually, autophagy dysfunction is reported to be associated with a variety of human pathologies, such as chronic infection, muscular disorders, cancer, and neurodegenerative disease (Ravikumar et al. 2010). Furthermore, autophagy blockade and mitochondrial damage were observed in alveolar macrophages of smokers. This blockade affects both pathogen phagocytosis and phagocytosed pathogen delivery to the lysosome, which could explain smokers' increased tendency to have bacterial infections (Monick et al. 2010). Furthermore, nanoscale particulates were reported to have a more important role in retarding lung particle clearance, inducing lung particle overload as compared to microscale particles of the same material (Oberdörster et al. 1994). This could be partially due to autophagy pathway blockade by nanoscale particles as clearance of pathogens and other immune processes were linked to the autophagy pathway (Levine 2005).

Accumulation of polyubiquitinated protein complexes and autophagy dysfunction were also observed in human vascular endothelial cells treated with fullerenes (Yamawaki and Iwai 2006).

Mitochondrial dysfunction could be introduced by treatment of alveolar macrophages from nonsmokers with proton pump inhibitors such as bafilomycin A1, which blocks autophagy by inhibition of the lysosomal proton pump (Monick et al. 2010). Furthermore, autophagy blockade and mitochondrial dysfunction in alveolar macrophages from nonsmokers treated with carbon black NPs, a component of cigarette smoke, suggests nanomaterial implication in these pathologies (Monick et al. 2010). The same results were observed in human umbilical vein endothelial cells treated with these NPs (Yamawaki and Iwai 2006). In our laboratory, we found that cytotoxicity is linked to autophagosome accumulation and mitochondrial damage in rat alveolar macrophages treated with polymeric NPs of Eudragit® RS (Figure 6.4; Eidi et al. 2012).

The pretreatment by superparamagnetic iron oxide NPs (IONPs) has been reported to enhance the toxicity of acrolein in H9c2 cardiomyocytes (Luo et al. 2015). This cytotoxicity was characterized by mitochondrial and lysosomal dysfunction, ROS generation, and necrotic cell death. Acrolein treatment induced an initial generation of ROS, which were catalyzed by the iron ions of degraded IONPs producing highly active hydroxyl radicals. These radicals induced mitochondrial dysfunction and lysosomal disruption leading to mitophagy blockade and necrosis activation (Figure 6.3). Thus, NPs can exacerbate the toxicity of other external factors and this observation should be taken into consideration in the systematic NPs toxicity assessment (Luo et al. 2015).

6.3.3 MECHANISMS OF AUTOPHAGY AND LYSOSOMAL DYSFUNCTION INDUCED BY NPS

Autophagy dysfunction-mediated apoptosis is explained by several mechanisms (Figure 6.5). Autophagy dysfunction is seen as a potential mechanism of apoptotic or autophagic cell death type (type II programmed cell death; Kroemer and Jaattela 2005). However, the role of autophagy in "type II of cell death" is still controversial as the majority of studies describes autophagy as a pro-survival pathway rather than a cell death one. Furthermore, autophagy implication in cell death was only reported in studies used artificial systems in which apoptosis is chemically or genetically inhibited (Kroemer and Jaattela 2005).

Lysosome membrane permeabilization (LMP) has been identified as a plausible mechanism of carbon nanotube and cationic polystyrene NPs toxicity in human

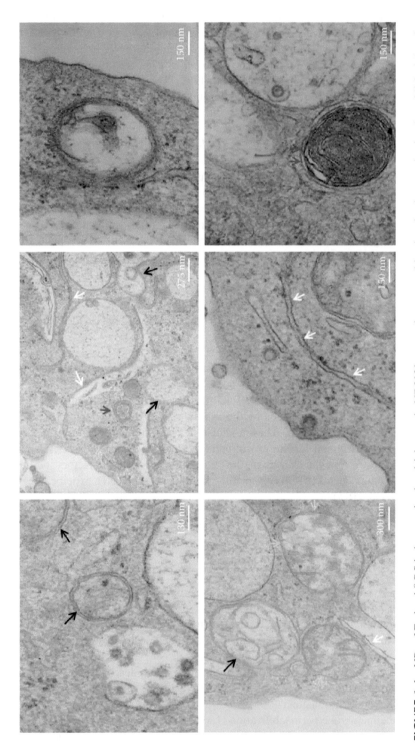

FIGURE 6.4 NPs of Eudragit® RS induce a mitochondrial stress in NR8383 macrophages, resulting in mitophagy activation (unpublished data from our laboratory). Cells were treated with NPs for 6 hours. Electron microscopy analysis show damaged mitochondria (yellow arrows), phagophors (white arrows), autophagosomes (black arrows), and autophagolysosomes (red arrows).

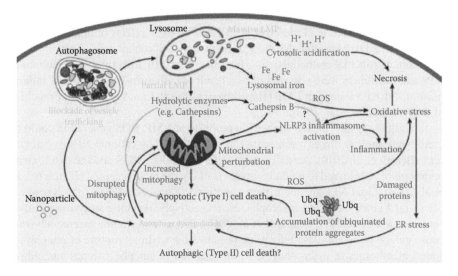

FIGURE 6.5 Toxicity mechanisms of autophagy and lysosomal dysfunction. Autophagy initiators and lysosomal dysfunction toxicity, displayed in light blue text in the figure, include blockade of vesicle trafficking, lysosomal membrane permeabilization (LMP), and autophagy blockade. NPs could cause autophagy dysfunction by overloading, directly damaging the lysosomal compartment, or altering the cell cytoskeleton, resulting in blockade of autophagosome–lysosome fusion. NPs could directly affect lysosomal stability by oxidative stress induction, alkalization, osmotic swelling, or causing detergent-like disruption of the lysosomal membrane itself, resulting in LMP. Toxic effectors (lysosomal iron, cytosolic acidification, hydrolytic enzymes, ROS, and the NLRP3 inflammasome) are displayed in dark blue. Conditions resulting from effector-mediated loss of homeostasis (oxidative stress, disrupted mitophagy, accumulation of ubiquitinated protein aggregates, and mitochondrial stress) are displayed in green. Homeostasis loss could lead to necrotic, apoptotic, or autophagic cell death (displayed in red). (Adapted from Stern, S. T. et al., *Part Fibre Toxicol* 9, 20, 2012.)

fibroblasts and macrophages (Sohaebuddin et al. 2010, Xia et al. 2008). In both cases, LMP was followed by mitochondrial damage and apoptotic cell death. As for the cationic polystyrene NPs, a "proton sponge" hypothesis has been adopted to understand the lysosomal dysfunction associated with a high proton buffering capacity of NPs surface amines, resulting in over proton pump activity and osmotic swelling (Xia et al. 2008). Cytotoxicity of cationic polyamidoamine dendrimers was also explained by a similar proton sponge mechanism, resulting in LMP induction, mitochondrial stress, and apoptosis (Thomas et al. 2009). LMP was also observed *in vivo* using mussel and oyster models treated with gold and silver NPs, respectively (Tedesco et al. 2010, Koehler et al. 2008, Ringwood et al. 2009). Additionally, zinc NPs were reported to induce lung injury in mice, which was also attributed to lysosomal dysfunction after their internalization by alveolar macrophages following by pH-mediated dissolution of zinc ion (Cho et al. 2011). This evidence is not only associated with nanoscale particles, as other studies have shown lysosomal dysfunction and apoptosis in alveolar macrophages treated by silica microparticles (Thibodeau et al. 2004). Nevertheless, comparative data between nano- and micro-gold particles suggested that "type II of cell death" nanoscale particles have a much greater tendency to LMP induction (Tedesco et al. 2010). Cytotoxic effects of titanium dioxide were attributed to lysosomal destabilization in mouse fibroblast cells (Jin et al. 2008) and human bronchial epithelial cells (Hussain et al. 2010). Inflammatory reactions to NPs and nanofibers were reported to be a result of cathepsin-B activation of inflammasome NLRP3 following LMP (Hamilton et al. 2009, Lunov et al. 2011, Franchi et al. 2009, Meunier et al. 2011).

In addition to the "proton sponge" hypothesis of LMP, ROS generation could be considered another direct mechanism to induced LMP by cationic NPs in cell culture (Berndt et al. 2010). Actually, many NPs can induce ROS and the cytotoxicity paradigm of NPs linked to oxidative stress is likely the most accepted (Figure 6.3; Li et al. 2008). Gold NPs and aluminum nanofibers (alum) could affect the lysosomal pH in rat kidney cells and macrophages, respectively, resulting in lysosomal dysfunction (Ma et al. 2011, Gherardi et al. 2015). Biopersistent alum vaccine adjuvant could induce lysosome-destabilization, possibly due to direct rupture of phagolysosomal membranes in macrophages. Alum overload in autophagosomes and subsequent fusion with repaired and re-acidified lysosomes will expose alum to lysosomal acidic pH resulting in alum particle solubilization (Gherardi et al. 2015).

Disruption of lysosomal trafficking also induces LMP susceptibility increase in cells (Huynh et al. 2004). In kidney cells treated with fullerenol, autophagy can be blocked by disruption of actin cytoskeleton-mediated lysosome trafficking (Johnson-Lyles et al. 2010). Indeed, disruption of lysosomal trafficking has a principal role in autophagy flux blockade, resulting in an accumulation of autophagosomes and lysosomal vacuoles in the cell. Several plausible mechanisms were reported to explain the role of nanoscale particulates in autophagy disruption and lysosomal trafficking (Figure 6.2). Lysosomal NP overload in alveolar macrophages treated by cigarette smoke was reported to be a mechanism of autophagy flux blockade (Monick et al. 2010). The lysosomal overload with indigestible particles in macrophages prevents lysosomal fusion with other cellular compartments, inducing a vacuole accumulation (Montgomery et al. 1991). Non-biodegradable and biopersistent NPs represent an important concern. Actually, smoke particulates, asbestos nanofibers, gold NPs, and aluminum nanofibers were reported to accumulate in macrophage lysosomes, resulting in their overload and blockade of autophagy machinery (Montgomery et al. 1991, Gherardi et al. 2015, Ma et al. 2011). This relationship between material biopersistence and intracellular vacuolation was already reported in rat kidneys and human livers receiving polyethylene-glycol conjugated proteins and polyvinyl, respectively (Bendele et al. 1998, Gall et al. 1953). Cytoskeleton disruption could be another plausible mechanism of autophagy blockade as autophagy and lysosomal compartments rely on cellular trafficking (Blankson et al. 1995, Seglen and Brinchmann 2010, Kochl et al. 2006, Xie et al. 2010). As the blockade of nanomaterial-induced autophagy seems to be linked to disruption of mitochondrial and protein quality control autophagy, actin cytoskeleton is suggested as a likely NP target (Stern et al. 2012). Actin is one of the most common proteins that bound silicon dioxide, titanium dioxide, and polystyrene NPs (Ehrenberg and McGrath 2005). Additionally, cationic dendrimers were reported to bind actin and induce autophagy blockade *in vitro* and *in vivo* (Li et al. 2009, Ruenraroengsak and Florence 2010). However, *in vivo* data of autophagy induction by NPs are still limited. Recently, silver NPs have been shown to have a pro-autophagic effect in rat liver following their intraperitoneal administration (Lee et al. 2013). The high level of autophagy induced by silver NPs is not linked to the presence of Ag^+ ions but to cellular NPs levels (Manshian et al. 2015). Another recent *in vivo* study showed that *Acheta domesticus* fed by nanodiamonds exhibit autophagy, especially mitophagy and reticulophagy, in gut epithelium cells (Karpeta-Kaczmarek et al. 2016).

Carbon nanotubes and gold NPs have been shown to induce actin cytoskeleton disruption and autophagy dysfunction in human aortic endothelial cells and primary human dermal fibroblasts, respectively (Walker et al. 2009, Mironava et al. 2010, Li et al. 2010, Liu et al. 2011). Additionally, iron oxide NPs were reported to induce disruption of actin and microtubule cytoskeletons, and autophagy blockade in human umbilical vein endothelial cells (Wu, Tan et al. 2010).

6.4 NPs AND MITOCHONDRIA

6.4.1 MITOCHONDRIA AS INTRACELLULAR TARGETS AND THEIR TARGETING BY NPs

Mitochondria and the endosomal–lysosomal system are the major cellular targets of engineered NPs in invertebrate organisms (Rocha et al. 2015). NPs can be freely dispersed in the cytoplasm, associated to the cytoskeleton, or be inside endocytic vesicles, lysosomes, mitochondria, or the nucleus (Ciacci et al. 2012, Couleau et al. 2012, Garcia-Negrete et al. 2013, Kadar et al. 2011, Katsumiti et al. 2014, Koehler et al. 2008, Trevisan et al. 2014).

Mitochondrial nanotargeting medicine has a long but exciting road to clinical applications, with many promising formulations currently under development (Milane et al. 2015). Furthermore, only a small minority of NPs based on metal oxides, gold NPs, dendrons, carbon nanotubes, and liposomes were engineered to target mitochondria. Most of these materials represent important challenges when administered *in vivo* due to their limited biocompatibility. Indeed, biodegradable polymeric nanoparticles were considered as eminent candidates for effective drug delivery (Pathak et al. 2015).

Mitochondria are reported to be a promising therapeutic target for treatment of various human diseases such as cancer (Biswas and Torchilin 2014, Heller et al. 2012), ischemia-reperfusion injury, diabetes type 2, and obesity (Wongrakpanich et al. 2014, Heller et al. 2012, Rodriguez-Nogales et al. 2016, Hyodo et al. 2014). As drug and DNA delivery systems (to lysosomes, mitochondria, nuclei and Golgi/endoplasmic reticulum), many types of NPs were developed to overcome the multiple barriers such as cell membrane and the double membrane of mitochondria (Verderio et al. 2014, Avti et al. 2013, Sakhrani and Padh 2013). However, sufficient penetration of the cell membrane barrier, which is necessary for the therapeutic drug delivery to intracellular targets, especially bringing pro-apoptotic drugs to mitochondria, is still far from being achieved (Biswas and Torchilin 2014). Thus, nanovectors with mitochondriotropic designs are made from lipids (liposomes), biodegradable polymers such as poly(lactic-co-glycolic acid; PLGA), or metals such as gold and titan dioxide NPs (Wongrakpanich et al. 2014). Carbon nanotubes have also been used for mitochondrial drug delivery applications. For example, formulations of multiwalled carbon nanotubes (MWCNTs) were prepared to deliver the anticancer cisplatin pro-drug (PtBz). These nanovectors protect delivered molecules from cellular elimination and metabolism *in vivo* before their arrival to their target, mitochondria, through the cellular and mitochondrial barriers (Milane et al. 2015). Since the 1990s, liposome formulations have been largely developed for pharmaceutical purposes, especially as mitochondria-targeting systems. Actually, liposomes are used in various clinical settings due to their surface amenable properties and their ability to host several kinds of molecules. Moreover, they are considered nontoxic nanovectors. Despite their advantages, which are similar to those of liposomes, use of polymeric NPs in mitochondria targeting, such as PLGA, is still relatively limited.

The use of metallic NPs seems promising as they are small in size and can be easily loaded with drug molecules. Up to now on the market, there are no pharma-ceutical formulations designed for drug delivery to mitochondria, but many NPs are seen as relevant therapeutic and diagnostic agents.

While mitochondria have an important role in vaccine modulation as unique tar-gets, mitochondria targeting vaccines using NPs delivery systems are still in their primary stages of development. This could be linked to the low availability of NPs formulation for vaccine designs (Stern et al. 2012).

Mitochondrial targeting is achieved by the incorporation of mitochondriotropic agents onto the nanovector surface, which can be designed to have the desired sizes and surface as well as the adequate molecular loading ratio (Wongrakpanich et al. 2014). One of the important approaches of mitochondrial targeting is to have a molecule/nanocarrier complex with a high affinity for mitochondria.

Several molecules could be nano-delivered to the mitochondria, such as RNA or DNA (e.g., antisense oligonucleotides, ribozymes, and plasmid DNA expressing mitochondrial genes), an approach that may be relevant for the treatment of mito-chondrial DNA diseases (Sakhrani and Padh 2013). One of these treatment strate-gies could be the delivery of antioxidant and proapoptotic drugs to mitochondria to protect them from oxidative stress and to trigger apoptotic cell death in tumor cells, respectively. Additionally, delivery of proteins and peptides to mitochondria could be also included in these treatment strategies for several mitochondrial disorders (Gruber et al. 2013, Weissig et al. 2004).

Dequalinium chloride is a mitochondriotropic cation that was reported to be selec-tively accumulated in the mitochondria of carcinoma cells (Weiss et al. 1987). Based on their experimental work, Weissig et al. (1998) proposed that dequalinium-based liposome-like vesicles (DQAsomes) could be the first colloidal drug and DNA deliv-ery system for mitochondria targeting. Positive surface charge and mitochondrio-tropic properties of DQAsomes could enable them to load or entrap drug molecules and DNA and deliver them to mitochondria (Weissig et al. 1998). In 2001, Weissig et al. further showed that DNA release could be achieved when DNA/DQA complex contact the mitochondrial surface. Paclitaxel has been encapsulated in DQA forming Paclitaxel–DQAsomes that induce apoptotic cell death *in vitro* (D'Souza et al. 2008).

It has been reported that high NP deposition within mitochondria is widely cor-related to several cellular processes, especially NP internalization. Twomey et al. (2016) suggested that macropinocytosis of conjugated polymer NPs allows them to escape of macropinosomes and to increase their trafficking to mitochondria as compared to an endocytosis form of internalization.

6.4.2 NPs Cause Mitochondrial Stress

Mitochondria play key roles in apoptosis and energy metabolism; the cell's survival is likely dependent on defined relationships between mitochondria and other cellular components. As there are several of such relationships, there are invariably several mitochondrial stress signals for these cellular components that will stimulate the cell for different cellular adaptions in response to various stress. However, this aspect of mitochondrial function is still unclear to date. Barbour and Turner (2014) suggested that when the cell is not able to identify and adequately respond to mitochondrial damage signals, mitochondrial dysfunction could occur. Mitochondrial dysfunction is generally involved in the pathologies of aging diseases and in the aging process itself (Bratic and Larsson 2013).

Recently, cell or mitochondria/NP interactions are considered as another possible cause of mitochondrial dysfunction as NPs affect mitochondrial biology either directly (physical interaction) or indirectly (biochemically). As mentioned above, mitochondria can be a specific intercellular target for several kinds of NPs, resulting in important morphological changes, such as a serious damage in the mitochondrial cristae structure and alteration of their double membrane integrity (Figure 6.6; Eidi et al. 2012). NPs that do not have any tendency to penetrate into mitochondria could affect mitochondria biology indirectly via different biochemical pathways, especially oxidative stress and gene expression. Mitochondrial morphology and membrane

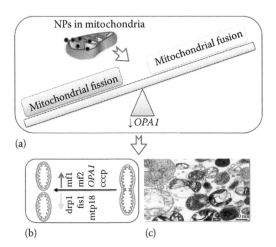

FIGURE 6.6 Nanoparticles affect mitochondrial dynamics and structure. (a) NPs induce *OPA1* down-regulation promoting mitochondrial network fragmentation rather than mitochondrial fusion. (b) Mitochondrial fission is controlled by some gens' expression such as mf1, mf2, *OPA1*, cccp, drp1, fis1, and mtp18. Gene up- and down-regulation is labeled by red and green arrows, respectively. (c) Fragmented and damaged mitochondria in NR8383 macrophages treated with Eudragit® NPs (55 nm) for 24 h (unpublished data from our laboratory).

integrity are important mitochondrial responses to stress signals. Furthermore, mitochondria are seen as dynamic intracellular organelles that continually undergo opposing morphological changes, fusion and fission, as a response to different signals (Barbour and Turner 2014). In the fusion process, several mitochondria form unique elongated mitochondria, while in fission, a single mitochondrion is fragmented into many smaller ones (Figure 6.6b). Mitochondrial morphology changes can be induced as a result of mitochondrial stress and may be a mechanism of homeostasis to regulate cell survival. Mitochondrial fusion generally is seen as a response to mitochondrial damage and elongated mitochondria are considered a pro-survival process resulting in prevention of apoptotic cell death and mitophagy (Barbour and Turner 2014). Mitochondrial fusion can be induced by oxidative stress (Barbour and Turner 2014) resulting in increased resistance to ROS (Wang et al. 2013). However, mitochondrial fission can be generated by different cell stressors, such as mitochondria/NPs interaction, inducing mitophagy and programmed cell death (Eidi et al. 2012).

Specific high surface reactivity of NPs is one of the major positive characteristics of NPs for nanotechnology applications. However, it causes mitochondria damage either by direct interaction with NPs or indirectly via different biochemical pathways. Additionally, surface engineering can widely improve NPs biocompatibility and stability in biological environments reducing cytotoxic and genotoxic effects. Indeed, surface passivation of silica-coated iron NPs reduces the oxidative stress and iron homeostasis alteration (Malvindi et al. 2014). Polyoxometalates NP–peptide conjugates are another example of NP surface modulation which affects their intracellular behavior. This surface engineering of NPs by various peptides enables them to target mitochondria after cellular uptake resulting in mitophagy (Zhang et al. 2015).

Almost all non-biodegradable and biopersistent NPs induce cytotoxic effects using different mechanisms. For example, non-degradable conjugated polymer NPs have been reported to be four times more cytotoxic than degradable ones in HeLa cell culture (Twomey et al. 2016). The lower toxicity of degradable conjugated polymer NPs could be linked to thiol components of the degraded oligomers that reduce the ROS production level, thus preventing mitochondrial stress (Zinchuk et al. 2007). Thus, to better understand structure/cytotoxicity relationships, more systematic investigations should be done (Twomey et al. 2016). Furthermore, the relationship between NP biodegradability and their cytotoxicity is still difficult to identify because this cytotoxicity may be achieved by NPs or their metabolites (Frohlich 2013).

As mentioned above, mitochondrial network morphology, which was reported to be affected by NPs (Eidi et al. 2012), depends on the fusion/fragmentation balance (Westermann 2002, Berman et al. 2008, Landes et al. 2010). NPs were reported to disrupt mitochondrial dynamics and expression of genes involved in this process (Figure 6.6). Indeed, mitochondrial dynamics are controlled by many proteins, especially *OPA1*, mfn1, and mfn2, which affect mitochondrial fusion; while drp1, fis1, and mtp18 control fragmentation. *OPA1* has a key role in maintaining the mitochondrial membrane integrity and its cristae structure (Landes et al. 2010, Liesa et al. 2009). *OPA1* down-regulation promotes mitochondrial network fragmentation, decreases mitochondrial respiration, and decreases the mitochondrial transmembrane potential activating the programmed cell death pathways (Figure 6.7). Polymeric Eudragit® NPs have been reported to induce *OPA1* down-regulation in alveolar macrophages

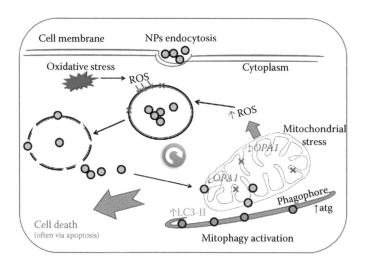

FIGURE 6.7 Hypothetical mechanism of the interaction between NPs and macrophages. After NPs internalization, ROS production increases, which alter the lysosomal membrane. Then, NPs could be seen free in cytoplasm and within mitochondria, resulting in their damage and alteration of their cristae structure (red crosses). *OPA1* down-regulation can be observed promoting mitochondrial fragmentation and stress. These signals could lead the cell to autophagic or apoptotic cell death.

in vitro resulting in aggregation of the mitochondrial network and cristae structure disorganization (Eidi et al. 2012). Interestingly, this study showed that apoptotic cell death pathways are inhibited in cells treated with Eudragit® RS NPs, suggesting that these NPs induce the autophagic cell death type.

The origin of mitochondrial damage could be linked to the mechanical effect of the NPs which penetrate the double membrane of mitochondria. It could also be the consequence of gene modulations, especially *OPA1*, the modulator gene of membrane integrity of mitochondria and their cristae structure. *OPA1* down-expression was reported to induce lysosomal perturbation (Arnoult et al. 2005), resulting in the release of internalized NPs from the phagolysosomes. The perturbation of the mitochondrial dynamics induced by NPs was considered as an important factor in ROS production and reduction of the mitochondrial membrane potential (Lee et al. 2007). In our laboratory, we have shown that oxidative stress affects autophagy's pathway and mitochondrial fusion/fission ratio (Figures 6.6 and 6.7). Based on these results, we propose that ROS production increases after NPs internalization, which alters the lysosomal membrane, leading to autophagic or apoptotic cell death (Figure 6.7).

Furthermore, the mitochondrial fusion/fragmentation ratio could be considered as a relevant biomarker of the cytotoxicity of NPs. Nevertheless, to date, there is no method to evaluate this ratio (Liesa et al. 2009). However, an indirect mitochondrial dynamic evaluation could be done by assessment of expression of the genes involved such as *OPA1*, mfn1, mfn2, drp1, and fis1. Furthermore, the use of this biomarker could also improve the understanding and diagnosis of several pathologies associated with mitochondrial dynamics disruption such as obesity, type 1 or 2 diabetes, Parkinson's disease, and Alzheimer's disease (Liesa et al. 2009). If this hypothesis of complex diseases could be confirmed, targeting mitochondrial proteins by nano-technology may represent a new therapeutic opportunity.

There is a balance between expression levels of genes involved in apoptosis and autophagy pathways. For example, the down-expression of the bcl pro-apoptotic gene family is associated with atg gene activation, a pro-autophagic gene family (Luo and Rubinsztein 2007, Shimizu et al. 2004). In addition to the mitochondrial fragmentation, down-regulation of *OPA1* promotes programmed cell death, making this gene an anti-apoptotic gene (Landes et al. 2010).

Mitochondrial dysfunction and cytotoxicity induced by NPs results in mitophagy or apoptosis (Eidi et al. 2012, El-Ansary et al. 2013). In addition to apoptotic cell death type, the autophagic or mitophagic cell death induced by NP was described by Eidi et al. (2012).

Mitochondria dysfunction and mitophagic cell death is one of the major positive aims of anticancer drug delivery systems using different nanovectors. However, this autophagy is considered a cytotoxic effect in normal cells. Endogenous selenite NPs (SeNPs) have been reported to induce cancer cell toxicity characterized by mitochondrial dysfunction, microtubule depolymerization, SeNPs-induced ROS, mitophagy inhibition, and apoptosis activation (Bao et al. 2015). Intracellular proteins were observed widely sequestered by SeNPs, including glycolytic enzymes, tubulin, and heat shock proteins (HSP), resulting in glycolysis inhibition, ATP depletion, and BAD dephosphorylation. Consequently, BAX translocation to mitochondria inducing mitochondrial damage, cytochrome *c* release, and morphological disruption of mitochondria can be observed in cancer cells (Bao et al. 2015).

Mitochondria were considered a target of quantum dot cytotoxicity and specific mitochondrial biomarkers could be useful parameters for quantum dot toxicity assessments (Lin et al. 2012, Zhan and Tang 2014). Additionally, Zhang et al. (2015) reported that mitophagy is the specific cellular response to the accumulation of NPs–peptide conjugates in mitochondria as an intracellular target. These processing steps hosted by cells have made important changes in the NP distribution through alternative intracellular trafficking. Nevertheless, some NPs were reported to have a protective role against mitophagy and mitochondrial stress, such as Cerieum oxide NPs (Dowding et al. 2014; Figure 6.8).

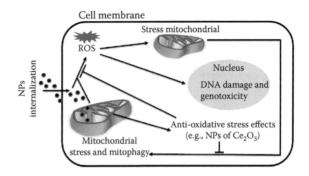

FIGURE 6.8 Some NPs, such as Cerieum oxide NPs, have a protective role against mitophagy and mitochondrial stress.

6.5 WHAT IS THE RELATIONSHIP BETWEEN VIRUSES, NPs, AND AUTOPHAGY?

The discovery of the first virus, tobacco mosaic virus (TMV), occurred by the end of the nineteenth century by Adolf Mayer. Dimitri Ivanoski in 1892 called it "filterable pathogens," thinking that it was a small bacteria. Martinus Beijerinck was the first to call it a "virus." However, viruses have played an important role in human evolution and have evolved diverse strategies to co-exist with their hosts.

TMV was the first virus observed by electron microscopy in 1939. Viral particles are rigid rods 150 to 300 nm long and 15 nm wide. A few years later in 1965, HeLa cells infected with poliovirus were examined in electron microscopy by George Palade's group (Dales et al. 1965). They observed the double-membraned autophagosomes that are characteristic of autophagy (Carlsson and Simonsen 2015) and C viruses (Lupfer et al. 2013, Kim, Syed et al. 2013). Beyond the replication power of viruses, we can imagine that the induction of autophagy might be due to their nanometric size. Indeed, nanomaterials in general, NPs or viruses, induce autophagy in different ways. The majority of the nanomaterials enter the intracellular medium by endocytosis, the lysosomes are therefore exposed to their toxicity, causing lysosome dysfunction, NP overload, and cytoskeletal disturbance (Wang et al. 2013, Stern et al. 2012). The introduction of autophagy can be initiated in response to diverse stress stimuli, essentially by the generation of ROS.

6.5.1 RETICULUM ENDOPLASMIC STRESS

The endoplasmic reticulum (ER) is involved in post-translational modifications, folding, and oligomerization of newly synthesized proteins. However, several endogenous imbalances in cells can contribute to an ER malfunction known as *ER stress*. ER stress activates a complex signaling network referred to the unfolded protein response (UPR) to reduce ER stress and restore homeostasis by the enhanced expression of several chaperones, such as GRP78/BiP, GRP94, calreticulin, and proteins involved in the disulfide bond formation (Kania et al. 2015, Luo and Lee 2013). However, if the UPR fails to reestablish the ER to normalcy, ER stress can either stimulate or inhibit autophagy (Rashid et al. 2015).

Some viruses have been demonstrated to increase autophagy following ER stress (Datan et al. 2016) and trigger UPR pathway in infected cells caused by the production of ROS. An increase in GRP78 protein levels was reported in Dengue virus– and West Nile virus–induced ER stress (Hou et al. 2014, Wati et al. 2009, Ambrose and Mackenzie 2011). It should be noted that many viruses count autophagy among their replication cycle.

As for NPs, the ROS generated, including metal oxide-based NPs, TiO_2 NPs, carbon fullerenes, and carbon nanotubes, are associated closely with cell damage, oxidative stress, and cell organelle disruption (Nel et al. 2006, Naqvi et al. 2010, Apopa et al. 2009). Diverse NPs, like zinc oxide, silver NPs, and iron oxide NPs, were shown to elevate ER stress events (Yang et al. 2015, Simard et al. 2015, Park et al. 2014); like viruses, this can either block or stimulate autophagy (Figure 6.9).

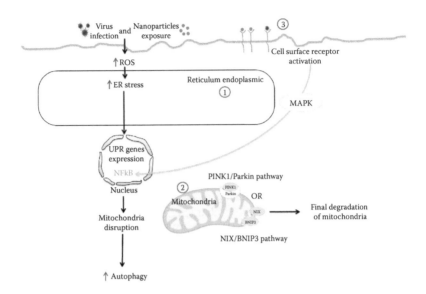

FIGURE 6.9 NPs and viruses induce autophagy. (1) Diverse NPs and some viruses were reported to elevate ER stress, autophagy activation, and trigger UPR pathway caused by ROS production. (2) Mitochondrial priming mediated either by the Pink1-Parkin signaling pathway or the mitophagic receptors Nix and Bnip3. (3) Viruses interact with cell surface receptors, leading to activation of intracellular signaling cascades. Thus, ROS formation will be increased, activating stress-dependent signaling pathways, such as mitogen-activated protein kinase (MAPK), and, ultimately, alter the gene expression of the antioxidant response by activating transcription factors, such as NF-kB.

6.5.2 MITOPHAGY

Mitochondria are considered the chief source of intracellular ROS production because mitochondrial ROS (mROS) have been directly linked to multiple physiological processes including immunity, differentiation, autophagy, and metabolic adaptation (Sena and Chandel 2012). The removal of damaged or excessive mitochondria through autophagy, a process called mitophagy, is thus critical for maintaining proper cellular functions. Recent progress in mitophagy studies reveals that mitochondrial priming is mediated either by the Pink1-Parkin signaling pathways or the mitophagic receptors Nix and Bnip3 (Ding and Yin 2012; Figure 6.9). Some viruses induce mitophagy (Kim, Khan et al. 2013, Kim, Syed et al. 2013). Studies suggest that this strategy might provide a replicative advantage for the virus against development of antiviral immune responses by the host (Xia et al. 2014). Indeed, viruses exploit the mitophagy pathway in order to increase mithophagy and thereby increase their replication (Xia et al. 2014). Also, some viruses can generate ROS via their oncogenic products: For example, the hepatitis B virus (HBV) X protein (HBx); hepatitis C virus (HCV) core, E1 and NS3; human papillomavirus 18 (HPV-18) E2; and the human T-cell leukemia virus 1 (HTLV-1) p13 and Tax (Dizdaroglu 1992, Lu et al. 2001, Demple and Harrison 1994). As viruses, NPs produce ROS causing mitochondrial damage which involves the disruption of the breathing chain and the formation of more ROS. Thus, damaged mitochondria will be degraded by mitophagy and the process of autophagy is put in place (Luo and Rubinsztein 2007, Yu et al. 2013).

6.5.3 VIRUS AND NP INTERACTION WITH MEMBRANE RECEPTORS

Espert et al. (2009) have revealed that autophagy is triggered following the binding of envelope glycoprotein (Env) to CXCR4 (chemokine receptor) in T cells and that autophagy is required for Env-induced apoptosis through CXCR4. Interestingly, Biard-Piechaczyk et al. demonstrated that HIV-infected cells that express Env-induced autophagy and accumulation of Beclin1 in uninfected CD4+ T lymphocytes via CXCR4 (Espert et al. 2006). For NPs, they interact with cell surface receptors, leading to the activation of intracellular signaling cascades that induce formation of ROS (Soenen et al. 2011). These ROS further activate stress-dependent signaling pathways, such as the mitogen-activated protein kinase (MAPK) or IκB kinase pathways, ultimately altering gene expression of the antioxidant response element via the activation of transcription factors, such as AP-1, NF-kB, or Nrf2. The end result of this signaling cascade is the ROS overproduction.

When the signal is issued, the LC3-I (cytosolic form) converts to LC3-II (conjugated form of LC3-phosphatidylethanolamine), which is recruited for the pre-autophagosomal to autophagosomal membranes. During the fusion of autophagosomes with lysosomes (autolysosomes), intra-autophagosomal LC3-II is also degraded by lysosomal proteases and it is recycled to LC3-I (Tanida et al. 2008; Figure 6.9). Indeed, infections with a wide range of DNA or RNA viruses increase abundance of autophagosomes or autophagic vesicles in infected cells (Jackson et al. 2005).

Finally, the autophagy process could be considered as an intracellular reaction due to cells' exposure to physical property of nanometric objects' physical properties rather than a response to their chemical properties (Zabirnyk et al. 2007). Yet, viruses would divert autophagy to their advantage to replicate. So, a high production of ROS induced by NPs or viruses would be extremely damaging to the cell, leading frequently to the autophagy process.

6.6 CONCLUSION

A new understanding of the mechanisms by which nanomaterials induce biological effects has to be adopted. A better insight is also needed on how a cellular response could affect the final fate of NPs by providing a different route to transport NPs between distinct types of cell organelles.

The huge expansion in the field of nanotechnology requires a deep understanding of the different mechanisms of nanomaterials toxicity to build an optimal assessment of safety and cytotoxicity biomarkers. More attention should be paid to the fact that nanomaterials affect autophagy and lysosomal pathways, affecting their biological effects.

The autophagy process could be considered an intracellular reaction due to a cell's exposure to nanometric object physical properties. Yet, viruses would divert autophagy to their advantage to promote replication. Thus, a high production of

ROS, induced by NPs or viruses, would be extremely damaging to the cell, leading frequently to the autophagy process.

Finally, the increasing knowledge of the activation or blockade pathway of autophagy and lysosomal dysfunction may well be a useful tool to improve our understanding of nanotoxicology so that we may work toward safe nanotechnology.

REFERENCES

Ambrose, R. L., and Mackenzie, J. M. 2011. West Nile virus differentially modulates the unfolded protein response to facilitate replication and immune evasion. *J Virol* 85:2723–2732.

Anderson, N., and Borlak, J. 2006. Drug-induced phospholipidosis. *FEBS Lett* 580:5533–5540.

Apopa, P. L., Qian, Y., Shao, R., Guo, N. L., Schwegler-Berry, D., Pacurari, M. et al. 2009. Iron oxide nanoparticles induce human microvascular endothelial cell permeability through reactive oxygen species production and microtubule remodeling. *Part Fibre Toxicol* 6:1.

Arnoult, D., Grodet, A., Lee, Y. J., Estaquier, J., and Blackstone, C. 2005. Release of OPA1 during apoptosis participates in the rapid and complete release of cytochrome c and subsequent mitochondrial fragmentation. *J Biol Chem* 280:35742–35750.

Avti, P. K., Maysinger, D., and Kakkar, A. 2013. Alkyne-azide "click" chemistry in designing nanocarriers for applications in biology. *Molecules* 18:9531–9549.

Bao, P., Chen, Z., Tai, R. Z., Shen, H. M., Martin, F. L., Zhu, Y. G. et al. 2015. Selenite-induced toxicity in cancer cells is mediated by metabolic generation of endogenous selenium nanoparticles. *J Proteome Res* 14:1127–1136.

Barbour, J. A., and Turner, N. 2014. Mitochondrial stress signaling promotes cellular adaptations. *Int J Cell Biol* 2014:156020.

Barth, S., Glick, D., and Macleod, K. F. 2010. Autophagy: Assays and artifacts. *J Pathol* 221:117–124.

Bendele, A., Seely, J., Richey, C., Sennello, G., and Shopp, G. 1998. Short communication: Renal tubular vacuolation in animals treated with polyethylene-glycol-conjugated proteins. *Toxicol Sci* 42:152–157.

Berman, S. B., Pineda, F. J., and Hardwick, J. M. 2008. Mitochondrial fission and fusion dynamics: The long and short of it. *Cell Death Differ* 15:1147–1152.

Berndt, C., Kurz, T., Selenius, M., Fernandes, A. P., Edgren, M. R., and Brunk, U. T. et al. 2010. Chelation of lysosomal iron protects against ionizing radiation. *Biochem J* 432:295–301.

Biswas, S., and Torchilin, V. P. 2014. Nanopreparations for organelle-specific delivery in cancer. *Adv Drug Deliv Rev* 66:26–41.

Blankson, H., Holen, I., and Seglen, P. O. 1995. Disruption of the cytokeratin cytoskeleton and inhibition of hepatocytic autophagy by okadaic acid. *Exp Cell Res* 218:522–530.

Boldogh, I., Albrecht, T., and Porter, D. D. 1996. Persistent viral infections. In Baron, S. ed., *Medical Microbiology*, 4th ed. Galveston, TX: Galveston University of Texas Medical Branch, Chapter 46.

Brandenberger, C., Clift, M. J., Vanhecke, D., Muhlfeld, C., Stone, V., Gehr, P. et al. 2010. Intracellular imaging of nanoparticles: Is it an elemental mistake to believe what you see? *Part Fibre Toxicol* 7:15.

Bratic, A., and Larsson, N. G. 2013. The role of mitochondria in aging. *J Clin Invest* 123:951–957.

Bruce, T. 1937. The occurrence of silicosis in the manufacture of silicon alloys. *J Indus Hyg and Tox* 19:155–162.

Budka, H., Aguzzi, A., Brown, P., Brucher, J. M., Bugiani, O., Gullotta, F. et al. 1995. Neuropathological diagnostic criteria for Creutzfeldt-Jakob disease (CJD) and other human spongiform encephalopathies (prion diseases). *Brain Pathol* 5:459–466.

Byron, P. R. 1986. Prediction of drug residence times in regions of the human respiratory tract following aerosol inhalation. *J Pharm Sci* 75:433–438.

Calzolai, L., Franchini, F., Gilliland, D., and Rossi, F. 2010. Protein—Nanoparticle interaction: Identification of the ubiquitin—Gold nanoparticle interaction site. *Nano Lett* 10:3101–3105.

Carlsson, S. R., and Simonsen, A. 2015. Membrane dynamics in autophagosome biogenesis. *J Cell Sci* 128:193–205.

Chen, L., Yokel, R. A., Hennig, B., and Toborek, M. 2008. Manufactured aluminum oxide nanoparticles decrease expression of tight junction proteins in brain vasculature. *J Neuroimmune Pharmacol* 3:286–295.

Chen, Y., Yang, L., Feng, C., and Wen, L. P. 2005. Nano neodymium oxide induces massive vacuolization and autophagic cell death in non-small cell lung cancer NCI-H460 cells. *Biochem Biophys Res Commun* 337:52–60.

Cho, W. S., Duffin, R., Howie, S. E., Scotton, C. J., Wallace, W. A., Macnee, W. et al. 2011. Progressive severe lung injury by zinc oxide nanoparticles; the role of Zn2+ dissolution inside lysosomes. *Part Fibre Toxicol* 8:27.

Ciacci, C., Canonico, B., Bilanicova, D., Fabbri, R., Cortese, K., Gallo, G. et al. 2012. Immunomodulation by different types of N-oxides in the hemocytes of the marine bivalve Mytilus galloprovincialis. *PLoS One* 7:e36937.

Comiskey, B., Albert, J. D., Yoshizawa, H., and Jacobson, J. 1998. An electrophoretic ink for all-printed reflective electronic displays. *Nature* 394:253–255.

Couleau, N., Techer, D., Pagnout, C., Jomini, S., Foucaud, L., Laval-Gilly, P. et al. 2012. Hemocyte responses of Dreissena polymorpha following a short-term in vivo exposure to titanium dioxide nanoparticles: Preliminary investigations. *Sci Total Environ* 438:490–497.

Courrier, H. M., Butz, N., and Vandamme, T. F. 2002. Pulmonary drug delivery systems: Recent developments and prospects. *Crit Rev Ther Drug Carrier Syst* 19:425–498.

D'Souza, G. G., Cheng, S. M., Boddapati, S. V., Horobin, R. W., and Weissig, V. 2008. Nanocarrier-assisted sub-cellular targeting to the site of mitochondria improves the pro-apoptotic activity of paclitaxel. *J Drug Target* 16:578–585.

Dales, S., Eggers, H. J., Tamm, I., and Palade, G. E. 1965. Electron microscopic study of the formation of poliovirus. *Virology* 26:379–389.

Datan, E., Roy, S. G., Germain, G., Zali, N., McLean, J. E., Golshan, G. et al. 2016. Dengue-induced autophagy, virus replication and protection from cell death require ER stress (PERK) pathway activation. *Cell Death Dis* 7:e2127.

De Duve, C. 1963. The lysosome. *Sci Am* 208:64–72.

De Matteis, V., Cascione, M., Brunetti, V., Toma, C. C., and Rinaldi, R. 2016. Toxicity assessment of anatase and rutile titanium dioxide nanoparticles: The role of degradation in different pH conditions and light exposure. *Toxicol In Vitro* 37:201–210.

Demple, B., and Harrison, L. 1994. Repair of oxidative damage to DNA: Enzymology and biology. *Annu Rev Biochem* 63:915–948.

Ding, W. X., and Yin, X. M. 2012. Mitophagy: Mechanisms, pathophysiological roles, and analysis. *Biol Chem* 393:547–564.

Dizdaroglu, M. 1992. Oxidative damage to DNA in mammalian chromatin. *Mutat Res* 275:331–342.

Dowding, J. M., Song, W., Bossy, K., Karakoti, A., Kumar, A., Kim, A. et al. 2014. Cerium oxide nanoparticles protect against Abeta-induced mitochondrial fragmentation and neuronal cell death. *Cell Death Differ* 21:1622–1632.

Dubas, S. T., Kumlangdudsana, P., and Potiyaraj, P. 2006. Layer-by-layer deposition of antimicrobial silver nanoparticles on textile fibers. *Coll & Surf A: Phys & Eng Asp* 289:105–109.

Ehrenberg, M., and McGrath, J. L. 2005. Binding between particles and proteins in extracts: Implications for microrheology and toxicity. *Acta Biomater* 1:305–315.

Eidi, H., Joubert, O., Nemos, C., Grandemange, S., Mograbi, B., Foliguet, B. et al. 2012. Drug delivery by polymeric nanoparticles induces autophagy in macrophages. *Int J Pharm* 422:495–503.

El-Ansary, A., Al-Daihan, S., Bacha, A. B., and Kotb, M. 2013. Toxicity of novel nanosized formulations used in medicine. *Methods Mol Biol* 1028:47–74.

Espert, L., Denizot, M., Grimaldi, M., Robert-Hebmann, V., Gay, B., Varbanov, M. et al. 2006. Autophagy is involved in T cell death after binding of HIV-1 envelope proteins to CXCR4. *J Clin Invest* 116:2161–2172.

Espert, L., Varbanov, M., Robert-Hebmann, V., Sagnier, S., Robbins, I., Sanchez, F. et al. 2009. Differential role of autophagy in CD4 T cells and macrophages during X4 and R5 HIV-1 infection. *PLoS One* 4:e5787.

Franchi, L., Eigenbrod, T., Munoz-Planillo, R., and Nunez, G. 2009. The inflammasome: A caspase-1-activation platform that regulates immune responses and disease pathogenesis. *Nat Immunol* 10:241–247.

Frohlich, E. 2013. Cellular targets and mechanisms in the cytotoxic action of non-biodegradable engineered nanoparticles. *Curr Drug Metab* 14:976–988.

Gall, E. A., Altemeier, W. A., Schiff, L., Hamilton, D. L., Braunstein, H., Guiseffi, Jr., J. et al. 1953. Liver lesions following intravenous administration of polyvinyl pyrrolidone. *Am J Clin Pathol* 23:1187–1198.

Garcia-Negrete, C. A., Blasco, J., Volland, M., Rojas, T. C., Hampel, M., Lapresta-Fernandez, A. et al. 2013. Behaviour of Au-citrate nanoparticles in seawater and accumulation in bivalves at environmentally relevant concentrations. *Environ Pollut* 174:134–141.

Gherardi, R. K., Eidi, H., Crepeaux, G., Authier, F. J., and Cadusseau, J. 2015. Biopersistence and brain translocation of aluminum adjuvants of vaccines. *Front Neurol* 6:4.

Gruber, J., Fong, S., Chen, C. B., Yoong, S., Pastorin, G., Schaffer, S. et al. 2013. Mitochondria-targeted antioxidants and metabolic modulators as pharmacological interventions to slow ageing. *Biotechnol Adv* 31:563–592.

Hamilton, R. F., Wu, N., Porter, D., Yoong, S., Pastorin, G., Schaffer, S. et al. 2009. Particle length-dependent titanium dioxide nanomaterials toxicity and bioactivity. *Part Fibre Toxicol* 6:35.

He, C., and Klionsky, D. J. 2009. Regulation mechanisms and signaling pathways of autophagy. *Annu Rev Genet* 43:67–93.

Heller, A., Brockhoff, G., and Goepferich, A. 2012. Targeting drugs to mitochondria. *Eur J Pharm Biopharm* 82:1–18.

Hendren, C. O., Mesnard, X., Droge, J., and Wiesner, M. R. 2011. Estimating production data for five engineered nanomaterials as a basis for exposure assessment. *Environ Sci Technol* 45:2562–2569.

Herd, H. L., Malugin, A., and Ghandehari, H. 2011. Silica nanoconstruct cellular toleration threshold in vitro. *J Control Release* 153:40–48.

Hou, L., Ge, X., Xin, L., Zhou, L., Guo, X., and Yang, H. et al. 2014. Nonstructural proteins 2C and 3D are involved in autophagy as induced by the encephalomyocarditis virus. *Virol J* 11:156.

Huang, T., Zhang, X., Ling, Z., Zhang, L., Gao, H., Tian, C. et al. 2016. Impacts of large-scale land-use change on the uptake of polycyclic aromatic hydrocarbons in the artificial three northern regions shelter forest across Northern China. *Environ Sci Technol* 50:12885–12893.

Hussain, S., Thomassen, L. C., Ferecatu, I. Borot, M. C., Andreau, K., Martens, J. A. et al. 2010. Carbon black and titanium dioxide nanoparticles elicit distinct apoptotic pathways in bronchial epithelial cells. *Part Fibre Toxicol* 7:10.

Huynh, C., Roth, D., Ward, D. M., Kaplan, J., and Andrews, N. W. 2004. Defective lysosomal exocytosis and plasma membrane repair in Chediak–Higashi/beige cells. *Proc Natl Acad Sci USA* 101:16795–16800.

Hyodo, M., Sakurai, Y., Akita, H., and Harashima, H. 2014. "Programmed packaging" for gene delivery. *J Control Release* 193:316–323.

Jackson, W. T., Giddings, T. H., Jr., Taylor, M. P., Mulinyawe, S., Rabinovitch, M., Kopito, R. R. et al. 2005. Subversion of cellular autophagosomal machinery by RNA viruses. *PLoS Biol* 3:e156.

Jin, C. Y., Zhu, B. S., Wang, X. F., and Lu, Q. H. 2008. Cytotoxicity of titanium dioxide nanoparticles in mouse fibroblast cells. *Chem Res Toxicol* 21:1871–1877.

Johnson-Lyles, D. N., Peifley, K., Lockett, S., Neun, B. W., Hansen, M., Clogston, J. et al. 2010. Fullerenol cytotoxicity in kidney cells is associated with cytoskeleton disruption, autophagic vacuole accumulation, and mitochondrial dysfunction. *Toxicol Appl Pharmacol* 248:249–258.

Kadar, E., Tarran, G. A., Jha, A. N., and Al-Subiai, S. N. 2011. Stabilization of engineered zero-valent nanoiron with Na-acrylic copolymer enhances spermiotoxicity. *Environ Sci Technol* 45:3245–3251.

Kamei, S., Chen-Kuo-Chang, M., Cazevieille, C., Lenaers, G., Olichon, A., Belenguer, P. et al. 2005. Expression of the Opa1 mitochondrial protein in retinal ganglion cells: Its downregulation causes aggregation of the mitochondrial network. *Invest Ophthalmol Vis Sci* 46:4288–4294.

Kania, E., Pajak, B., and Orzechowski, A. 2015. Calcium homeostasis and ER stress in control of autophagy in cancer cells. *Biomed Res Int* 2015:352794.

Karpeta-Kaczmarek, J., Augustyniak, M., and Rost-Roszkowska, M. 2016. Ultrastructure of the gut epithelium in Acheta domesticus after long-term exposure to nanodiamonds supplied with food. *Arthropod Struct Dev* 45:253–264.

Katsumiti, A., Gilliland, D., Arostegui, I., and Cajaraville, M. P. 2014. Cytotoxicity and cellular mechanisms involved in the toxicity of CdS quantum dots in hemocytes and gill cells of the mussel Mytilus galloprovincialis. *Aquat Toxicol* 153:39–52.

Kim, S. J., Khan, M., Quan, J., Till, A., Subramani, S., and Siddiqui, A. et al. 2013. Hepatitis B virus disrupts mitochondrial dynamics: Induces fission and mitophagy to attenuate apoptosis. *PLoS Pathog* 9:e1003722.

Kim, S. J., Syed, G. H., and Siddiqui, A. 2013. Hepatitis C virus induces the mitochondrial translocation of Parkin and subsequent mitophagy. *PLoS Pathog* 9:e1003285.

Klionsky, D. J. 2007. Autophagy: From phenomenology to molecular understanding in less than a decade. *Nat Rev Mol Cell Biol* 8:931–937.

Klionsky, D. J., Abeliovich, H., Agostinis, P., Agrawal, D. K., Aliev, G., Askew, D. S. et al. 2008. Guidelines for the use and interpretation of assays for monitoring autophagy in higher eukaryotes. *Autophagy* 4:151–175.

Kochl, R., Hu, X. W., Chan, E. Y., and Tooze, S. A. 2006. Microtubules facilitate autophagosome formation and fusion of autophagosomes with endosomes. *Traffic* 7:129–145.

Koehler, A., Marx, U., Broeg, K., Bahns, S., and Bressling, J. 2008. Effects of nanoparticles in Mytilus edulis gills and hepatopancreas—A new threat to marine life? *Mar Environ Res* 66:12–14.

Koivisto, A. J., Lyyranen, J., Auvinen, A., Vanhala, E., Hameri, K., Tuomi, T. et al. 2012. Industrial worker exposure to airborne particles during the packing of pigment and nanoscale titanium dioxide. *Inhal Toxicol* 24:839–849.

Kroemer, G., and Jaattela, M. 2005. Lysosomes and autophagy in cell death control. *Nat Rev Cancer* 5:886–897.

Landes, T., Leroy, I., Bertholet, A., Diot, A., Khosrobakhsh, F., Daloyau, M. et al. 2010. OPA1 (dys)functions. *Semin Cell Dev Biol* 21:593–598.

Lee, S., Jeong, S. Y., Lim, W. C., Kim, S., Park, Y. Y., Sun, X. et al. 2007. Mitochondrial fission and fusion mediators, hFis1 and OPA1, modulate cellular senescence. *J Biol Chem* 282:22977–22983.

Lee, T. Y., Liu, M. S., Huang, L. J., Lue, S. I., Lin, L. C., Kwan, A. L. et al. 2013. Bioenergetic failure correlates with autophagy and apoptosis in rat liver following silver nanoparticle intraperitoneal administration. *Part Fibre Toxicol* 10:40.

Levine, B. 2005. Eating oneself and uninvited guests: Autophagy-related pathways in cellular defense. *Cell* 120:159–162.

Levrero, M. 2006. Viral hepatitis and liver cancer: The case of hepatitis C. *Oncogene* 25:3834–3847.

Li, C., Liu, H., Sun, Y., Wang, H., Guo, F., Rao, S. et al. 2009. PAMAM nanoparticles promote acute lung injury by inducing autophagic cell death through the Akt-TSC2-mTOR signaling pathway. *J Mol Cell Biol* 1:37–45.

Li, H., Li, Y., Jiao, J., and Hu, H. M. 2011. Alpha-alumina nanoparticles induce efficient autophagy-dependent cross-presentation and potent antitumour response. *Nat Nanotechnol* 6:645–650.

Li, J. J., Hartono, D., Ong, C. N., Bay, B. H., and Yung, L. Y. 2010. Autophagy and oxidative stress associated with gold nanoparticles. *Biomaterials* 31:5996–6003.

Li, N., Xia, T., and Nel, A. E. 2008. The role of oxidative stress in ambient particulate matter-induced lung diseases and its implications in the toxicity of engineered nanoparticles. *Free Radic Biol Med* 44:1689–1699.

Liesa, M., Palacin, M., and Zorzano, A. 2009. Mitochondrial dynamics in mammalian health and disease. *Physiol Rev* 89:799–845.

Lin, C. H., Chang, L. W., Wei, Y. H., Wu, S. B., Yang, C. S., Chang, W. H. et al. 2012. Electronic microscopy evidence for mitochondria as targets for Cd/Se/Te-based quantum dot 705 toxicity in vivo. *Kaohsiung J Med Sci* 28:S53–S62.

Liu, H. L., Zhang, Y. L., Yang, N., Zhang, Y. X., Liu, X. Q., Li, C. G. et al. 2011. A functionalized single-walled carbon nanotube-induced autophagic cell death in human lung cells through Akt-TSC2-mTOR signaling. *Cell Death Dis* 2:e159.

Lu, A. L., Li, X., Gu, Y., Wright, P. M., and Chang, D. Y. 2001. Repair of oxidative DNA damage: Mechanisms and functions. *Cell Biochem Biophys* 35:141–170.

Lunov, O., Syrovets, T., Loos, C., Nienhaus, G. U., Mailander, V., Landfester, K. et al. 2011. Amino-functionalized polystyrene nanoparticles activate the NLRP3 inflammasome in human macrophages. *ACS Nano* 5:9648–9657.

Luo, B., and Lee, A. S. 2013. The critical roles of endoplasmic reticulum chaperones and unfolded protein response in tumorigenesis and anticancer therapies. *Oncogene* 32:805–818.

Luo, C., Li, Y., Yang, L., Wang, X., Long, J., and Liu, J. et al. 2015. Superparamagnetic iron oxide nanoparticles exacerbate the risks of reactive oxygen species-mediated external stresses. *Arch Toxicol* 89:357–369.

Luo, S., and Rubinsztein, D. C. 2007. Atg5 and Bcl-2 provide novel insights into the interplay between apoptosis and autophagy. *Cell Death Differ* 14:1247–1250.

Lupfer, C., Thomas, P. G., Anand, P. K., Vogel, P., Milasta, S., Martinez, J. et al. 2013. Receptor interacting protein kinase 2-mediated mitophagy regulates inflammasome activation during virus infection. *Nat Immunol* 14:480–488.

Ma, X., Wu, Y., Jin, S., Tian, Y., Zhang, X., Zhao, Y. et al. 2011. Gold nanoparticles induce autophagosome accumulation through size-dependent nanoparticle uptake and lysosome impairment. *ACS Nano* 5:8629–8639.

Malvindi, M. A., De Matteis, V., Galeone, A., Brunetti, V., Anyfantis, G. C., Athanassiou, A. et al. 2014. Toxicity assessment of silica coated iron oxide nanoparticles and biocompatibility improvement by surface engineering. *PLoS One* 9:e85835.

Manshian, B. B., Pfeiffer, C., Pelaz, B., Heimerl, T., Gallego, M., Moller, M. et al. 2015. High-content imaging and gene expression approaches to unravel the effect of surface functionality on cellular interactions of silver nanoparticles. *ACS Nano* 9:10431–10444.

Manunta, M., Izzo, L., Duncan, R., and Jones, A. T. 2007. Establishment of subcellular fractionation techniques to monitor the intracellular fate of polymer therapeutics II. Identification of endosomal and lysosomal compartments in HepG2 cells combining single-step subcellular fractionation with fluorescent imaging. *J Drug Target* 15:37–50.

Meunier, E., Coste, A., Olagnier, D., Authier, H., Lefevre, L., Dardenne, C. et al. 2011. Double-walled carbon nanotubes trigger IL-1beta release in human monocytes through Nlrp3 inflammasome activation. *Nanomedicine* 8:987–995.

Milane, L., Trivedi, M., Singh, A., Talekar, M., and Amiji, M. 2015. Mitochondrial biology, targets, and drug delivery. *J Control Release* 207:40–58.

Mironava, T., Hadjiargyrou, M., Simon, M., Jurukovski, V., and Rafailovich, M. H. 2010. Gold nanoparticles cellular toxicity and recovery: Effect of size, concentration and exposure time. *Nanotoxicology* 4:120–137.

Mohanraj, V. J., and Chen, Y. 2006. Nanoparticles–A review. *Trop J Pharm* 5:561–573.

Monick, M. M., Powers, L. S., Walters, K., Lovan, N., Zhang, M., Gerke, A. et al. 2010. Identification of an autophagy defect in smokers' alveolar macrophages. *J Immunol* 185:5425–5435.

Montgomery, R. R., Webster, P., and Mellman, I. 1991. Accumulation of indigestible substances reduces fusion competence of macrophage lysosomes. *J Immunol* 147:3087–3095.

Naqvi, S., Samim, M., Abdin, M., Ahmed, F. J., Maitra, A., Prashant, C. et al. 2010. Concentration-dependent toxicity of iron oxide nanoparticles mediated by increased oxidative stress. *Int J Nanomedicine* 5:983–989.

Nel, A., Xia, T., Madler, L., and Li, N. 2006. Toxic potential of materials at the nanolevel. *Science* 311:622–627.

Oberdörster, G., Ferin, J., Soderholm, S., Gelein, R., Cox, C., Baggs, R. et al. 1994. Increased pulmonary toxicity of inhaled ultrafine particles: Due to lung overload alone? *Ann Occup Hyg* 38:295–302.

Oberdorster, G., Oberdorster, E., and Oberdorster, J. 2005. Nanotoxicology: An emerging discipline evolving from studies of ultrafine particles. *Environ Health Perspect* 113:823–839.

Padgett, B. L., Walker, D. L., ZuRhein, G. M., Hodach, A. E., and Chou, S. M. 1976. JC Papovavirus in progressive multifocal leukoencephalopathy. *J Infect Dis* 133:686–690.

Palikaras, K., Lionaki, E., and Tavernarakis, N. 2016. Mitophagy: In sickness and in health. *Mol Cell Oncol* 3:e1056332.

Park, E. J., Choi, D. H., Kim, Y., Lee, E. W., Song, J., Cho, M. H. et al. 2014. Magnetic iron oxide nanoparticles induce autophagy preceding apoptosis through mitochondrial damage and ER stress in RAW264.7 cells. *Toxicol In Vitro* 28:1402–1412.

Pathak, R. K., Kolishetti, N., and Dhar, S. 2015. Targeted nanoparticles in mitochondrial medicine. *Wiley Interdiscip Rev Nanomed Nanobiotechnol* 7:315–329.

Piccinno, F., Gottschalk, F., Seege, S., and Nowack, B. 2012. Industrial production quantities and uses of ten engineered nanomaterials in Europe and the world. *J Nanopart Res* 14:1109–1119.

Powell, A. C., Paciotti, G. F., and Libutti, S. K. 2010. Colloidal gold: A novel nanoparticle for targeted cancer therapeutics. *Methods Mol Biol* 624:375–384.

Rashid, H. O., Yadav, R. K., Kim, H. R., and Chae, H. J. 2015. ER stress: Autophagy induction, inhibition and selection. *Autophagy* 11:1956–1977.

Ravikumar, B., Sarkar, S., Davies, J. E., Futter, M., Garcia-Arencibia, M., Green-Thompson, Z. W. et al. 2010. Regulation of mammalian autophagy in physiology and pathophysiology. *Physiol Rev* 90:1383–1435.

Ringwood, A. H., Levi-Polyachenko, N., and Carroll, D. L. 2009. Fullerene exposures with oysters: Embryonic, adult, and cellular responses. *Environ Sci Technol* 43:7136–7141.

Roberts, J. C., Bhalgat, M. K., and Zera, R. T. 1996. Preliminary biological evaluation of polyamidoamine (PAMAM) Starburst dendrimers. *J Biomed Mater Res* 30:53–65.

Rocha, T. L., Gomes, T., Sousa, V. S., Mestre, N. C., and Bebianno, M. J. 2015. Ecotoxicological impact of engineered nanomaterials in bivalve molluscs: An overview. *Mar Environ Res* 111:74–88.

Rodriguez-Nogales, C., Garbayo, E., Carmona-Abellan, M. M., Luquin, M. R., and Blanco-Prieto, M. J. 2016. Brain aging and Parkinson's disease: New therapeutic approaches using drug delivery systems. *Maturitas* 84:25–31.

Ruenraroengsak, P., and Florence, A. T. 2010. Biphasic interactions between a cationic dendrimer and actin. *J Drug Target* 18:803–811.

Ruiz, P. A., Moron, B., Becker, H. M., Lang, S., Atrott, K., Spalinger, M. R. et al. 2016. Titanium dioxide nanoparticles exacerbate DSS-induced colitis: Role of the NLRP3 inflammasome. *Gut* 0:1–9.

Sakhrani, N. M., and Padh, H. 2013. Organelle targeting: Third level of drug targeting. *Drug Des Devel Ther* 7:585–599.

Schneider, P., Korolenko, T. A., and Busch, U. 1997. A review of drug-induced lysosomal disorders of the liver in man and laboratory animals. *Microsc Res Tech* 36:253–275.

Seglen, P. O., and Brinchmann, M. F. 2010. Purification of autophagosomes from rat hepatocytes. *Autophagy* 6:542–547.

Seib, F. P., Jones, A. T., and Duncan, R. 2006. Establishment of subcellular fractionation techniques to monitor the intracellular fate of polymer therapeutics I. Differential centrifugation fractionation B16F10 cells and use to study the intracellular fate of HPMA copolymer—Doxorubicin. *J Drug Target* 14:375–390.

Seleverstov, O., Zabirnyk, O., Zscharnack, M., Bulavina, L., Nowicki, M., Heinrich, J. M. et al. 2006. Quantum dots for human mesenchymal stem cells labeling. A size-dependent autophagy activation. *Nano Lett* 6:2826–2832.

Sena, L. A., and Chandel, N. S. 2012. Physiological roles of mitochondrial reactive oxygen species. *Mol Cell* 48:158–167.

Shelby, B. D., Nelson, A., and Morris, C. 2005. Gamma-herpesvirus neoplasia: A growing role for COX-2. *Microsc Res Tech* 68:120–129.

Shimizu, S., Kanaseki, T., Mizushima, N., Mizuta, T., Arakawa-Kobayashi, S., Thompson, C. B. et al. 2004. Role of Bcl-2 family proteins in a non-apoptotic programmed cell death dependent on autophagy genes. *Nat Cell Biol* 6:1221–1228.

Simard, J. C., Vallieres, F., de Liz, R., Lavastre, V., and Girard, D. 2015. Silver nanoparticles induce degradation of the endoplasmic reticulum stress sensor activating transcription factor-6 leading to activation of the NLRP-3 inflammasome. *J Biol Chem* 290:5926–5939.

Soenen, S. J., Rivera-Gil, P., Montenegro, J.-M., Parak, W. J., De Smedt S. C., Braeckmans K. et al. 2011. Cellular toxicity of inorganic nanoparticles: Common aspects and guidelines for improved nanotoxicity evaluation. *Nanotoday* 6:446–465.

Sohaebuddin, S. K., Thevenot, P. T., Baker, D., Eaton, J. W., and Tang, L. 2010. Nanomaterial cytotoxicity is composition, size, and cell type dependent. *Part Fibre Toxicol* 7:22.

Stern, S. T., Adiseshaiah, P. P., and Crist, R. M. 2010. Autophagy and lysosomal dysfunction as emerging mechanisms of nanomaterial toxicity. *Part Fibre Toxicol* 9:20.

Stern, S. T., Zolnik, B. S., McLeland, C. B., Clogston J., Zheng J., McNeil, S. E. et al. 2008. Induction of autophagy in porcine kidney cells by quantum dots: A common cellular response to nanomaterials? *Toxicol Sci* 106:140–152.

Tanida, I., Ueno, T., and Kominami, E. 2008. LC3 and autophagy. *Methods Mol Biol* 445:77–88.

Tedesco, S., Doyle, H., Blasco, J., Redmond, G., and Sheehan, D. 2010. Oxidative stress and toxicity of gold nanoparticles in Mytilus edulis. *Aquat Toxicol* 100:178–186.

Thibodeau, M. S., Giardina, C., Knecht, D. A., Helble, J., and Hubbard, A. K. 2004. Silica-induced apoptosis in mouse alveolar macrophages is initiated by lysosomal enzyme activity. *Toxicol Sci* 80:34–48.

Thomas, T. P., Majoros, I., Kotlyar, A. et al. 2009. Cationic poly(amidoamine) dendrimer induces lysosomal apoptotic pathway at therapeutically relevant concentrations. *Biomacromolecules* 10:3207–3214.

Trevisan, R., Delapedra, G., Mello, D. F., Arl, M., Schmidt, E. C., Meder, F. et al. 2014. Gills are an initial target of zinc oxide nanoparticles in oysters *Crassostrea gigas*, leading to mitochondrial disruption and oxidative stress. *Aquat Toxicol* 153:27–38.

Twomey, M., Mendez, E., Manian, R. K., Lee, S., and J. H. Moon. 2016. Mitochondria-specific conjugated polymer nanoparticles. *Chem Commun (Camb)* 52:4910–4913.

Verderio, P., Avvakumova, S., Alessio, G. Bellini, M., Colombo, M., Galbiati, E. et al. 2014. Delivering colloidal nanoparticles to mammalian cells: A nano-bio interface perspective. *Adv Healthc Mater* 3:957–976.

Walker, V. G., Li, Z., Hulderman, T. et al. 2009. Potential in vitro effects of carbon nanotubes on human aortic endothelial cells. *Toxicol Appl Pharmacol* 236:319–328.

Wang, F., Bexiga, M. G., Anguissola, S., Boya, P., Simpson, J. C., Salvati, A. et al. 2013. Time resolved study of cell death mechanisms induced by amine-modified polystyrene nanoparticles. *Nanoscale* 5:10868–10876.

Wang, Z. L., and Feng, X. 2003. Polyhedral shapes of CeO_2 nanoparticles. *J Phys Chem B* 107:13563–13566.

Wati, S., Soo, M. L., Zilm, P., Li, P., Paton, A. W., Burrell, C. J. et al. 2009. Dengue virus infection induces upregulation of GRP78, which acts to chaperone viral antigen production. *J Virol* 83:12871–12880.

Watson, A. S., Mortensen, M., and Simon, A. K. 2011. Autophagy in the pathogenesis of myelodysplastic syndrome and acute myeloid leukemia. *Cell Cycle* 10:1719–1725.

Weiss, M. J., Wong, J. R., Ha, C. S., Bleday, R., Salem, R. R., Steele, Jr., G. D. et al. 1987. Dequalinium, a topical antimicrobial agent, displays anticarcinoma activity based on selective mitochondrial accumulation. *Proc Natl Acad Sci USA* 84:5444–5448.

Weissig, V., Cheng, S. M., and D'Souza, G. G. 2004. Mitochondrial pharmaceutics. *Mitochondrion* 3:229–244.

Weissig, V., D'Souza, G. G., and Torchilin, V. P. 2001. DQAsome/DNA complexes release DNA upon contact with isolated mouse liver mitochondria. *J Control Release* 75: 401–408.

Weissig, V., Lasch, J., Erdos, G., Meyer, H. W., Rowe, T. C., and Hughes, J. et al. 1998. DQAsomes: A novel potential drug and gene delivery system made from Dequalinium. *Pharm Res* 15:334–337.

Westermann, B. 2002. Merging mitochondria matters: Cellular role and molecular machinery of mitochondrial fusion. *EMBO Rep* 3:527–531.

Wild, T. F. 1981. Measles virus and chronic infections. *Pathol Biol (Paris)* 29:429–433.

Wongrakpanich, A., Geary, S. M., Joiner, M. L., Anderson, M. E., and Salem, A. K. 2014. Mitochondria-targeting particles. *Nanomedicine (Lond)* 9:2531–2543.

Wu, H. F., Kailasa, S. K., and Shastri, L. 2010. Electrostatically self-assembled azides on zinc sulfide nanoparticles as multifunctional nanoprobes for peptide and protein analysis in MALDI-TOF MS. *Talanta* 82:540–547.

Wu, J., and Xie, H. 2014. Effects of titanium dioxide nanoparticles on alpha-synuclein aggregation and the ubiquitin-proteasome system in dopaminergic neurons. *Artif Cells Nanomed Biotechnol* 44:690–694.

Wu, X., Tan, Y., Mao, H., and Zhang, M. 2010. Toxic effects of iron oxide nanoparticles on human umbilical vein endothelial cells. *Int J Nanomedicine* 5:385–399.

Xia, M., Gonzalez, P., Li, C., Meng, G., Jiang, A., Wang, H. et al. 2014. Mitophagy enhances oncolytic measles virus replication by mitigating DDX58/RIG-I-like receptor signaling. *J Virol* 88:5152–5164.

Xia, T., Kovochich, M., Liong, M., Zink, J. I., and Nel, A. E. 2008. Cationic polystyrene nanosphere toxicity depends on cell-specific endocytic and mitochondrial injury pathways. *ACS Nano* 2:85–96.

Xie, R., Nguyen, S., McKeehan, W. L., and Liu, L. 2010. Acetylated microtubules are required for fusion of autophagosomes with lysosomes. *BMC Cell Biol* 11:89.

Xie, Z., and Klionsky, D. J. 2007. Autophagosome formation: Core machinery and adaptations. *Nat Cell Biol* 9:1102–1109.

Yamawaki, H., and Iwai, N. 2006. Cytotoxicity of water-soluble fullerene in vascular endothelial cells. *Am J Physiol Cell Physiol* 290:C1495–1502.

Yang, X., Shao, H., Liu, W., Gu, W., Shu, X., Mo, Y. et al. 2015. Endoplasmic reticulum stress and oxidative stress are involved in ZnO nanoparticle-induced hepatotoxicity. *Toxicol Lett* 234:40–49.

Yu, K. N., Yoon, T. J., Minai-Tehrani, A., Kim, J. E., Park, S. J., Jeong, M. S. et al. 2013. Zinc oxide nanoparticle induced autophagic cell death and mitochondrial damage via reactive oxygen species generation. *Toxicol In Vitro* 27:1187–1195.

Yu, L., Lu, Y., Man, N., Yu, S. H., and Wen, L. P. 2009. Rare earth oxide nanocrystals induce autophagy in HeLa cells. *Small* 5:2784–2787.

Zabirnyk, O., Yezhelyev, M., and Seleverstov, O. 2007. Nanoparticles as a novel class of autophagy activators. *Autophagy* 3:278–281.

Zhan, Q., and Tang, M. 2014. Research advances on apoptosis caused by quantum dots. *Biol Trace Elem Res* 161:3–12.

Zhang, Z., Zhou, L., Zhou, Y., Liu, J., Xing, X., Zhong, J. et al. 2015. Mitophagy induced by nanoparticle-peptide conjugates enabling an alternative intracellular trafficking route. *Biomaterials* 65:56–65.

Zinchuk, V., Zinchuk, O., and Okada, T. 2007. Quantitative colocalization analysis of multicolor confocal immunofluorescence microscopy images: Pushing pixels to explore biological phenomena. *Acta Histochem Cytochem* 40:101–111.

Zuccheri, T., Colonna, M., Stefanini, I., Santini, C., and Di Gioia, D. 2013. Bactericidal activity of aqueous acrylic paint dispersion for wooden substrates based on TiO2 nanoparticles activated by fluorescent light. *Materials* 6:3270–3283.

Section III

Safety Assessment
for Human Use

7 Rodent Inhalation Studies in Nanomaterial Risk Assessment

Laurent Gaté, Frédéric Cosnier, and Flemming R. Cassee

CONTENTS

7.1 INTRODUCTION

Due to their physical and chemical properties, the use of nanomaterials is constantly increasing. According to the Nanotechnology Consumer Products Inventory of the Project on Emerging Nanotechnologies, more than 1,800 products are already on the market (Vance et al. 2015; http://www.nanotechproject.org/cpi/). The occupational exposure to such compounds may occur during their use in many industrial processes. They may get aerosolized and it is expected that the main occupational route of exposure is inhalation. In the general population, the risks are still likely to be low but exposures may occur if nanomaterials are released from consumer products during spray application. In addition, it is currently not very clear how combined exposure to processes generating ultrafine particles such as combustion-derived nanoparticles will add to the total health risk of exposure to nanomaterials.

The assessment of their toxicological properties can be achieved by *in vitro* assays and *in vivo* experiments by various administration routes and different experimental models, including rodents. Due to the lack of data from epidemiological studies and ethical issues regarding experiments performed with human volunteers, inhalation experiments in which animals (mainly rodents) are exposed to a well-characterized aerosol are the gold standard since they respect human exposure route and allow the distribution of inhaled nanomaterials throughout the entire respiratory system in a physiological manner. In addition, rodents share similarities with humans in terms of anatomy, physiology, and susceptibility to diseases. Even though the extrapolation of experimental inhalation toxicity data to humans needs to be addressed with caution, in the absence of sufficient epidemiological results regarding the toxicity of nanomaterials, they are of great value for setting recommendations regarding occupational exposure limits (NIOSH 2013, 2011).

7.2 AEROSOL GENERATION AND CHARACTERIZATION

7.2.1 AEROSOL GENERATION

Over the years, many methods have been used to generate stable nanostructured aerosols for toxicity testing. They could be divided into three groups: (1) wet-based methods, (2) dry-based methods, and (3) direct synthesis methods (Figure 7.1; Morimoto et al. 2013). Each of them has its advantages and disadvantages (Table 7.1).

7.2.1.1 From Nanopowder

7.2.1.1.1 Wet-Based Methods

These methods involve devices such as atomizers, nebulizers, electrospray generators, or ultrasonic atomizers, for examples. Most of the time, nanomaterials are dispersed in an aqueous solution using sonication. This may also require the use of surfactant (often in small amount).

The size of particle agglomerates in the aerosol depends on the size of the droplets produced by the generator, the particle concentration, and the level of particle dispersion (Noel, Charbonneau et al. 2013; Noel, Cloutier et al. 2013; Figure 7.1). It is

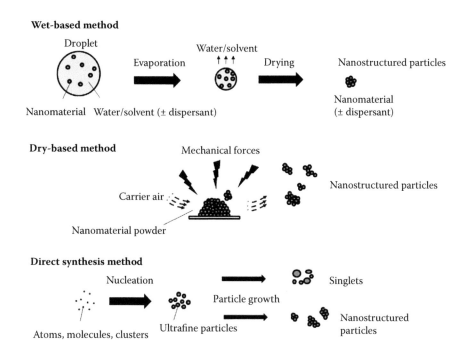

FIGURE 7.1 Illustration of methods for preparing aerosolized test nanomaterials. (Adapted with permission from Morimoto, Y. et al., *Acc Chem Res*, 46(3), 770–781, 2013. Copyright 2013, American Chemical Society.)

therefore possible to produce large (>100 nm) or small (<100 nm) monodispersed nanostructured agglomerates, but also aerosols made of primary particles (especially with an electrospray generator; Figure 7.2c).

Since the suspension treatment can change the physiochemical properties of nanomaterials in their aerosol form, these wet-based methods should be reserved for "hazard-oriented" inhalation studies. In addition, because of its tremendous impact on the size of the produced aerosol and the stability of the generation process over time, the suspension preparation is a crucial step that deserves special care.

The main issue with this approach is the possible presence of contaminants in the solvent used to disperse the nanomaterial (like salts originating from the aqueous solution) but also in some cases the use of surfactant that may affect the physical properties of the nanomaterials. As an example, Iskandar et al. (2003) observed that during the generation of nanostructured particles of silica with a spray-drying method they obtained either solid and dense particles or doughnut-shaped particles based on the generation condition and the presence of surfactant (Iskandar et al. 2003). This may also have consequences on the biological response induced by particles. In order to evaluate the impact of the aqueous solution on the toxicological properties of nanostructured aerosols, it is also required to expose the control group using the same aerosolization method to the same aqueous solution as the one used to disperse the particles.

TABLE 7.1

Aerosol Generation Methods

Methods	Example of Generators	Advantages	Disadvantages	References
Dry-based method	Rotating brush generator Wright dust feeder Jet mill Fluidized bed aerosol generator Acoustical based computer controlled system	Dispersion of nanopowder without treatment Long period of generation	Production of nanostructured particles larger than 100 nm	Li et al. 2007, Ma-Hock et al. 2007, McKinney, Chen, and Frazer 2009, Mitchell et al. 2007, Nurkiewicz et al. 2008, Pauluhn 2009, Porter et al. 2013, Cosnier et al. 2016, Geraets et al. 2012
Wet-based method	Atomizer/nebulizer Electrospray generator Ultrasonic atomizer	Production of nanostructured particles larger than or below 100 nm	Possible impurities from solvent used (water, ethanol) Possible change of nanomaterial initial properties due to suspension preparation (surfactant, sonification)	Fujita et al. 2009, Kwon et al. 2008, Takenaka et al. 2004
Direct synthesis methods	Hot plate generator Spark generator Furnace/flame	Generation of pure metal, metal oxide, or alloy Homogeneous monodisperse aerosol Production of nanostructured particles below 100 nm Generation of radioactive particles[a]	Not representative of manufactured nanomaterials and occupational exposure Not suitable for all nanomaterials (carbon nanotubes)	Geiser et al. 2005, Kreyling et al. 2009, Sung et al. 2008, Zhou et al. 2003

[a] Spark generator.

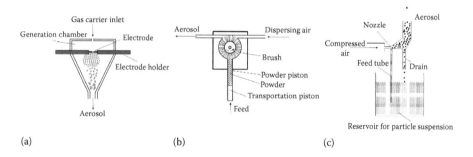

FIGURE 7.2 Examples of aerosol generators. (a) Schematic representation of a spark generator. (Adapted with permission from Messing, M. A. et al., *J Phys Chem C*, 114(20), 9257–9263, 2010. Copyright 2010, American Chemical Society.) (b) Schematic representation of a rotating brush generator. (Adapted with permission from Palas GmbH, Germany.) (c) Schematic representation of an atomizer.

7.2.1.1.2 Dry-Based Methods

Aerosol is produced from a nanostructured powder which is aerosolized by a combination of mechanical forces and air carriers (Table 7.1 and Figure 7.1). Available dispersion techniques include rotating brush generator, Wright dust feeder, small-scale powder disperser, jet mill, fluidized bed aerosol generator, and acoustical-based computer controlled system (Figure 7.2b). These devices, which are often easy-to-use and inexpensive, allow the dispersion of (nano) materials without prior treatment and the generation of high concentrations of nanostructured aerosols if necessary.

With this approach, it is, however, difficult to generate nanostructured aerosols composed of primary nano-objects or small agglomerates below 100 nm due to their agglomeration/aggregation state in the starting powder or formed during aerosol generation (Noel, Cloutier et al. 2013). The agglomeration process, which is also seen with other methods, is fast and mostly dependent on the size and concentration of primary particles in the aerosol. In addition, it is difficult to disperse agglomerates consisting of small particles since the forces applied to the powder by the generator are often not strong enough (Kim et al. 2010, Valverde and Castellanos 2007). Even though starting from nanopowder usually gives off relatively large airborne agglomerates in the micrometric range, they are believed to be representative of aerosols from realistic occupational exposure scenarios. Despite the fact that few data are available, one would assume that the handling of nanopowder in industrial processes would lead to the production of nanostructured aerosols within the same size ranges as those obtained with dry-based aerosolization methods (Curwin and Bertke 2011, Pelclova et al. 2016). Thus, these dry-based methods are more suitable for "risk-oriented" inhalation studies.

7.2.1.2 Direct Synthesis Methods

Aerosols can also be generated directly from nanoparticle precursors, which could be under different states: Solid (spark generator), liquid (hot plate), or gas (flame; Figure 7.2a). Nanoparticles are then produced by nucleation of the atoms or molecules present into the precursor (Geiser et al. 2005, Ji et al. 2007, Ostraat et al. 2008; Figure 7.1; Table 7.1).

Such methods allow the production of monodispersed aggregates/agglomerates of nano-objects below 100 nm and which are then much smaller than the ones obtained with the two previously mentioned techniques. However, by this approach, the properties of the aerosol and the achievable concentrations (often much lower than for the other methods) are very dependent on the nature of the precursor material. In addition, one may argue that such aerosols are not representative of an occupational exposure. Nonetheless, such experiments might be suited for better understanding the toxicological properties of nanoparticles and their interactions with biological macromolecules.

7.2.2 AEROSOL CHARACTERIZATION

Primary particle and aerosol characterizations are essential in inhalation toxicology studies in order to determine the aerosol respirability and the estimated deposited dose throughout the respiratory system and subsequently its toxicological properties. This is essential for risk assessment and the comparison of the results for different studies. The Organization for Economic Cooperation and Development (OECD 2016b) and the International Organization of Standardization (ISO 2016) have been actively involved in this field in order to provide international guidelines that would facilitate the work of scientists and regulators in nanomaterial risk assessment.

Before starting any inhalation study, it is mandatory to perform a thorough characterization of the nanopowder that will be used (when not using a direct synthesis method). The list of the main physical and chemical parameters that may appear relevant for risk assessment are listed in Table 7.2 (ISO 2013, OECD 2016a, ISO 2012). Even though it is still difficult to draw definite conclusions regarding all the parameters that would be important for assessing the toxicity of nanomaterials, some of them have drawn attention (Braakhuis et al. 2014). For instance, specific surface area has been identified as one of the most important players in the toxicity of

---

TABLE 7.2

Main Physicochemical Characterization of Nanomaterials for Toxicology Studies

Physical and Chemical Parameters

Agglomeration/aggregation state
Composition, including impurities
Primary particle size/distribution
Shape/aspect ratio
Solubility/dispersibility
Porosity/specific surface area
Surface chemistry/reactivity
Surface charge

---

nanomaterials. It has been observed for titanium dioxide and carbon black that comparable mass concentrations of nanoparticles induce a greater pulmonary inflammatory response in animals than their counterparts in the submicronic/micronic size range. However, when the results were reported according to the particle surface area, the pulmonary inflammatory effects of these materials were similar (Elder et al. 2005, Ferin et al. 1992, Oberdorster et al. 2005, Stoeger et al. 2006). In a recent review of the literature analyzing the pulmonary toxicity of intratracheally instilled nanomaterials in rodents, the authors also suggest that specific surface area was an important dose metric in particle toxicity assessment, but other parameters, such as particle number or volume, should not be neglected either (Schmid and Stoeger 2016).

The instrumentation used for aerosol characterization is a constantly growing market. There are several categories of pieces of equipment, such as real time instruments and aerosol samplers (offline), which may allow discriminating measures in size for accessing different metrics directly or by calculation associated with assumptions. They are based on different technologies (sometimes combined): Filter collection, dynamic mass and surface area measurements, inertial, condensation, diffusion, optical, electrical techniques, and so on (Kulkarni et al. 2011). Since the size distribution of an aerosol could be wide and could greatly differ from one nanopowder to another, it is not that simple to select suitable pieces of equipment to use. Indeed, it is important to be aware of the limitations of the different instruments; for example, their size-range measurement capabilities. As an example, for number–size distribution, one can use a Scanning Mobility Particle Sizer Spectrometer (SMPS) and an Aerodynamic Particle Sizer Spectrophotometer (APS); however, while the former is measuring the particle mobility diameter of particles from about 1 nm to 1 μm, the latter is measuring their aerodynamic diameter ranging from around 0.5 to 20 μm. In addition, one should understand that based on the physical properties of the particles and the measurement technology of the analytical instrument, their size could be expressed according to different parameters (mobility or aerodynamic diameter for example) which would only give an estimate of the "true size" of the nanostructured particles. Furthermore, for the measurement of its size, an agglomerate or aggregate would be often described as an equivalent spherical particle with the same diameter, which is also an issue since agglomerates rarely have a spherical shape. Finally, depending on the measurement method used, the median diameter of particles detected varies widely based on the parameter measured by the analytical instrument. For example, the median size of an aerosol 21-nm TiO_2 nanoparticles varies between 0.25 (electrical mobility analyzer, SMPS) and 1.1 μm (cascade impactor) because of the parameters measured (number size distribution vs. mass size distribution, respectively; Ma-Hock et al. 2007). It is then important to use a combination of different analytical instruments to get the best estimate of the aerosol to which animals are exposed (Table 7.3; Cosnier et al. 2016).

It is also necessary to make a critical analysis of the metrological results obtained throughout the generation to ensure that the particle size determined by the instruments is the most representative of that of the aerosol truly present inside the exposure chamber.

TABLE 7.3

Minimal Aerosol Characterization

Parameters	Laboratory Equipment	Observations
Total mass concentration	Membrane filter sampling	Off-line
(mg/m^3)	Tapered Element Oscillating Microbalance (TEOM®)	Real-time
Mass size distribution	Cascade Impactor	Off-line
Total number concentration ($part/cm^3$)	Condensation Particle Counter (CPC)	Real-time
Number size distribution	Scanning Mobility Particle Sizer (SMPS) (Differential Mobility Analyser +CPC)	Real-time
	Electrical Low Pressure Impactor (ELPI)	
	Aerodynamic Particle Sizer (APS)	
Electrical state of charge	Electrometer	Real-time
	Electrical Low Pressure Impactor (ELPI)	
Morphology	Transmission and Scanning Electron Microscopy	Off-line

If the in-depth characterization of the aerosol is obviously important, the full set of instruments does not necessarily need to be deployed during the animal exposure phase. An aerosol characterization strategy must however be developed that allows monitoring continuously of the aerosol delivered to the animals and ensuring its quality and stability. The key parameters that need to be followed are the mass and the number concentrations which should not deviate from the means by more than 20 percent (worst cases) for aerosols (OECD 2009a,b).

7.3 ANIMAL EXPOSURE

7.3.1 REGULATIONS IN ANIMAL RESEARCH

Because of the capacity of laboratory animals to sense and express pain, suffering, distress, and lasting harm, it is mandatory to ensure their welfare and avoid or minimize their pain, discomfort, and distress throughout inhalation studies. In addition, in scientific research, in order to limit the biological variations due to the use of animals and increase the reproducibility of the assays, it is essential to work with homogeneous animal populations. For this, there is a need to use rodents with known genetic backgrounds which are bred and housed in standardized conditions. In order to meet these goals, legislations for the protection and the welfare of animals used in research have been enforced all around the world (EU 2010).

Finally, any animal experiment should be performed with respect to the principle of the "three Rs" (replacement, reduction, and refinement; Russell and Burch 1959) and whenever possible, alternative methods should be used or developed (Burden et al. 2017).

7.3.2 Environmental Conditions

As mentioned above, since these experiments are performed with live animals, for ethical and scientific reasons it is mandatory to control the temperature and the relative humidity of the air to which animals are exposed in order to minimize their discomfort and distress as well as the variability in the results. For mice and rats, temperatures should be kept between 20 and 24°C and the relative humidity kept between around 45 and 65 percent (EU 2010). In addition, in order to ensure the appropriate breathing of the animals, the air flow and renewal must continuously be verified to meet the animal physiological requirements.

7.3.3 Exposure Methods

7.3.3.1 Nose-Only Inhalation

Animals are placed in restraining tubes and only their noses and snouts are exposed to the aerosol (Figure 7.3a). This method ensures that inhalation is almost the only exposure route; however, the restraint is a source of stress that may induce an increase in corticosterone blood level (Scherer et al. 2011). This hormone has immunomodulary activities on macrophages and the immune system in general (Rickard and Young 2009) that may decrease the inflammatory response induced by inhaled particles. Restraint may also affect the animals' breathing parameters and increase their body temperatures. Since the tail of the rodent plays a critical role in thermoregulation, it should be maintained outside the tube or in a cooler area (Narciso et al. 2003). Nonetheless, the acclimatization of the animals to the restraining tubes minimizes the stress induced by the procedure (Narciso et al. 2003). It is therefore essential to acclimatize the animals to the restraining tubes before starting their exposure to nanostructured aerosols. The design of the tubes and the inhalation chambers should also guarantee that the animals are continuously breathing the aerosol.

Using specially designed head-out plethysmography tubes, it is also possible to measure respiratory and even cardiovascular parameters during animal exposure to aerosols. These experimental systems allow assessing of the impact of inhaled nanomaterials on lung function and their ability to induce sensory irritation (Hoymann

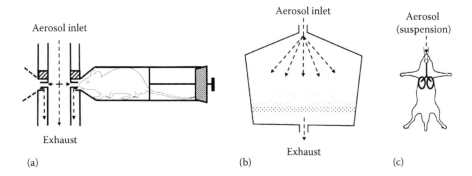

FIGURE 7.3 Schematic representations of inhalation exposure models for rodents. (a) Nose-only inhalation system. (b) Whole body inhalation system. (c) Endotracheal intubation.

2012). The respiratory parameters measured with these tubes may also be useful for particle deposition calculations (cf. § 4.1 deposition models).

Another advantage of the nose-only systems is that the amount of test substance is reduced since the inner volume of inhalation chambers is often smaller than that of whole-body chambers.

7.3.3.2 Whole-Body Inhalation

Animals are placed in chambers with limited restraint, which limits the stress of the animals and the need for acclimatization (Figure 7.3b). The use of such experimental setup is also less labor-intensive since it requires less animal handling. This design is then more suitable for long-term studies. However, in addition to inhalation; other routes of exposure, including dermal and oral, are possible. It was indeed estimated that 60 to 80 percent of a ^{99}Tc radiolabeled aerosol deposited to the fur could reach the gastrointestinal tract of some of the exposed animals (Griffis et al. 1979).

The dose reaching the respiratory system of the animal is also less controllable since it is not excluded that their behavior may affect the amount of inhaled particles (Phalen 2009). As compared to nose-only chambers, where aerosol sampling and monitoring could be easily performed in the breathing zone of the animal since it corresponds to the inhalation port, in whole body chambers aerosol monitoring is done inside the chamber but not directly in the breathing zone of the animals. One must also ensure that the aerosol is homogenously distributed within the chamber.

7.3.3.3 Endotracheal Intubation

Animal are anesthetized and an endotracheal tube is placed into the mouth of the animal. The aerosol is then directly administered to the lung (Figure 7.3c). This method, like intratracheal instillation (Driscoll et al. 2000), bypasses the upper respiratory system and does not respect the natural and physiological route of entry of aerosols. However, it allows a better control of the dose delivered to the lungs. Because of the efficient containment of the test aerosol, it is a good model for working with radioactive nanomaterials or highly dangerous test substances. However, on the downside, anesthesia leads to a modification of the animal respiratory parameters and may influence the deposition rate of particles (Kreyling et al. 2002, Kreyling et al. 2009, Kreyling 2016).

7.4 DEPOSITED DOSE

7.4.1 DEPOSITION MODELS

Once inhaled, nanoparticles have a high probability of deposition in the lungs. This deposition occurs primarily by diffusion and secondarily by thermophoretic effects in the first few airways of the lung during exhalation. Fibers and platelets like graphene that are nanosized in at least one dimension are also deposited in the lower respiratory tract, mainly by interception due to their small size and elongated shape. Once deposited, the physicochemical properties, including surface reactivity and dissolution rates, are the driving forces for toxicity. Often, the toxicity is driven by oxidative stress, leading to inflammatory responses and tissue damage as well as lung cancer including mesothelioma related to persistent fibers. Particles can be translocated to other organs, through the blood, where they can also lead to adverse health outcomes. As much of physics can be captured in mathematical equations and the morphology and the functional parameters can be assessed, computational modeling will allow calculations of the deposited dose in various area of the respiratory tract. One the most advanced models is the Multiple-Path Particle Dosimetry Model (MPPD v3.04) which is freely available (via www.ara.com; Anjilvel and Asgharian 1995, RIVM 2002). The MPPD model is a computational model that can be used for estimating human and rat airway particle dosimetry. The model is applicable to risk assessment, research, and education.

The MPPD model calculates the deposition and clearance of monodisperse and polydisperse aerosols in the respiratory tracts of mice, rats, and human adults and children, among others, for particles ranging in size from 0.01 μm to 20 μm. The models are based on single-path and multiple-path methods for tracking air flow and calculating aerosol deposition in the lung. The single-path method calculates deposition in a typical path per airway generation, while the multiple-path method calculates particle deposition in all airways of the lung and provides lobar-specific and airway-specific information. Within each airway, deposition is calculated using theoretically derived efficiencies for deposition by diffusion, sedimentation, and impaction within the airway or airway bifurcation. Filtration of aerosols by the nose and mouth is determined using empirical efficiency functions. The MPPD model includes calculations of particle clearance in the lung following deposition.

Even though deposition models give a good estimate of the pulmonary deposited dose, it is essential whenever possible to measure directly the amount of nanomaterials deposited into the lung since the toxicological properties of a given nanomaterial cannot be determined from the atmospheric concentration but from the amount of material in contact with target tissues. In addition, it is crucial to evaluate the retention time of the particles into the lung since their toxicity may depend on it.

However, to make sense, it is also essential to know particle solubility, which could be obtained by performing *in vitro* solubilization assay in artificial interstitial fluid (Gamble's solution, pH 7.4) and artificial lysosomal fluid (pH 4.5), for example, to mimic the dissolution events that may occur in contact with lung lining fluid or lysosomal content after phagocytosis by macrophages, respectively. It is also important to confirm by microscopy methods (electronic microscopy, hyperspectral microscopy) that what has been measured is coming from material and not ions; these methods also allow determination of the status of the particle (shape, agglomeration, etc.).

7.4.2 Lung Particle Deposition, Retention, and Clearance

After inhalation, particles with low solubility will deposit throughout the respiratory tract according to their size (ICRP 1994). Once deposited into the lung, different clearance mechanisms may occur: (1) Phagocytosis by alveolar macrophages and migration either to the ciliated airways for clearance through the mucociliary escalator and subsequent swallowing into the gastro-intestinal tract or transported toward the lung-associated lymph nodes; and (2) translocation into the blood stream and accumulation in secondary organs. Efficient phagocytosis of particles by macrophages depends greatly on particle size and surface properties. It has been suggested that particle phagocytosis was inversely proportional to their size; indeed, about 20 percent of the lung deposited 20-nm iridium particles was found associated with alveolar macrophages while this fraction reached 80 percent with polystyrene particles in the micrometric range (Kreyling et al. 2013). This may be explained by the fact that deposited nanoparticles interact with the epithelial lining fluid and then may translocate into the lung interstitium (Ferin et al. 1992) where they are less accessible for macrophage phagocytosis and clearance (Geiser 2010). However, if nanoparticles are inhaled as agglomerates or aggregates with an overall median diameter in the micro-size range, their deposition profile would be similar to that of equivalent spherical particles with the same aerodynamic diameter; in addition, in such a nanostructured form they are easily recognized by macrophages. However, a question remains about the toxicity and the fate of these agglomerates, and it seems that the probability of deagglomeration within the lung fluid is low (Creutzenberg et al. 2012) and the likelihood for primary particles originating from these agglomerates to escape classical clearance pathways is small (Landsiedel et al. 2012). In addition, the pulmonary retention of particles depends on their deposition site: Indeed, if they are deposited in conducting airways (bronchi and bronchioles) they are efficiently cleared through the mucociliary escalator within hours or days and are often swallowed and transferred to the gastro-intestinal tract. However, if they go deeper into the lung and reach gas exchange airways and alveoli, the mucus transport is less efficient and the retention time increased (Kreyling et al. 2013). This is particularly true for particles or agglomerates between 10 and 100 nm (ICRP 1994).

Therefore, decreased phagocytosis and clearance of nanoparticles may lead to long-term toxic effects even though the particles have a low toxic potential.

7.5 PULMONARY TOXICITY OF NANOMATERIALS

7.5.1 Pulmonary Inflammation

Inflammation is a physiological defense mechanism involved in host response against exogenous bodies, including microorganisms and particles. Its purpose is to eliminate the cause of cell injury and initiate the repair process (Wong et al. 2016). Alveolar influx of neutrophilic granulocytes is a hallmark of particle-induced inflammation, which is triggered by the production of pro-inflammatory cytokines and chemokines produced by alveolar macrophages and epithelial cells. Among those, the most prominent initiating cytokines are TNFα and IL-1β, which stimulate their own production but also the synthesis of other chemokines including IL-8, CXCL1 and 2, and CCL2. Inflammation also leads to the production and release of reactive nitrogen species and reactive oxygen species that could damage lung epithelial cells (Folkerts et al. 2001) with physiopathological consequences, such as chronic obstructive pulmonary disease and fibrosis. Exposure to crystalline silica or asbestos has been clearly linked to lung fibrosis (Kawasaki 2015, Sayan and Mossman 2016). Such toxicological properties have also been reported for some carbon nanotubes (Labib et al. 2016, Vietti et al. 2016). Following inhalation of nanomaterials, acute inflammation is a physiological mechanism. However, concerns may arise if the inflammatory response is persistent over time.

7.5.2 GENOTOXICITY

Genotoxicity of nanomaterials may occur through different mechanisms. One of them, called *primary genotoxicity*, is driven either by the direct interaction of particles with DNA, or by their ability to induce the production of cellular reactive oxygen species due to their surface reactivity or the release of pro-oxidant molecules (Pati et al. 2016, Wang et al. 2012, Schins and Knaapen 2007). Another one, called *secondary genotoxicity*, is associated with the production of reactive nitrogen species and reactive oxygen species during prolonged inflammation. *In vivo*, this could be due to the surface reactivity of the particles but also as a result of high pulmonary particle load (Borm et al. 2015, Schins and Knaapen 2007). Nanomaterial-induced genotoxicity has been observed in cell culture as well as in rodents. More data are available from *in vitro* models, which assess mainly primary genotoxicity and seem to be more sensitive than animal models (Magdolenova et al. 2014); however, it is still unclear whether regular genotoxicity assays developed for soluble chemicals are appropriate for nanomaterial testing.

7.5.3 CARCINOGENICITY

Due to a lack of studies, the capability of nanomaterials to induce lung tumors in animal models has been described for only a limited number of them. It has been shown that one type of nanometric titanium dioxide–induced lung tumor in rats but not in mice after inhalation (7.2 mg/m^3 for 4 month [both species], 14.8 mg/m^3 for 4 months [both species], and 9.4 mg/m^3 for 5.5 months [mice], or 16 months [rats]) and intratracheal instillation, but one may discuss whether the toxicity of this titanium dioxide sample is related to the intrinsic properties of the particles or an "overload mechanism" since tumors were observed at relatively high doses (Baan 2007). Similarly, carbon black nanoparticles (Printex 90) induced lung tumors following inhalation in rats but not mice (18 hours/day, 5 days/week, 7.4 mg/m^3 for 4 months followed by 12.2 mg/m^3; IARC 2010). Because of these results and the inadequate evidence of the carcinogenicity these nanomaterials in humans; they were classified by the International Agency for Research on Cancer (IARC) as "possibly carcinogenic for humans" (Group 2B; IARC 2010).

Since carbon nanotubes are high aspect ratio nanomaterials that make them resemble fibers such as asbestos, concerns have been raised regarding their capabilities to induce lung tumors and mesotheliomas (Donaldson et al. 2013). However, until now only two carbon nanotubes have been identified as carcinogenic in rodent models (Kasai et al. 2016, Suzui et al. 2016). Following whole-body inhalation, MWNT-7 induced lung tumors but not mesothelioma in rats in a recently published two-year study (starting at 0.2 mg/m^3; 6 hours/day, 5 days/week for 104 weeks; Kasai et al. 2016). In addition, inhalation of this carbon nanotube (5 mg/m^3, 5 hours/day, 5 days/week for 15 days) promoted mouse lung adenocarcinomas following an initial exposure by intraperitoneal injection to initiator methylcholanthrene (10 μg/g

body weight; Sargent et al. 2014). A second carbon nanotube sample was also shown to induce lung tumors and mesothelioma following intratracheal instillation in rats (cumulative dose of 1 mg/rat; Suzui et al. 2016).

Carbon nanotubes have also been classified by the IARC. It was agreed to classify specifically the MWNT-7 sample as "possibly carcinogenic to humans" (Group 2B). But because of a lack of sufficient data, it was not possible to generalize from one type of carbon nanotubes to the others. Therefore, the other carbon nanotube samples were categorized as "not classifiable as to their carcinogenicity to humans" (Group 3; Grosse et al. 2014).

Carcinogenicity data are only available for few nanomaterials because of the cost and the time needed for such studies. Hence, it is required to develop alternative methods to predict the carcinogenicity of such compounds.

7.6 BIODISTRIBUTION OF INHALED NANOMATERIALS

Depending on their size and state of agglomeration/aggregation, nanoparticles can enter into cells through different endocytic mechanisms including phagocytosis, macropinocytosis, clathrin-dependent and clathrin-independent endocytosis, and caveolae-dependent endocytosis (Yameen et al. 2014). While the four first internalization mechanisms of particles lead to their sequestration into lysosomes, the caveolae-dependent mechanism is believed to allow nanoparticles being distributed within the cell but also crossing the cell by transcytosis (Oh et al. 2007), and consequently passing through air–blood barrier (George et al. 2015, Wang et al. 2011). Particle internalization is highly dependent on their surface properties, such as charge and protein corona, but also their shape and size (Kettler et al. 2014, Bannunah et al. 2014, Chithrani 2010, Zhang et al. 2015). However, since it is often in the literature that the influence of only one parameter on particle uptake is reported, it is still too early to draw conclusions about which properties are influencing their uptake and transport.

Translocation into the blood stream and distribution into extrapulmonary organs have been reported in many studies (Elder et al. 2005, Geraets et al. 2012, Kreyling 2016, Kreyling et al. 2009, Gaté et al. 2017, Czarny et al. 2014). However, the level of translocation appears to be low. In an experiment, where ^{192}Ir nanoparticles with aggregated size of 20 and 80 nm were administered by endotracheal inhalation to rats for one hour, it was observed twenty-four hours after animal exposure that 0.1 to 1 percent of the ^{192}Ir lung-deposited fraction was found in the liver, spleen, kidneys, heart, and brain, and 1 to 5 percent was found in the remaining carcass consisting of soft tissues and bones. In addition, the fraction of 20 nm particles was higher in secondary organs than the larger 80 nm particles, suggesting a possible size-dependent translocation of nanoparticles from the lung to the blood stream (Kreyling et al. 2009). However, this size effect was not observed with ceria particles. Indeed, when rats were exposed by nose-only inhalation for six hours to cerium oxide aerosols composed of particles with a nominal primary size of 5–10 nm, 40 nm, and <5000 nm, but with similar mass median aerodynamic diameter, it was shown that the pulmonary deposited fraction was slightly different for the three samples (about 10 percent of the inhaled dose), but the faction of particles found in secondary organs, including liver, kidneys, spleen, brain, and testis, were similar. The amounts found in extra-pulmonary tissues were also very low (<0.2 percent of inhaled dose; Geraets et al. 2012). Translocation of gold, silver, and cadmium nanoparticles to secondary organs has also been reported, but as for the other studies presented here, the fraction of the pulmonary deposited dose reaching these tissues was really small (less than 0.1%; Takenaka et al. 2006, Takenaka et al. 2004, Takenaka et al. 2001).

These results were obtained in animal models exposed to relatively high amounts of nanomaterials as compared to what would be expected with humans during occu-pational or environmental exposure. Experiments performed with human subjects have shown that inhalation of 35 or 100 nm ^{99m}Tc-labeled carbonaceous particles by healthy subjects may not lead to a significant translocation of nanoparticles to extra-pulmonary organs (Wiebert, Sanchez-Crespo, Falk et al. 2006, Wiebert, Sanchez-Crespo, Seitz et al. 2006).

In addition, Oberdorster et al. (2004) observed a significant increase in ^{13}C con-tent in the olfactory bulb cerebrum and cerebellum of rats exposed for six hours by inhalation to ^{13}C nanoparticles aerosol (count median diameter 36 nm). More recently, in an experiment where rats were exposed for one hour by either nose-only inhalation or endotracheal intubation to a 20 nm-sized, ^{192}Ir radiolabeled iridium nanoparticle aerosol, it was observed that the fraction of ^{192}Ir found in the brain was nine times higher after inhalation than endotracheal intubation which bypassed the upper respiratory tract (Kreyling 2016). These results suggest that the translocation of nanoparticle from the nasal mucosa to the central nervous system is possible and probably occurs through the olfactory and the trigeminal pathways. These paths con-nect directly the nasal mucosa and the brain and thus bypass the blood–brain barrier. Nanoparticles can then pass through the nasal epithelium by the intercellular spaces. Moreover, as mentioned above, nanoparticles may also be transported across the nasal epithelium by transcytosis. After crossing the epithelium, nanoparticles can use nerve pathways to reach deeper regions of the brain (Lochhead and Thorne 2012, Lochhead et al. 2015).

7.7 EXTRAPULMONARY TOXICITY OF NANOMATERIALS

7.7.1 NEUROTOXICITY

The neurological consequences of the nasal passage of nanomaterials to the brain have not been well-studied yet (Heusinkveld et al. 2016). Nanoparticles could also reach the central nervous system by a way other than by the nasal passage. Indeed, once into the blood stream, nanoparticles may come in contact with the blood–brain barrier (BBB). Using *in vitro* models, it was shown that TiO_2 nanoparticles may cross the BBB but also deregulate its permeability as well as its integrity and induce the expression of inflammatory cytokines (Brun et al. 2012). Following intra-venous injection of TiO_2 nanoparticles to rats, such an impact on the blood–brain barrier function was not observed but a brain inflammation was noticed that can be due to the production of cellular mediators (Disdier et al. 2015). The impact of inhaled nanoparticles on the blood–brain barrier are, however, believed to be more subtle since the amount reaching the blood stream will be very low as compared to intravenous injection. Nonetheless, the physiopathological consequences have to be addressed in order to prevent any potential neurodegenerative disease associated with nanomaterial exposure.

7.7.2 REPRODUCTIVE TOXICITY

The contact of nanoparticles with the placenta and their transplacental transport are also of concern (Hougaard et al. 2015). *In vitro* and ex vivo models have shown that nanoparticles, however in small amount, can cross this barrier (Correia Carreira et al. 2015, Myllynen et al. 2008, Poulsen et al. 2015). *In vivo* experiments have also shown that CuO, CdO, and TiO_2 inhaled nanoparticles could induce some significant effects on the fetus as well as the dams. Inhalation by pregnant mice 4 hours/day of a 35-nm aerosol of CuO nanoparticles (3.5 mg/m^3) from gestational day 3 to 19 leads to a significant pulmonary inflammation in dams and a strong immunomodulation in the spleen of pups. However, no increase of Cu was detected in pups (Adamcakova-Dodd et al. 2015). In addition, inhalation by pregnant mice 2.5 hours/day of a 15-nm aerosol of CdO nanoparticles (230 µg/m^3) from postcoitus day 4.5 to 16.5 leads to a decrease of maternal body weight and a delayed weight gain during pregnancy. Such an exposure also alters placental weight and fetal crown to rump length as well as leads to a delayed neonatal growth which is associated with a significant increase of cadmium in neonates tissues (Blum et al. 2012). Inhalation by pregnant Sprague Dawley rats 5 hours/week, 4 days/week of a 171-nm titanium dioxide aerosol (10.4 mg/m^3) from gestational day 7 to 20 leads also to an alteration in behavior and cognitive functions of male offspring measured 5 months after birth (Engler-Chiurazzi et al. 2016). Similar results were observed in mice exposed by inhalation to a 97-nm TiO_2 aerosol (40.2 mg/m^3), 1 hour/day from gestational days 8 to 18 (Hougaard et al. 2010)

7.7.3 CARDIOVASCULAR TOXICITY

Epidemiological and toxicological studies have clearly shown a link between ultra-fine particle airborne pollution and cardiovascular diseases (Simkhovich et al. 2008). Experimental data showing a link between inhaled engineered nanomaterials and cardiovascular dysfunctions are also available, but they are still scarce. Inhalation of nanometric titanium dioxide and multiwalled carbon nanotubes leads to an alteration of the cardiac autonomic neuron activity and consequently heart rate rhythm (Kan et al. 2014, Zheng et al. 2016). Inhalation of nanometric titanium dioxide also induces endothelial dysfunction and alters vasoreactivity (Knuckles et al. 2012, LeBlanc et al. 2010, Nurkiewicz et al. 2008, Nurkiewicz et al. 2009). In addition, inhalation of 80 µg/m^3 for 5 months of nickel hydroxide nanoparticles can also promote atherosclerosis in the susceptible Apo E deficient mouse model (Kang et al. 2011). Similar results were also obtained following intratracheal instillation of carbon black (Niwa et al. 2007).

Thrombogenic effects were also observed in mice following acute inhalation of nanosized carbon black, such as platelet accumulation and fibrinogen deposition in hepatic microvessels (Khandoga et al. 2010).

7.8 FROM EXPERIMENTAL DATA TO OCCUPATIONAL EXPOSURE LIMIT

While intratracheal instillation and short term inhalation studies (up to 28 days) could be used for hazard assessment and toxicity ranking, sub-chronic (90 days), and chronic (2 years) inhalation assays have been of great value for risk assessment and threshold limit value (TLV) determination. To date there is no regulatory occupational exposure limit (OEL) specifically calculated for nanomaterials. The National Institute for Occupational Safety and Health in the United States (NIOSH) has proposed an occupational exposure limit of 0.3 mg/m^3 for respirable nanostructured titanium aerosol (NIOSH 2011). This value was derived from inflammation and carcinogenicity experimental data generated during inhalation studies in rats. Since it seems that rats are more sensitive than humans to pro-inflammatory response induced by a prolonged exposure to inhaled nanomaterials, it could be assumed that rat data already integrate a safety margin. The NIOSH has also observed that the rat is the most appropriated species to perform quantitative risk assessment for titanium dioxide and nanomaterials in general. Despite the scarce data available, it seems that inhalation of particles increases the pulmonary inflammatory response which if persistent may increase the risk of cancer. Of note, the OEL proposed by the NIOSH for nanoparticles is lower than the one for their micrometric counterparts (2.4 mg/m^3). This is linked to the fact that for the same mass, the risk increases with the diminution of the particle size and the increase of their specific surface area. In addition, it is assumed that low doses of particles with low solubility and low toxicity that are not able to trigger sustained inflammation won't be able to induce any lung cancer. This hypothesis reflects in the quantitative risk assessment approach in which the dose/response curve predicts that low exposure doses induced risks considerably lower than those observed with higher doses (NIOSH 2011). Since titanium dioxide belongs to the family of particles with low solubility and low toxicity, it would be worth evaluating whether these OELs could be generalized to the other particulates not otherwise regulated. Based on the same approach, NIOSH has determined a recommended OEL of 1 $\mu g/m^3$ for carbon nanotubes (NIOSH 2013).

7.9 NANOMATERIAL GROUPING

Due to the ever-growing production of new nanomaterials, it is not conceivable, for ethical (animal welfare) as well as economic reasons, to perform *in vivo* and even *in vitro* experiments on all of these compounds to assess their human health effects. It is then crucial to develop new approaches to predict the toxicity of a given nanomaterial from data obtained with other particulate matters. This read-across and grouping methodology recommended by the REACH legislation (ECHA 2013) consists of classifying as a group, chemicals (and nanomaterials) whose physicochemical, toxicological, and ecotoxicological properties are likely to be similar or follow a pattern as a result of structural similarity. The European Centre for Ecotoxicology and Toxicology of Chemicals (ECETOC) Nano Task Force has proposed a decision-making framework for the grouping and testing of nanomaterials (DF4nanoGrouping) to fulfill this goal (Arts et al. 2014, 2015, 2016). Other grouping and read-across approaches have also been described (Braakhuis et al. 2016, Oomen et al. 2015) as well as quantitative structure activity relationship (QSAR) methodologies adapted to nanomaterials (Gajewicz et al. 2015, Tantra et al. 2015).

7.10 CONCLUSIONS

Inhalation studies in rodents are of great value for assessing hazards and risks associated with the exposure to nanostructured aerosols. However, in order to generate exploitable data for legislators and regulators it is important to perform a thorough characterization of the aerosol and whenever possible to make sure it is representative of an occupational or environmental exposure in terms of aerosol size distribution but also concentration. In addition, it is clear that the lung retained dose is far more important than the aerosol concentration in nanomaterial toxicity evaluation. However, the most relevant dose metric is still in debate, but it seems to be in favor of specific surface area, even though others such as particle number, volume, and mass should not be neglected.

Because of the ever-growing production of new nanomaterials, it will not be possible for ethical and economic reasons to perform *in vivo* experiments for each and every one of them. New approaches, including read-across, nanomaterial grouping, and nanoQSAR, are required to tackle this tremendous task. Nonetheless, inhalation studies remain the gold standard in nanomaterial risk assessment and these alternative methods would need to be validated or to take into consideration the experimental data generated from animal studies.

Inhalation studies would remain important in the toxicology field, but the development of these in silico approaches as well as new physiologically relevant cell culture models would help to develop decision trees in order to use *in vivo* models only with the most preoccupying materials.

REFERENCES

Adamcakova-Dodd, A., M. M. Monick, L. S. Powers, K. N. Gibson-Corley, and P. S. Thorne. 2015. Effects of prenatal inhalation exposure to copper nanoparticles on murine dams and offspring. *Part Fibre Toxicol* 12:30. doi: 10.1186/s12989-015-0105-5.

Anjilvel, S., and B. Asgharian. 1995. A multiple-path model of particle deposition in the rat lung. *Fundam Appl Toxicol* 28(1):41–50.

Arts, J. H., M. Hadi, M. A. Irfan, A. M. Keene, R. Kreiling, D. Lyon, M. Maier, K. Michel, T. Petry, U. G. Sauer, D. Warheit, K. Wiench, W. Wohlleben, and R. Landsiedel. 2015. A decision-making framework for the grouping and testing of nanomaterials (DF4nanoGrouping). *Regul Toxicol Pharmacol* 71(2 Suppl):S1–S27. doi: 10.1016/j.yrtph.2015.03.007.

Arts, J. H., M. Hadi, A. M. Keene, R. Kreiling, D. Lyon, M. Maier, K. Michel, T. Petry, U. G. Sauer, D. Warheit, K. Wiench, and R. Landsiedel. 2014. A critical appraisal of existing concepts for the grouping of nanomaterials. *Regul Toxicol Pharmacol* 70(2):492–506. doi: 10.1016/j.yrtph.2014.07.025.

Arts, J. H., M. A. Irfan, A. M. Keene, R. Kreiling, D. Lyon, M. Maier, K. Michel, N. Neubauer, T. Petry, U. G. Sauer, D. Warheit, K. Wiench, W. Wohlleben, and R. Landsiedel. 2016. Case studies putting the decision-making framework for the grouping and testing of nanomaterials (DF4nanoGrouping) into practice. *Regul Toxicol Pharmacol* 76:234–261. doi: 10.1016/j.yrtph.2015.11.020.

Baan, R. A. 2007. Carcinogenic hazards from inhaled carbon black, titanium dioxide, and talc not containing asbestos or asbestiform fibers: Recent evaluations by an IARC Monographs Working Group. *Inhal Toxicol* 19 Suppl 1:213–228. doi: 10.1080/08958370701497903.

Bannunah, A. M., D. Vllasaliu, J. Lord, and S. Stolnik. 2014. Mechanisms of nanoparticle internalization and transport across an intestinal epithelial cell model: Effect of size and surface charge. *Mol Pharm* 11(12):4363–4373. doi: 10.1021/mp500439c.

Blum, J. L., J. Q. Xiong, C. Hoffman, and J. T. Zelikoff. 2012. Cadmium associated with inhaled cadmium oxide nanoparticles impacts fetal and neonatal development and growth. *Toxicol Sci* 126(2):478–486. doi: 10.1093/toxsci/kfs008.

Borm, P., F. R. Cassee, and G. Oberdorster. 2015. Lung particle overload: Old school—New insights? *Part Fibre Toxicol* 12:10. doi: 10.1186/s12989-015-0086-4.

Braakhuis, H. M., A. G. Oomen, and F. R. Cassee. 2016. Grouping nanomaterials to predict their potential to induce pulmonary inflammation. *Toxicol Appl Pharmacol* 299:3–7. doi: 10.1016/j.taap.2015.11.009.

Braakhuis, H. M., M. V. Park, I. Gosens, W. H. De Jong, and F. R. Cassee. 2014. Physicochemical characteristics of nanomaterials that affect pulmonary inflammation. *Part Fibre Toxicol* 11:18. doi: 10.1186/1743-8977-11-18.

Brun, E., M. Carriere, and A. Mabondzo. 2012. In vitro evidence of dysregulation of blood–brain barrier function after acute and repeated/long-term exposure to TiO(2) nanoparticles. *Biomaterials* 33(3):886–896. doi: 10.1016/j.biomaterials.2011.10.025.

Burden, N., K. Aschberger, Q. Chaudhry, M. J. D. Clift, S. H. Doak, P. Fowler, H. Johnston, R. Landsiedel, J. Rowland, and V. Stone. 2017. The 3Rs as a framework to support a 21st century approach for nanosafety assessment. *Nano Today* 12:10–13. doi:10.1016/j.nantod.2016.06.007.

Chithrani, D. B. 2010. Intracellular uptake, transport, and processing of gold nanostructures. *Mol Membr Biol* 27(7):299–311. doi: 10.3109/09687688.2010.507787.

Correia Carreira, S., L. Walker, K. Paul, and M. Saunders. 2015. The toxicity, transport and uptake of nanoparticles in the in vitro BeWo b30 placental cell barrier model used within NanoTEST. *Nanotoxicology* 9 Suppl 1:66–78. doi: 10.3109/17435390.2013.833317.

Cosnier, F., S. Bau, S. Grossmann, H. Nunge, C. Brochard, S. Viton, R. Payet, O. Witschger, and L. Gaté. 2016. Design and characterization of an inhalation system to expose rodents to nanoaerosols. *Aerosol and Air Qual Res* 16:2989–3000. doi: 10.4209/aaqr.2016.01.0034.

Creutzenberg, O., B. Bellmann, R. Korolewitz, W. Koch, I. Mangelsdorf, T. Tillmann, and D. Schaudien. 2012. Change in agglomeration status and toxicokinetic fate of various nanoparticles in vivo following lung exposure in rats. *Inhal Toxicol* 24(12):821–830. doi: 10.3109/08958378.2012.721097.

Curwin, B., and S. Bertke. 2011. Exposure characterization of metal oxide nanoparticles in the workplace. *Journal of Occupational and Environmental Hygiene* 8(10):580–587.

Czarny, B., D. Georgin, F. Berthon, G. Plastow, M. Pinault, G. Patriarche, A. Thuleau, M. M. L'Hermite, F. Taran, and V. Dive. 2014. Carbon nanotube translocation to distant organs after pulmonary exposure: Insights from in situ (14)C-radiolabeling and tissue radioimaging. *ACS Nano* 8(6):5715–5724. doi: 10.1021/nn500475u.

Disdier, C., J. Devoy, A. Cosnefroy, M. Chalansonnet, N. Herlin-Boime, E. Brun, A. Lund, and A. Mabondzo. 2015. Tissue biodistribution of intravenously administrated titanium dioxide nanoparticles revealed blood-brain barrier clearance and brain inflammation in rat. *Part Fibre Toxicol* 12:27. doi: 10.1186/s12989-015-0102-8.

Donaldson, K., C. A. Poland, F. A. Murphy, M. MacFarlane, T. Chernova, and A. Schinwald. 2013. Pulmonary toxicity of carbon nanotubes and asbestos—Similarities and differences. *Adv Drug Deliv Rev* 65(15):2078–2086. doi: 10.1016/j.addr.2013.07.014.

Driscoll, K. E., D. L. Costa, G. Hatch, R. Henderson, G. Oberdorster, H. Salem, and R. B. Schlesinger. 2000. Intratracheal instillation as an exposure technique for the evaluation of respiratory tract toxicity: Uses and limitations. *Toxicol Sci* 55(1):24–35.

ECHA. 2013 (April). Grouping of substances and read-across approach. Part I. Introductory note. European Chemicals Agency, ECHA-13-R-02-EN, p. 11.

Elder, A., R. Gelein, J. N. Finkelstein, K. E. Driscoll, J. Harkema, and G. Oberdorster. 2005. Effects of subchronically inhaled carbon black in three species. I. Retention kinetics, lung inflammation, and histopathology. *Toxicol Sci* 88(2):614–629.

Engler-Chiurazzi, E. B., P. A. Stapleton, J. J. Stalnaker, X. Ren, H. Hu, T. R. Nurkiewicz, C. R. McBride, J. Yi, K. Engels, and J. W. Simpkins. 2016. Impacts of prenatal nanomaterial exposure on male adult Sprague-Dawley rat behavior and cognition. *J Toxicol Environ Health A* 79(11):447–452. doi: 10.1080/15287394.2016.1164101.

EU. 2010. Directive 2010/63/EU of the European Parliament and of the Council of 22 September 2010 on the protection of animals used for scientific purposes.

Ferin, J., G. Oberdorster, and D. P. Penney. 1992. Pulmonary retention of ultrafine and fine particles in rats. *Am J Respir Cell Mol Biol* 6(5):535–542.

Folkerts, G., J. Kloek, R. B. Muijsers, and F. P. Nijkamp. 2001. Reactive nitrogen and oxygen species in airway inflammation. *Eur J Pharmacol* 429(1–3):251–262.

Fujita, K., Y. Morimoto, A. Ogami, T. Myojyo, I. Tanaka, M. Shimada, W. N. Wang, S. Endoh, K. Uchida, T. Nakazato, K. Yamamoto, H. Fukui, M. Horie, Y. Yoshida, H. Iwahashi, and J. Nakanishi. 2009. Gene expression profiles in rat lung after inhalation exposure to C(60) fullerene particles. *Toxicology* 258(1):47–55.

Gajewicz, A., N. Schaeublin, B. Rasulev, S. Hussain, D. Leszczynska, T. Puzyn, and J. Leszczynski. 2015. Towards understanding mechanisms governing cytotoxicity of metal oxides nanoparticles: Hints from nano-QSAR studies. *Nanotoxicology* 9(3):313–325. doi: 10.3109/17435390.2014.930195.

Gaté, L., C. Disdier, F. Cosnier, F. Gagnaire, J. Devoy, W. Saba, E. Brun, M. Chalansonnet, and A. Mabondzo. 2017. Biopersistence and translocation to extrapulmonary organs of titanium dioxide nanoparticles after subacute inhalation exposure to aerosol in adult and elderly rats. *Toxicology Lett* 265:61–69. doi: 10.1016/j.toxlet.2016.11.009.

Geiser, M. 2010. Update on macrophage clearance of inhaled micro- and nanoparticles. *J Aerosol Med Pulm Drug Deliv* 23(4):207–217. doi: 10.1089/jamp.2009.0797.

Geiser, M., B. Rothen-Rutishauser, N. Kapp, S. Schurch, W. Kreyling, H. Schulz, M. Semmler, V. Im Hof, J. Heyder, and P. Gehr. 2005. Ultrafine particles cross cellular membranes by nonphagocytic mechanisms in lungs and in cultured cells. *Environ Health Perspect* 113(11):1555–1560.

George, I., G. Naudin, S. Boland, S. Mornet, V. Contremoulins, K. Beugnon, L. Martinon, O. Lambert, and A. Baeza-Squiban. 2015. Metallic oxide nanoparticle translocation across the human bronchial epithelial barrier. *Nanoscale* 7(10):4529–4544. doi: 10.1039/c4nr07079h.

Geraets, L., A. G. Oomen, J. D. Schroeter, V. A. Coleman, and F. R. Cassee. 2012. Tissue distribution of inhaled micro- and nano-sized cerium oxide particles in rats: Results from a 28-day exposure study. *Toxicol Sci* 127(2):463–473. doi: 10.1093/toxsci/kfs113.

Griffis, L. C., R. E. Wolff, R. L. Beethe, C. H. Hobbs, and R. O. McClellan. 1979. Pulmonary deposition of a 99mTc labeled aerosol in a whole-body exposure, in *Inhalation Toxicology Research Institute Annual Report*, pp. 259–266. Albuquerque, NM: Lovelace Biomedical Environmental Research Institute.

Grosse, Y., D. Loomis, K. Z. Guyton, B. Lauby-Secretan, F. El Ghissassi, V. Bouvard, L. Benbrahim-Tallaa, N. Guha, C. Scoccianti, H. Mattock, and K. Straif. 2014. Carcinogenicity of fluoro-edenite, silicon carbide fibres and whiskers, and carbon nanotubes. *Lancet Oncol* 15(13):1427–1428. doi: 10.1016/S1470-2045(14)71109-X.

Heusinkveld, H. J., T. Wahle, A. Campbell, R. H. Westerink, L. Tran, H. Johnston, V. Stone, F. R. Cassee, and R. P. Schins. 2016. Neurodegenerative and neurological disorders by small inhaled particles. *Neurotoxicology* 56:94–106. doi: 10.1016/j.neuro.2016.07.007.

Hougaard, K. S., L. Campagnolo, P. Chavatte-Palmer, A. Tarrade, D. Rousseau-Ralliard, S. Valentino, M. V. Park, W. H. de Jong, G. Wolterink, A. H. Piersma, B. L. Ross, G. R. Hutchison, J. S. Hansen, U. Vogel, P. Jackson, R. Slama, A. Pietroiusti, and F. R. Cassee. 2015. A perspective on the developmental toxicity of inhaled nanoparticles. *Reprod Toxicol* 56:118–140. doi: 10.1016/j.reprotox.2015.05.015.

Hougaard, K. S., P. Jackson, K. A. Jensen, J. J. Sloth, K. Loschner, E. H. Larsen, R. K. Birkedal, A. Vibenholt, A. M. Boisen, H. Wallin, and U. Vogel. 2010. Effects of prenatal exposure to surface-coated nanosized titanium dioxide (UV-Titan). A study in mice. *Part Fibre Toxicol* 7:16. doi: 10.1186/1743-8977-7-16.

Hoymann, H. G. 2012. Lung function measurements in rodents in safety pharmacology studies. *Front Pharmacol* 3:156. doi: 10.3389/fphar.2012.00156.

IARC. 2010. ARC Monographs on the Evaluation of Carcinogenic Risks to Humans. Carbon Black, Titanium Dioxide, and Talc, 93.

ICRP. 1994. ICRP Publication 66: Human respiratory tract model for radiobiological protection. *Ann ICRP* 24(1–3):482.

Iskandar, F., L. Gradon, and K. Okuyama. 2003. Control of the morphology of nanostructured particles prepared by the spray drying of a nanoparticle sol. *J Colloid Interface Sci* 265:296–303.

ISO. 2012. ISO/TR 13014 (2012). Nanotechnologies—Guidance on physicochemical characterization of engineered nanoscale materials for toxicologic assessment.

ISO. 2013. ISO/TS 17200 (2013). Nanotechnology—Nanoparticles in powder form—Characteristics and measurements.

ISO. 2016. ISO/TC 229—Nanotechnologies. Accessed from http://www.iso.org/iso/fr/home/store /catalogue_tc/catalogue_tc_browse.htm?commid=381983&published=on&includesc=true.

Ji, J. H., J. H. Jung, S. S. Kim, J. U. Yoon, J. D. Park, B. S. Choi, Y. H. Chung, I. H. Kwon, J. Jeong, B. S. Han, J. H. Shin, J. H. Sung, K. S. Song, and I. J. Yu. 2007. Twenty-eight-day inhalation toxicity study of silver nanoparticles in Sprague-Dawley rats. *Inhal Toxicol* 19(10):857–871.

Kan, H., Z. Wu, Y. C. Lin, T. H. Chen, J. L. Cumpston, M. L. Kashon, S. Leonard, A. E. Munson, and V. Castranova. 2014. The role of nodose ganglia in the regulation of cardiovascular function following pulmonary exposure to ultrafine titanium dioxide. *Nanotoxicology* 8(4):447–454. doi: 10.3109/17435390.2013.796536.

Kang, G. S., P. A. Gillespie, A. Gunnison, A. L. Moreira, K. M. Tchou-Wong, and L. C. Chen. 2011. Long-term inhalation exposure to nickel nanoparticles exacerbated atherosclerosis in a susceptible mouse model. *Environ Health Perspect* 119(2):176–81. doi:10.1289/ehp.1002508.

Kasai, T., Y. Umeda, M. Ohnishi, T. Mine, H. Kondo, T. Takeuchi, M. Matsumoto, and S. Fukushima. 2016. Lung carcinogenicity of inhaled multi-walled carbon nanotube in rats. *Part Fibre Toxicol* 13(1):53. doi: 10.1186/s12989-016-0164-2.

Kawasaki, H. 2015. A mechanistic review of silica-induced inhalation toxicity. *Inhal Toxicol* 27(8):363–377. doi: 10.3109/08958378.2015.1066905.

Kettler, K., K. Veltman, D. van de Meent, A. van Wezel, and A. J. Hendriks. 2014. Cellular uptake of nanoparticles as determined by particle properties, experimental conditions, and cell type. *Environ Toxicol Chem* 33(3):481–492. doi: 10.1002/etc.2470.

Khandoga, A., T. Stoeger, A. G. Khandoga, P. Bihari, E. Karg, D. Ettehadieh, S. Lakatos, J. Fent, H. Schulz, and F. Krombach. 2010. Platelet adhesion and fibrinogen deposition in murine microvessels upon inhalation of nanosized carbon particles. *J Thromb Haemost JTH* 8(7):1632–1640.

Kim, S. C., D.-R. Chen, C. Qi, R. M. Gelein, J. N. Finkelstein, A. Elder, K. Bentley, G. Oberdörster, and D. Y. H. Pui. 2010. A nanoparticle dispersion method for in vitro and in vivo nanotoxicity study. *Nanotoxicology* 4(1):42–51.

Knuckles, T. L., J. Yi, D. G. Frazer, H. D. Leonard, B. T. Chen, V. Castranova, and T. R. Nurkiewicz. 2012. Nanoparticle inhalation alters systemic arteriolar vasoreactivity through sympathetic and cyclooxygenase-mediated pathways. *Nanotoxicology* 6(7):724–735. doi: 10.3109/17435390.2011.606926.

Kreyling, W. G. 2016. Discovery of unique and ENM- specific pathophysiologic pathways: Comparison of the translocation of inhaled iridium nanoparticles from nasal epithelium versus alveolar epithelium towards the brain of rats. *Toxicol Appl Pharmacol* 299:41–46. doi: 10.1016/j.taap.2016.02.004.

Kreyling, W. G., M. Semmler-Behnke, J. Seitz, W. Scymczak, A. Wenk, P. Mayer, S. Takenaka, and G. Oberdorster. 2009. Size dependence of the translocation of inhaled iridium and carbon nanoparticle aggregates from the lung of rats to the blood and secondary target organs. *Inhal Toxicol* 21 Suppl 1:55–60. doi: 10.1080/08958370902942517.

Kreyling, W. G., M. Semmler-Behnke, S. Takenaka, and W. Moller. 2013. Differences in the biokinetics of inhaled nano- versus micrometer-sized particles. *Acc Chem Res* 46(3):714–722. doi: 10.1021/ar300043r.

Kreyling, W. G., M. Semmler, F. Erbe, P. Mayer, S. Takenaka, H. Schulz, G. Oberdörster, and A. Ziesenis. 2002. Translocation of ultrafine insoluble iridium particles from lung epithelium to extrapulmonary organs is size dependent but very low. *J Toxicol Environ Health A* 65(20):1513–1530. doi: 10.1080/00984100290071649.

Kulkarni, P., P. A. Baron, and K. Willeke. 2011. *Aerosol Measurement: Principles, Techniques, and Applications.* Hoboken, NJ: John Wiley & Sons.

Kwon, J. T., S. K. Hwang, H. Jin, D. S. Kim, A. Minai-Tehrani, H. J. Yoon, M. Choi, T. J. Yoon, D. Y. Han, Y. W. Kang, B. I. Yoon, J. K. Lee, and M. H. Cho. 2008. Body distribution of inhaled fluorescent magnetic nanoparticles in the mice. *J Occup Health* 50 (1):1–6.

Labib, S., A. Williams, C. L. Yauk, J. K. Nikota, H. Wallin, U. Vogel, and S. Halappanavar. 2016. Nano-risk science: Application of toxicogenomics in an adverse outcome pathway framework for risk assessment of multi-walled carbon nanotubes. *Part Fibre Toxicol* 13:15. doi: 10.1186/s12989-016-0125-9.

Landsiedel, R., E. Fabian, L. Ma-Hock, B. van Ravenzwaay, W. Wohlleben, K. Wiench, and F. Oesch. 2012. Toxico-/biokinetics of nanomaterials. *Arch Toxicol* 86(7):1021–1060. doi: 10.1007/s00204-012-0858-7.

LeBlanc, A. J., A. M. Moseley, B. T. Chen, D. Frazer, V. Castranova, and T. R. Nurkiewicz. 2010. Nanoparticle inhalation impairs coronary microvascular reactivity via a local reactive oxygen species-dependent mechanism. *Cardiovasc Toxicol* 10(1):27–36. doi: 10.1007/s12012-009-9060-4.

Li, J. G., W. X. Li, J. Y. Xu, X. Q. Cai, R. L. Liu, Y. J. Li, Q. F. Zhao, and Q. N. Li. 2007. Comparative study of pathological lesions induced by multiwalled carbon nanotubes in lungs of mice by intratracheal instillation and inhalation. *Environ Toxicol* 22(4):415–421.

Lochhead, J. J., and R. G. Thorne. 2012. Intranasal delivery of biologics to the central nervous system. *Adv Drug Deliv Rev* 64(7):614–628. doi: 10.1016/j.addr.2011.11.002.

Lochhead, J. J., D. J. Wolak, M. E. Pizzo, and R. G. Thorne. 2015. Rapid transport within cerebral perivascular spaces underlies widespread tracer distribution in the brain after intranasal administration. *J Cereb Blood Flow Metab* 35(3):371–381. doi: 10.1038/jcbfm.2014.215.

Ma-Hock, L., A. O. Gamer, R. Landsiedel, E. Leibold, T. Frechen, B. Sens, M. Linsenbuehler, and B. van Ravenzwaay. 2007. Generation and characterization of test atmospheres with nanomaterials. *Inhal Toxicol* 19(10):833–848.

Magdolenova, Z., A. Collins, A. Kumar, A. Dhawan, V. Stone, and M. Dusinska. 2014. Mechanisms of genotoxicity. A review of in vitro and in vivo studies with engineered nanoparticles. *Nanotoxicology* 8(3):233–278. doi: 10.3109/17435390.2013.773464.

McKinney, W., B. Chen, and D. Frazer. 2009. Computer controlled multi-walled carbon nanotube inhalation exposure system. *Inhal Toxicol* 21(12):1053–1061. doi: 10.1080/08958370802712713.

Messing, M. E., R. Westerström, B. O. Meuller, S. Blomberg, J. Gustafson, J. N. Andersen, E. Lundgren, R. van Rijn, O. Balmes, H. Bluhm, and K. Deppert. 2010. Generation of pd model catalyst nanoparticles by spark discharge. *J Phys Chem C* 114(20):9257–9263. doi: 10.1021/jp101390a.

Mitchell, L. A., J. Gao, R. V. Wal, A. Gigliotti, S. W. Burchiel, and J. D. McDonald. 2007. Pulmonary and systemic immune response to inhaled multiwalled carbon nanotubes. *Toxicol Sci* 100(1):203–214. doi: 10.1093/toxsci/kfm196.

Morimoto, Y., M. Horie, N. Kobayashi, N. Shinohara, and M. Shimada. 2013. Inhalation toxicity assessment of carbon-based nanoparticles. *Acc Chem Res* 46(3):770–781. doi: 10.1021/ar200311b.

Myllynen, P. K., M. J. Loughran, C. V. Howard, R. Sormunen, A. A. Walsh, and K. H. Vahakangas. 2008. Kinetics of gold nanoparticles in the human placenta. *Reprod Toxicol* 26(2):130–137. doi: 10.1016/j.reprotox.2008.06.008.

Narciso, S. P., E. Nadziejko, L. C. Chen, T. Gordon, and C. Nadziejko. 2003. Adaptation to stress induced by restraining rats and mice in nose-only inhalation holders. *Inhal Toxicol* 15(11):1133–1143. doi: 10.1080/08958370390228592.

NIOSH. 2011. Current Intelligence Bulletin 63: Occupational Exposure to Titanium Dioxide.

NIOSH. 2013. Current Intelligence Bulletin 65: Occupational Exposure to Carbon Nanotubes and Nanofibers.

Niwa, Y., Y. Hiura, T. Murayama, M. Yokode, and N. Iwai. 2007. Nano-sized carbon black exposure exacerbates atherosclerosis in LDL-receptor knockout mice. *Circ J* 71(7):1157–1161.

Noel, A., M. Charbonneau, Y. Cloutier, R. Tardif, and G. Truchon. 2013. Rat pulmonary responses to inhaled nano-TiO(2): Effect of primary particle size and agglomeration state. *Part Fibre Toxicol* 10:48. doi: 10.1186/1743-8977-10-48.

Noel, A., Y. Cloutier, K. J. Wilkinson, C. Dion, S. Halle, K. Maghni, R. Tardif, and G. Truchon. 2013. Generating nano-aerosols from TiO(2) (5 nm) nanoparticles showing different agglomeration states. Application to toxicological studies. *J Occup Environ Hyg* 10(2):86–96. doi: 10.1080/15459624.2012.748340.

Nurkiewicz, T. R., D. W. Porter, A. F. Hubbs, J. L. Cumpston, B. T. Chen, D. G. Frazer, and V. Castranova. 2008. Nanoparticle inhalation augments particle-dependent systemic microvascular dysfunction. *Part Fibre Toxicol* 5:1. doi: 10.1186/1743-8977-5-1.

Nurkiewicz, T. R., D. W. Porter, A. F. Hubbs, S. Stone, B. T. Chen, D. G. Frazer, M. A. Boegehold, and V. Castranova. 2009. Pulmonary nanoparticle exposure disrupts systemic microvascular nitric oxide signaling. *Toxicol Sci* 110(1):191–203. doi: 10.1093/toxsci/kfp051.

Oberdorster, G., E. Oberdorster, and J. Oberdorster. 2005. Nanotoxicology: An emerging discipline evolving from studies of ultrafine particles. *Environ Health Perspect* 113(7):823–839.

Oberdorster, G., Z. Sharp, V. Atudorei, A. Elder, R. Gelein, W. Kreyling, and C. Cox. 2004. Translocation of inhaled ultrafine particles to the brain. *Inhal Toxicol* 16(6–7):437–445. doi: 10.1080/08958370490439597.

OECD. 2009a. OECD Guidelines for the Testing of Chemicals. Test No. 412: Subacute Inhalation Toxicity: 28-Day Study.

OECD. 2009b. OECD Guidelines for the Testing of Chemicals. Test No. 413: Subchronic Inhalation Toxicity: 90-day Study.

OECD. 2016a. Physical-chemical parameters: Measurements and methods relevant for the regulation of nanomaterials, OECD Workshop Report. Series on the Safety of Manufactured Nanomaterials No. 63.

OECD. 2016b. Publications in the Series on the Safety of Manufactured Nanomaterials. Accessed from http://www.oecd.org/env/ehs/nanosafety/publications-series-safety-manu factured-nanomaterials.htm.

Oh, P., P. Borgstrom, H. Witkiewicz, Y. Li, B. J. Borgstrom, A. Chrastina, K. Iwata, K. R. Zinn, R. Baldwin, J. E. Testa, and J. E. Schnitzer. 2007. Live dynamic imaging of caveolae pumping targeted antibody rapidly and specifically across endothelium in the lung. *Nat Biotechnol* 25(3):327–337. doi: 10.1038/nbt1292.

Oomen, A. G., E. A. Bleeker, P. M. Bos, F. van Broekhuizen, S. Gottardo, M. Groenewold, D. Hristozov, K. Hund-Rinke, M. A. Irfan, A. Marcomini, W. J. Peijnenburg, K. Rasmussen, A. S. Jimenez, J. J. Scott-Fordsmand, M. van Tongeren, K. Wiench, W. Wohlleben, and R. Landsiedel. 2015. Grouping and read-across approaches for risk assessment of nanomaterials. *Int J Environ Res Public Health* 12(10):13415–13434. doi: 10.3390/ijerph121013415.

Ostraat, M. L., K. A. Swain, and J. J. Krajewski. 2008. SiO$_2$ aerosol nanoparticle reactor for occupational health and safety studies. *J Occup Environ Hyg* 5(6):390–398.

Pati, R., I. Das, R. K. Mehta, R. Sahu, and A. Sonawane. 2016. Zinc-oxide nanoparticles exhibit genotoxic, clastogenic, cytotoxic, and actin depolymerization effects by inducing oxidative stress responses in macrophages and adult mice. *Toxicol Sci* 150(2):454–472. doi: 10.1093/toxsci/kfw010.

Pauluhn, J. 2009. Pulmonary toxicity and fate of agglomerated 10 and 40 nm aluminum oxy-hydroxides following 4-week inhalation exposure of rats: Toxic effects are determined by agglomerated, not primary particle size. *Toxicol Sci* 109(1):152–167.

Pelclova, D., V. Zdimal, Z. Fenclova, S. Vlckova, F. Turci, I. Corazzari, P. Kacer, J. Schwarz, N. Zikova, O. Makes, K. Syslova, M. Komarc, J. Belacek, T. Navratil, M. Machajova, and S. Zakharov. 2016. Markers of oxidative damage of nucleic acids and proteins among workers exposed to TiO2 (nano) particles. *Occup Environ Med* 73(2):110–118. doi: 10.1136/oemed-2015-103161.

Phalen, R. F. 2009. *Inhalation studies: Foundations and Techniques*, 2nd ed. London: Informa Healthcare.

Porter, D. W., A. F. Hubbs, B. T. Chen, W. McKinney, R. R. Mercer, M. G. Wolfarth, L. Battelli, N. Wu, K. Sriram, S. Leonard, M. Andrew, P. Willard, S. Tsuruoka, M. Endo, T. Tsukada, F. Munekane, D. G. Frazer, and V. Castranova. 2013. Acute pulmonary dose-responses to inhaled multi-walled carbon nanotubes. *Nanotoxicology* 7(7):1179–1194. doi: 10.3109/17435390.2012.719649.

Poulsen, M. S., T. Mose, L. L. Maroun, L. Mathiesen, L. E. Knudsen, and E. Rytting. 2015. Kinetics of silica nanoparticles in the human placenta. *Nanotoxicology* 9 Suppl 1:79–86. doi: 10.3109/17435390.2013.812259.

Rickard, A. J., and M. J. Young. 2009. Corticosteroid receptors, macrophages and cardiovascular disease. *J Mol Endocrinol* 42(6):449–459. doi: 10.1677/JME-08-0144.

RIVM. 2002. National Institute for Public Health and the Environment (RIVM). Multiple Path Particle Dosimetry Model (MPPD v 1.0): A Model for Human and Rat Airway Particle Dosimetry. RIVA Report 650010030.

Russell, W. M. S., and R. L. Burch. 1959. *The Principles of Humane Experimental Technique.* London: Methuen.

Sargent, L. M., D. W. Porter, L. M. Staska, A. F. Hubbs, D. T. Lowry, L. Battelli, K. J. Siegrist, M. L. Kashon, R. R. Mercer, A. K. Bauer, B. T. Chen, J. L. Salisbury, D. Frazer, W. McKinney, M. Andrew, S. Tsuruoka, M. Endo, K. L. Fluharty, V. Castranova, and S. H. Reynolds. 2014. Promotion of lung adenocarcinoma following inhalation exposure to multi-walled carbon nanotubes. *Part Fibre Toxicol* 11:3. doi: 10.1186/1743-8977-11-3.

Sayan, M., and B. T. Mossman. 2016. The NLRP3 inflammasome in pathogenic particle and fibre-associated lung inflammation and diseases. *Part Fibre Toxicol* 13(1):51. doi: 10.1186/s12989-016-0162-4.

Scherer, I. J., P. V. Holmes, and R. B. Harris. 2011. The importance of corticosterone in mediating restraint-induced weight loss in rats. *Physiol Behav* 102(2):225–233. doi: 10.1016/j.physbeh.2010.11.014.

Schins, R. P., and A. M. Knaapen. 2007. Genotoxicity of poorly soluble particles. *Inhal Toxicol* 19 Suppl 1:189–198. doi: 10.1080/08958370701496202.

Schmid, O., and T. Stoeger. 2016. Surface area is the biologically most effective dose metric for acute nanoparticle toxicity in the lung. *J Aerosol Sci* 99:133–143.

Simkhovich, B. Z., M. T. Kleinman, and R. A. Kloner. 2008. Air pollution and cardiovascular injury epidemiology, toxicology, and mechanisms. *J Am Coll Cardiol* 52(9):719–726. doi: 10.1016/j.jacc.2008.05.029.

Stoeger, T., C. Reinhard, S. Takenaka, A. Schroeppel, E. Karg, B. Ritter, J. Heyder, and H. Schulz. 2006. Instillation of six different ultrafine carbon particles indicates a surface area threshold dose for acute lung inflammation in mice. *Environ Health Perspect* 114(3):328–333.

Sung, J. H., J. H. Ji, J. U. Yoon, D. S. Kim, M. Y. Song, J. Jeong, B. S. Han, J. H. Han, Y. H. Chung, J. Kim, T. S. Kim, H. K. Chang, E. J. Lee, J. H. Lee, and I. J. Yu. 2008. Lung function changes in Sprague-Dawley rats after prolonged inhalation exposure to silver nanoparticles. *Inhal Toxicol* 20(6):567–574.

Suzui, M., M. Futakuchi, K. Fukamachi, T. Numano, M. Abdelgied, S. Takahashi, M. Ohnishi, T. Omori, S. Tsuruoka, A. Hirose, J. Kanno, Y. Sakamoto, D. B. Alexander, W. T. Alexander, X. Jiegou, and H. Tsuda. 2016. Multiwalled carbon nanotubes intratracheally instilled into the rat lung induce development of pleural malignant mesothelioma and lung tumors. *Cancer Sci* 107(7):924–935. doi: 10.1111/cas.12954.

Takenaka, S., E. Karg, W. G. Kreyling, B. Lentner, W. Moller, M. Behnke-Semmler, L. Jennen, A. Walch, B. Michalke, P. Schramel, J. Heyder, and H. Schulz. 2006. Distribution pattern of inhaled ultrafine gold particles in the rat lung. *Inhal Toxicol* 18(10):733–740. doi: 10.1080/08958370600748281.

Takenaka, S., E. Karg, W. G. Kreyling, B. Lentner, H. Schulz, A. Ziesenis, P. Schramel, and J. Heyder. 2004. Fate and toxic effects of inhaled ultrafine cadmium oxide particles in the rat lung. *Inhal Toxicol* 16 Suppl 1:83–92. doi: 10.1080/08958370490443141.

Takenaka, S., E. Karg, C. Roth, H. Schulz, A. Ziesenis, U. Heinzmann, P. Schramel, and J. Heyder. 2001. Pulmonary and systemic distribution of inhaled ultrafine silver particles in rats. *Environ Health Perspect* 109 Suppl 4:547–551.

Tantra, R., C. Oksel, T. Puzyn, J. Wang, K. N. Robinson, X. Z. Wang, C. Y. Ma, and T. Wilkins. 2015. Nano(Q)SAR: Challenges, pitfalls and perspectives. *Nanotoxicology* 9(5):636–642. doi: 10.3109/17435390.2014.952698.

Valverde, J. M., and A. Castellanos. 2007. Fluidization, bubbling and jamming of nanoparticle agglomerates. *Chem Eng Sci* 62(23):6947–6956.

Vance, M. E., T. Kuiken, E. P. Vejerano, S. P. McGinnis, M. F. Hochella, Jr., D. Rejeski, and M. S. Hull. 2015. Nanotechnology in the real world: Redeveloping the nanomaterial consumer products inventory. *Beilstein J Nanotechnol* 6:1769–1780. doi: 10.3762/bjnano.6.181.

Vietti, G., D. Lison, and S. van den Brule. 2016. Mechanisms of lung fibrosis induced by carbon nanotubes: Towards an Adverse Outcome Pathway (AOP). *Part Fibre Toxicol* 13:11. doi: 10.1186/s12989-016-0123-y.

Wang, Z., N. Li, J. Zhao, J. C. White, P. Qu, and B. Xing. 2012. CuO nanoparticle interaction with human epithelial cells: Cellular uptake, location, export, and genotoxicity. *Chem Res Toxicol* 25(7):1512–1521. doi: 10.1021/tx3002093.

Wang, Z., C. Tiruppathi, J. Cho, R. D. Minshall, and A. B. Malik. 2011. Delivery of nanoparticle: Complexed drugs across the vascular endothelial barrier via caveolae. *IUBMB Life* 63(8):659–667. doi: 10.1002/iub.485.

Wiebert, P., A. Sanchez-Crespo, R. Falk, K. Philipson, A. Lundin, S. Larsson, W. Moller, W. G. Kreyling, and M. Svartengren. 2006. No significant translocation of inhaled 35-nm carbon particles to the circulation in humans. *Inhal Toxicol* 18(10):741–747. doi: 10.1080/08958370600748455.

Wiebert, P., A. Sanchez-Crespo, J. Seitz, R. Falk, K. Philipson, W. G. Kreyling, W. Moller, K. Sommerer, S. Larsson, and M. Svartengren. 2006. Negligible clearance of ultrafine particles retained in healthy and affected human lungs. *Eur Respir J* 28(2):286–290. doi: 10.1183/09031936.06.00103805.

Wong, J., B. E. Magun, and L. J. Wood. 2016. Lung inflammation caused by inhaled toxicants: A review. *Int J Chron Obstruct Pulmon Dis* 11:1391–1401. doi: 10.2147/COPD.S106009.

Yameen, B., W. I. Choi, C. Vilos, A. Swami, J. Shi, and O. C. Farokhzad. 2014. Insight into nanoparticle cellular uptake and intracellular targeting. *J Control Release* 190:485–499. doi: 10.1016/j.jconrel.2014.06.038.

Zhang, S., H. Gao, and G. Bao. 2015. Physical principles of nanoparticle cellular endocytosis. *ACS Nano* 9(9):8655–8671. doi: 10.1021/acsnano.5b03184.

Zheng, W., W. McKinney, M. Kashon, R. Salmen, V. Castranova, and H. Kan. 2016. The influence of inhaled multi-walled carbon nanotubes on the autonomic nervous system. *Part Fibre Toxicol* 13:8. doi: 10.1186/s12989-016-0119-7.

Zhou, Y. M., C. Y. Zhong, I. M. Kennedy, and K. E. Pinkerton. 2003. Pulmonary responses of acute exposure to ultrafine iron particles in healthy adult rats. *Environ Toxicol* 18(4):227–235.

8 *In Vivo* Evaluation of the Hepatonephrotoxicity of Polymeric Nanoparticles in Rats

Mosaad A. Abdel-Wahhab, Olivier Joubert,
Aziza A. El-Nekeety, Khaled G. Abdel-Wahhab,
Carole Ronzani, Ramia Safar, Ahmed A. El-Kady,
Nabila S. Hassan, Fathia A. Mannaa,
and Bertrand Henri Rihn

CONTENTS

8.1 INTRODUCTION

During the last two decades, considerable attention has been given to the development of a novel drug delivery system (Tamizhrasi et al. 2009). A novel method applicable to synthesize water-soluble drugs in the form of nanoparticles (NPs) is reported, since NPs made of drugs below 100 nm in size enhances the transport properties across biological cell membranes to reach a target site (Ravikumar et al. 2010). The toxicity of NPs depends greatly, however, upon the particular arrangement of their many atoms. Considering all the possible variations in shape and chemistry of even the smallest NPs, with only tens of atoms, yields a huge number of distinct materials with potentially very different physical and toxological properties (Buzea et al. 2007).

Eudragit® is a well-known pharmaceutical excipient and has been widely used for the formation of different sustained and controlled release formations (Jose et al. 2011). Different techniques used for the preparation of enteric nanoparticles include aerosol flow reactor method (Raula et al. 2004), emulsification diffusion method (Dai et al. 2004), self-organized method (Palena et al. 2012), and oil-in-oil emulsification method (Oliveira et al. 2009). There are also several methods for the preparation of enteric-coated NPs, such as electrospray deposition and emulsification methods (Zhang et al. 2011). Eudragit® nanoparticles (ENPs) prepared by nanoprecipitation or by double emulsion techniques containing ibuprofen and cyclosporine (Pignatello et al. 2002), indomethacin (Bhardwaj et al. 2010), melatonin (Schaffazick et al. 2008), DNA plasmid (Gargouri et al. 2009), or molecular weight heparin (LMWH; Jiao et al. 2002) have been obtained and suggested for therapeutic usage. However, Eidi et al. (2010) reported that unloaded Eudragit® RS (ERS) nanoparticles, at concentrations of 25–400 µg/mL showed cytotoxic effects on the rat monocyte cell line. Hoffart et al. (2006) reported that NPs reach the blood stream after oral administration and Hasovits and Clarke (2012) reported that the intraperitoneal route is widely used for chemotherapy in patients with gastrointestinal and gynecological cancers. Consequently, the current study was preformed to evaluate whether empty Eudragit® RL nanoparticles (ENPs) prepared by the double emulsion/solvent evaporation technique induces toxicity or oxidative stress on the liver and kidney of rats after PO or IP exposure for different time points.

8.2 MATERIALS AND METHODS

8.2.1 CHEMICALS AND KITS

Eudragit® RL PO (MW = 150,000 Da [CAS: 33434-24-1]), an acrylic polycationic copolymer of acrylic and methacrylic acid esters with a proportion of quaternary ammonium groups comprised between 0.5 and 0.8 percent, was a generous gift from Evonik polymers (Darmstadt, Germany). Pluronic F68 [11104-97-5] used as a surfactant, was obtained from Sigma Aldrich (Saint-Quentin Fallavier, France) and dichloromethane (DCM) [75-09-2] from Laurylab (Saint Fons, France). Kits of Transaminase (ALT, AST) were purchased from RANDOX Laboratories Ltd. (United Kingdom). Kits of alkaline phosphatase (ALP) were purchased from QCA (AMPOSTA, Spain). Urea and creatinine were purchased from FAR Diagnostics Company (Italy). TNF-α enzyme-linked immunosorbent assay (ELISA) kits were purchased from Assaypro Co. (Michigan, United States). Interleukin 1-α (IL-α) ELISA biokits were purchased from Orgenium Laboratories Business Unit (Finland). Malondialdehyde (MDA), Total Antioxidant Capacity (TAC), and glucose kits were purchased from Biodiagnostic (Giza, Egypt). Other chemicals were of the highest purity commercially available.

8.2.2 Preparation of Eudragit RL Nanoparticles

Eudragit® RL NPs (ENPs) were prepared using the double emulsion/solvent evaporation technique as described in our previous work (Abdel-Wahhab et al. 2014). The obtained nanoparticles were then re-suspended in an appropriate medium for further investigations. The weight of ENPs was calculated based on polymer concentration in the prepared NP suspension considering the density of Eudragit polymer: 1 μg Eudragit polymer corresponds to 8.23×10^7 of nanoparticles. Nile Red–labeled ENPs were prepared using the same protocol, except that 6.25 mg of Nile Red were dissolved in the organic phase.

8.2.3 Physical Characterization of Nanoparticles

Particle sizes were determined using dynamic light scattering (DLS; Zetasizer™ 3000E, Malvern Instruments Worcestershire, UK). To avoid multiscattering events, each sample was diluted with double-distilled water until the appropriate concentration of particles, the concentration, and dilution were kept constant for all samples. The particle size (z-average) and size distribution of equivalent hydrodynamic spheres were calculated using the associated Malvern Software by the exponential sampling method. The size of prepared ENPs was tested at natural (pH 7) and acidic (pH 3) conditions and each measurement was performed in triplicate. Zeta potential measurement was based on nanoparticles' electrophoretic mobility and calculated from Smoluchowski's equation (Sze et al. 2003). All measurements were performed in triplicate at 25°C.

8.2.4 Morphological Determination

Morphological determination of ENPs was analyzed by transmission electron microscopy (2100-HR, JEOL, California, United States). Briefly, a drop of the fresh ENP sample was placed onto a carbon-coated copper grid, forming a thin liquid film, which was negatively stained by the addition of a drop of uranyl acetate. The excess of the staining solution was removed with filter paper and then air-dried before the observation. Image acquisition was done with an Orius 1000 CCD camera (GATAN, Warrendale, Pennsylvania, United States).

8.2.5 Experimental Rats

Three-month-old male Sprague Dawley rats (150–180 g, purchased from Animal House Colony, Giza, Egypt) were maintained on a standard lab diet (protein: 160.4; fat: 36.3; fiber: 41 g/kg; namely, 12.1 MJ of metabolized energy) purchased from Meladco Feed Co. (Aubor City, Cairo, Egypt). Rats were housed in filter-top polycarbonate cages in a room free from any source of chemical contamination, artificially illuminated and thermally controlled, at the Animal House Lab, National Research Center, Dokki, Cairo, Egypt. All rats received humane care in compliance with the guidelines of the Animal Care and Use Committee of the National Research Center, Dokki, Cairo, Egypt, and the National Academy of Sciences (NIH publication 86-23 revised 1985).

8.2.6 EXPERIMENTAL DESIGN

After an acclimatization period of one week, the rats were divided into two main groups (50 rats/group): Groups A and B were exposed PO or IP, respectively. Group A was further divided into five subgroups (10 rats/subgroup), including the control group (received vehicle only), and the groups were treated orally with a single dose of ENPs (50 mg/kg bw). The experimentation was terminated as follows: after 4 hours, 48 hours, 1 week and 3 weeks for the control and PO-exposed subgroups.

Rats in Group B were also divided into five subgroups (10 rats/subgroup) as follows: the control group, the groups treated with IP via a single dose of ENPs (50 mg/kg bw), and the experiments were terminated at the same time points as in Group A (i.e., 4 hours, 48 hours, 1 week, and 3 weeks). At each time period, blood samples were collected after 4 hours of vehicle exposure from the control subgroups in Groups A and B, after 4 hours, 48 hours, 1 week, and 3 weeks of exposure from all ENPs-exposed rats under diethylether anesthesia. The blood samples were centrifuged at 3000 rpm for 15 minutes and the sera were separated and stored at $-20°C$ until analysis. The serum biochemical analyses included ALT AST, ALP, urea, creatinine, TNF-α, IL-1α, TAC, and glucose and were carried out according to kit instructions. After the collection of blood samples, all rats were euthanized and samples of the liver and kidney tissue were removed and washed with saline, weighed, and homogenized in a phosphate buffer (pH 7.4) to give 20 percent w/v homogenate. This homogenate was centrifuged at 1700 rpm and $4°C$ for 10 minutes and the supernatant was stored at $-70°C$ for the determination of lipid peroxidation by measuring the formed malondialdehyde (MDA) using thiobarbituric acid reactive substances method according to kit instructions. The level of lipid peroxidation was expressed as nmol MDA per g tissue. The liver homogenate was further diluted to give 5 percent homogenate (w/v), centrifuged at 3000 rpm for 5 minutes at $0°C$ and used for the determination of TAC according to kit instructions. Other samples of liver and kidney were excised and fixed in natural formalin and were hydrated in ascending grades of ethanol, cleared in xylene, and embedded in paraffin. Sections 5 μm thick were cut and stained with hematoxylin and eosin (H&E) for histological examination (Drury and Wallington 1980). The distribution of Nile Red–labeled ENPs in the liver and kidney tissues after different time periods in the PO- and IP-treated rats was detected by fluorescent microscopy examination.

8.2.7 STATISTICAL ANALYSIS

All data were statistically analyzed using the General Linear Models Procedure of the Statistical Analysis System SAS (1982). The significance of the differences among exposure groups was determined by Waller–Duncan k-ratio. All statements of significance were based on probability of $P \leq 0.05$.

8.3 RESULTS

Transmission electron microscopy (TEM) images showed nearly spherical shape for the prepared ENPs (Figure 8.1) with average size of 300.0 ± 18.5 nm. The ENPs also showed a positive zeta potential value of 57.5 ± 5.47 mV.

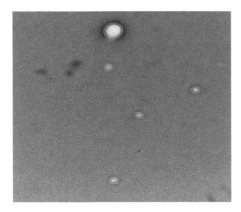

FIGURE 8.1   TEM image of the prepared Eudragit® L (Eudragit® RL) nanoparticles.

The effects of ENPs on serum biochemical parameters after different periods are depicted in Table 8.1. The results revealed that PO exposure to ENPs resulted in a significant decrease in AST activity accompanied with a significant increase in ALT and ALP activity after 4 and 48 hours; however, it was comparable to the control after 1 and 3 weeks. IP exposure resulted in a significant decrease in AST after 4 hours and 48 hours, then increased significantly and reached the normal range at 1 week or 3 weeks. On the other hand, ALT showed a significant decrease at 4 hours, 48 hours, and 1 week, and then returned to the normal range after 3 weeks. However, ALP did not significantly change at any period after IP exposure (Table 8.1). No significant changes were observed in urea and creatinine in PO- or IP-treated rats except a significant increase in urea after 4 hours and creatinine after 48 hours (Table 8.1). Treatment with ENPs, either PO or IP, did not induce any significant changes in serum TAC at all tested time periods except after 1 week and 4 weeks in IP-treated animals, which showed a significant increase in TAC.

Data presented in Table 8.2 reveals that both route of treatments showed a significant decrease in MDA in the liver tissue after 4 hours, 48 hours, and 1 week, although the MDA value was comparable to the control by the third week of treatment. The same table showed that no significant changes were observed in liver TAC at all time periods for either PO or IP treatment. In the same concern, animals treated with ENPs, either PO or IP, showed a significant decrease in kidney MDA level at 4 hours, 48 hours, and 1 week, but these values returned to the normal value of the control at the 3rd week (Table 8.3). TAC in the kidney tissue in animals treated with PO exposure to ENPs showed a significant increase at all time periods tested; however, TAC was comparable to the control group at all periods except at 4 hours, which showed a significant decrease (Table 8.3).

Rats treated orally with ENPs showed a significant increase of TNF-α level after 4 hours and IL-1α after 48 hours, but no significant changes were observed in these parameters at the other tested periods (Table 8.4). Moreover, these data also indicated that IP exposure resulted in a significant increase in TNF-α after 4 hours, 48 hours, and 1 week, but it showed a significant decrease after 3 weeks of treatment. As for

TABLE 8.1

Effect of Oral Administration or IP Injection of ENP on Liver and Kidney Function Parameters and TAC of Rats

Parameters	AST (U/L)		ALT (U/L)		ALP (U/L)	
Groups	Oral	IP	Oral	IP	Oral	IP
Control	46.67 ± 2.3[a]	45.26 ± 3.2[a]	50.67 ± 1.67[a]	53.5 ± 3.5[b]	115.9 ± 2.21[a]	119.78 ± 0.86[a]
4 hours	43.33 ± 3.28[b]	42.33 ± 1.27[b]	53.67 ± 1.70[b]	51.43 ± 2.29[b]	117.84 ± 0.88[b]	122.64 ± 0.46[a]
48 hours	43.33 ± 2.67[b]	43.33 ± 1.67[c]	54.43 ± 2.29[b]	50.33 ± 1.67[c]	117.39 ± 4.38[c]	119.12 ± 1.39[a]
1 week	46.67 ± 1.89[a]	46.67 ± 1.67[a]	52.5 ± 2.5[a]	53.67 ± 1.67[a]	114.31 ± 1.73[a]	120.68 ± 1.21[a]
3 weeks	46.33 ± 2.67[a]	45.33 ± 2.67[a]	51.33 ± 2.33[a]	53.33 ± 1.33[a]	113.86 ± 2.31[a]	118.25 ± 0.92[a]

Note: Within each column, means superscript with different letters are significantly different ($P \leq 0.05$).

(Continued)

IL-1α, its level was increased only at 48 hours in IP-treated rats and was comparable to the control at the other time periods tested (Table 8.4).

It is of interest to mention that rats treated PO with ENPs showed a significant decrease in serum glucose after 3 weeks of exposure (Figure 8.2). However, serum glucose was not significantly affected at other time points. Rats treated with IP ENPs showed insignificant changes in serum glucose after 4 hours, but glucose levels started to decrease significantly after 48 hours until 3 weeks. This decrease was more pronounced after 1 week of exposure (Figure 8.2).

Microscopic examination of the liver revealed that hepatocytes, central vein, and portal tracts displayed no differences in the control or in the rats treated PO with ENPs after 4 hours (Figure 8.3a,b). The liver section of the rats treated PO with ENPs after 48 hours showed nearly normal hepatocytes with vesiculated nuclei, central veins, and portal tracts (Figure 8.3c). However, liver sections in the PO group showed nearly normal hepatocytes with vesiculated nuclei, central veins, and marked fibrosis around the portal tracts after 1 week (Figure 8.3d). The examination of the liver sections of rats treated PO with ENPs after 3 weeks also showed nearly normal hepatocytes with vesiculated nuclei and normal central veins, but with marked fibrosis and congested portal tracts (Figure 8.3e).

In the rats IP injected with ENPs, the examination of the liver section in the control group showed unmodified hepatocytes, central veins, and portal tracts (Figure 8.4a). Liver sections of the IP-injected rats showed nearly unmodified hepatocytes with vesiculated nuclei and normal central veins after 4 hours (Figure 8.4b). Their liver sections showed nearly normal hepatocytes with vesiculated nuclei, normal central vein with some nuclear necrosis and pycnosis around portal tracts whether after 48 hours (Figure 8.4c) or 1 week (Figure 8.4d). Furthermore, fibrous tissues and necrosis around portal tracts appeared after 3 weeks (Figure 8.4e).

The histological examination of the kidney sections of control rats showed normal distal and convoluted tubules and glomeruli (G) with preserved renal space (Figure 8.5a). The kidney sections of the rats treated orally with ENPs after 4 hours showed nearly normal distal and convoluted tubules and glomeruli with preserved renal space (Figure 8.5b). The kidney sections of rats treated orally with ENPs after 48 hours showed

TABLE 8.1 (CONTINUED)
Effect of Oral Administration or IP Injection of ENP on Liver and Kidney Function Parameters and TAC of Rats

Parameters	Urea (mg/dl)		Creatinine (mg/dl)		Serum TAC (mM/L)	
Groups	Oral	IP	Oral	IP	Oral	IP
Control	109.78 ± 10.91^a	43.42 ± 2.75^a	0.58 ± 0.05^a	1.37 ± 0.38^a	1.97 ± 0.09^a	1.89 ± 0.09^a
4 hours	114.32 ± 7.90^b	45.87 ± 3.14^b	0.32 ± 0.05^a	1.7 ± 0.28^a	1.97 ± 0.20^a	2.03 ± 0.02^b
48 hours	117.6 ± 4.14^a	49.2 ± 3.35^a	0.60 ± 0.07^b	1.87 ± 0.25^b	1.95 ± 0.08^a	1.79 ± 0.1^a
1 week	117.27 ± 20.17^a	44.38 ± 6.44^a	0.40 ± 0.06^a	1.02 ± 0.28^c	1.90 ± 0.08^a	2.07 ± 0.02^b
3 weeks	117.19 ± 6.28^a	48.05 ± 5.49^a	0.41 ± 0.03^a	1.73 ± 0.38^a	1.90 ± 0.18^a	1.86 ± 0.07^a

Note: Within each column, means superscript with different letters are significantly different ($P \leq 0.05$).

TABLE 8.2
Effect of Oral Administration or IP Injection of ENP on Hepatic Lipid Peroxidation (MDA) and Total Antioxidant Capacity (TAC) of Rats

Parameter	MDA (n mol/g Liver Tissue)		TAC (µmol/g Liver Tissue)	
Group	Oral	IP	Oral	IP
Control	113.63 ± 11.06^a	118.86 ± 15.29^a	20.15 ± 0.41^a	20.07 ± 0.40^a
4 hours	112.80 ± 15.95^b	113.01 ± 18.05^b	20.79 ± 0.99^a	21.53 ± 0.29^a
48 hours	115.76 ± 18.74^c	116.3 ± 16.26^c	19.04 ± 1.34^a	19.25 ± 0.81^a
1 week	115.90 ± 16.03^d	117.78 ± 11.05^d	20.27 ± 1.41^a	21.43 ± 0.24^a
3 weeks	116.07 ± 10.71^a	118.89 ± 14.55^a	21.81 ± 0.27^a	21.60 ± 0.19^a

Note: Within each column, means superscript with different letters are significantly different ($P \leq 0.05$).

TABLE 8.3
Effect of Oral Administration or IP Injection of ENP on Renal Lipid Peroxidation (MDA) and Total Antioxidant Capacity (TAC) of Rats

Parameter	MDA (n mol/g Kidney Tissue)		TAC (µmol/g Kidney Tissue)	
Group	Oral	IP	Oral	IP
Control	158.86 ± 5.29^a	153.63 ± 4.06^a	15.91 ± 0.44^a	17.15 ± 0.34^a
4 hours	153.01 ± 8.05^b	151.79 ± 5.94^b	16.55 ± 0.50^b	14.93 ± 1.05^b
48 hours	156.37 ± 6.25^c	152.76 ± 8.74^b	16.23 ± 0.35^b	16.34 ± 0.78^a
1 week	156.78 ± 2.05^c	152.89 ± 6.03^b	16.31 ± 0.11^b	16.86 ± 0.43^a
3 weeks	158.89 ± 14.55^a	153.07 ± 2.71^a	17.05 ± 0.10^b	16.67 ± 0.98^a

Note: Within each column, means superscript with different letters are significantly different ($P \leq 0.05$).

TABLE 8.4

Effect of Oral Administration or IP Injection of ENP on Serum Cytokines

Parameter	TNF-α (pg/ml)		IL-1α (pg/ml)	
Group	Oral	IP	Oral	IP
Control	9.57 ± 0.35^a	9.57 ± 0.35^a	1.7 ± 0.20^a	1.37 ± 0.38^a
4 hours	10.9 ± 1.98^b	11.77 ± 1.84^b	1.98 ± 0.18^a	1.7 ± 0.28^a
48 hours	9.1 ± 1.45^a	10.67 ± 0.96^c	2.83 ± 0.14^b	2.87 ± 0.25^b
1 week	9.57 ± 1.41^a	10.067 ± 0.96^c	2.01 ± 0.14^a	1.22 ± 0.28^a
3 weeks	9.87 ± 1.84^a	8.47 ± 0.33^d	1.51 ± 0.39^a	1.73 ± 0.38^a

Note: Within each column, means superscript with different letters are significantly different ($P \leq 0.05$).

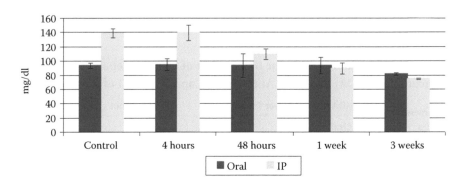

FIGURE 8.2 Effect of oral administration or IP injection of ENP on serum glucose level in rats after different tested time period.

vacuolar degeneration in the epithelial cells of renal tubules and in some glomeruli, with interstitial fibrosis and congestion also present (Figure 8.5c). The kidney sections of rats treated orally with ENPs after 1 week showed focal vacuolar degeneration in the epithelial cells of some renal tubules and in some glomeruli; mild interstitial fibrosis and congestion were also present (Figure 8.5d). The kidney sections of rats treated orally with ENPs after 3 weeks showed most renal tubules as nearly normal, some glomeruli as abnormal, and interstitial fibrosis and congestion also present (Figure 8.5e). Moreover, the examination of kidney sections in the groups IP injected showed normal distal and convoluted tubules and glomeruli with preserved renal space in the control rats injected with saline (Figure 8.6a). The kidneys of rats IP injected with ENPs after 4 hours showed most of the renal tubules as nearly normal and some glomeruli as abnormal, with dilated congested blood vessels also present (Figure 8.6b). However, the kidney sections of rats IP injected with ENPs after 48 hours showed renal tubular dilatation and increase in the size of glomeruli with dense nucleus (Figure 8.6c). Kidney sections of rats IP injected with ENPs after 1 week showed loss of normal architecture of renal tubules cells with exfoliated parts and congested blood vessels and the glomeruli as segmented or damaged (Figure 8.6e). The kidney sections of rats IP injected with ENPs

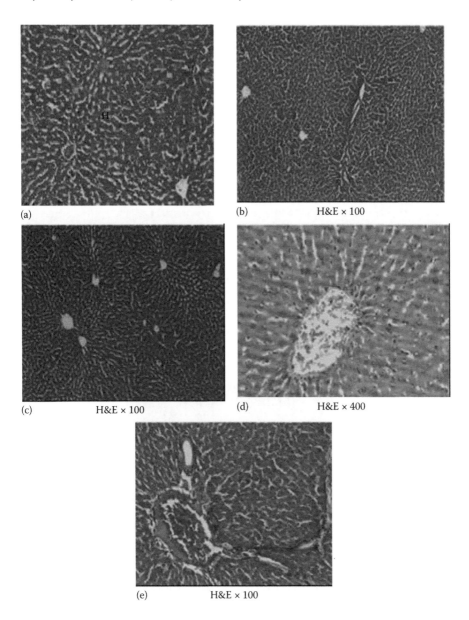

(a)

(b) H&E × 100

(c) H&E × 100

(d) H&E × 400

(e) H&E × 100

FIGURE 8.3 Liver sections from (a) control rats showing the normal hepatocytes, central vein, and portal tracts; (b) rats treated orally with ENP after 4 hours showing nearly normal hepatocytes, central vein, and portal tracts; (c) rats treated orally with ENP after 48 hours showing nearly normal hepatocytes with vesiculated nuclei, central vein, and portal tracts; (d) rats treated orally with ENP after 1 week showing nearly normal hepatocytes with vesiculated nuclei, central vein, and marked fibrosis around the portal tracts; and (e) rats treated orally with ENP after 3 weeks showing nearly normal hepatocytes with vesiculated nuclei, normal central vein, marked fibrosis, and congested portal tracts.

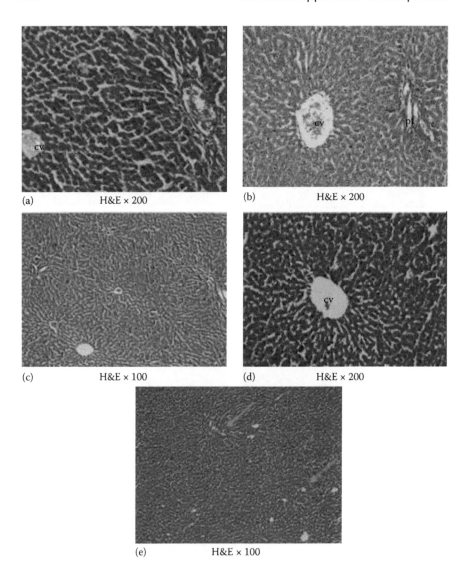

FIGURE 8.4 Liver sections from (a) control rats showing normal hepatocytes, central vein, and portal tracts; (b) rats treated IP with ENP after 4 hours showing nearly normal hepatocytes with vesiculated nuclei and normal central vein; (c) rats treated IP with ENP after 48 hours showing nearly normal hepatocytes with vesiculated nuclei, normal central vein, and nuclear necrosis and pyknosis; (d) rats treated IP with ENP after 1 week showing nearly normal hepatocytes with vesiculated nuclei, normal central vein, and nuclear necrosis and pyknosis around portal tract; and (e) rats treated IP with ENP after 3 weeks showing nearly normal hepatocytes with vesiculated nuclei, normal central vein, increased in fibrous tissues, and necrosis around the portal tract.

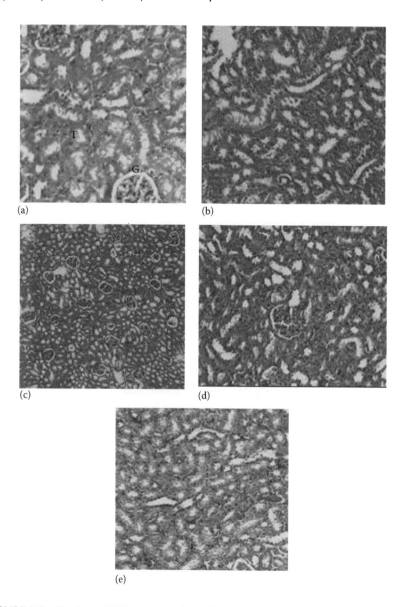

FIGURE 8.5 Sections of kidney cortex from (a) control rat showing normal distal and convoluted tubules and glomeruli (G) with preserved renal space; (b) rats treated orally with ENP after 4 h showing nearly normal distal and convoluted tubules and glomeruli (G) with preserved renal space; (c) rats treated orally with ENP after 48 hours showing vacuolar degeneration in the epithelial cells of renal tubules and in some glomeruli, interstitial fibrosis, and congestion also present; (d) rats treated orally with ENP after one week showing focal vacuolar degeneration in the epithelial cells of some renal tubules and in some glomeruli, mild interstitial fibrosis, and congestion also present. Sections of kidney cortex from (e) rats treated orally with ENP after three week showing most of renal tubules nearly normal, some glomeruli are abnormal, and the interstitial fibrosis and congestion also present (H&E × 200).

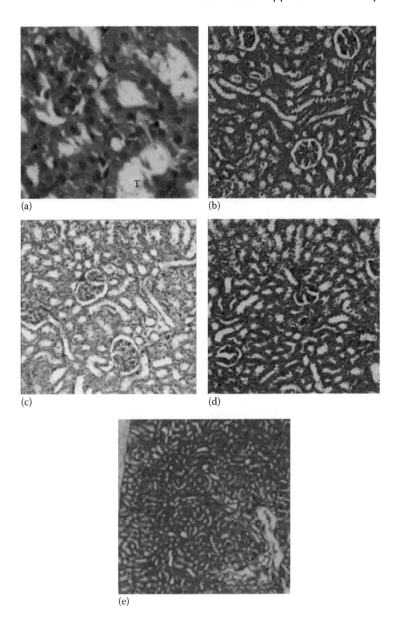

FIGURE 8.6 Sections of kidney cortex from (a) control rats showing normal distal and convoluted tubules and glomeruli (G) with preserved renal space; (b) rats IP injected with ENP after 4 hours showing most of renal tubules nearly normal, some glomeruli are abnormal with dilated congested blood vessels also present; (c) rats IP injected with ENP after 48 hours showing renal tubular dilatation and increase in the size of glomeruli with dense nucleus; (d) rats IP injected with ENP after 1 week showing loss of normal architecture of renal tubules cells with exfoliated parts, congested blood vessels, and the glomeruli are segmented or damaged Sections of kidney cortex from (e) rats IP injected with ENP after 3 weeks showing nearly normal renal tubules and increase in the size of renal corpuscle with congested and dilated glomerular capillaries.

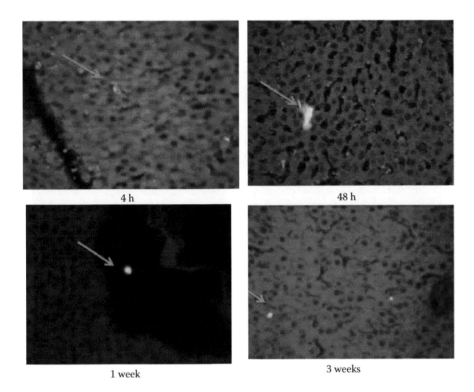

4 h

48 h

1 week

3 weeks

FIGURE 8.7   The distribution of ENP in liver tissues of PO-treated rats.

after 3 weeks showed nearly normal renal tubules and an increase in the size of the renal corpuscle with congested and dilated glomerular capillaries (Figure 8.6e).

It is of interest to mention that Nile Red–labeled ENPs were detected by fluorescent microscopy after various tested periods in both exposed groups, indicating that ENPs were found in the liver during all periods of PO- (Figure 8.7) or IP-exposed (Figure 8.8) rats. Moreover, the fluorescent microscopy examination revealed the distribution of Nile Red in the kidney tissues after different tested periods in the animals treated PO (Figure 8.9) or those IP injected (Figure 8.10) with ENPs.

8.4   DISCUSSION

In biological systems, nanosized particles may play an ambivalent role. On one hand, they may elicit toxic side effects (Boczkowski and Hoet 2010); on the other hand, novel nanoscaled diagnostics and drug-delivery vehicles hold great promise for better medical treatment (Kim et al. 2010). Especially the targeting of tumors and inflammatory cells for diagnostic or therapeutic reasons are of prime interest. Recently, we developed Eudragit® RL nanoparticles (ENPs) as a drug delivery and concluded that the prepared ENPs induced a slight oxidative stress on hematological parameters *in vivo* (Abdel-Wahhab et al. 2014). In the current study, we evaluated the oxidative stress in liver of rats exposed PO or IP-injected with ENPs. The

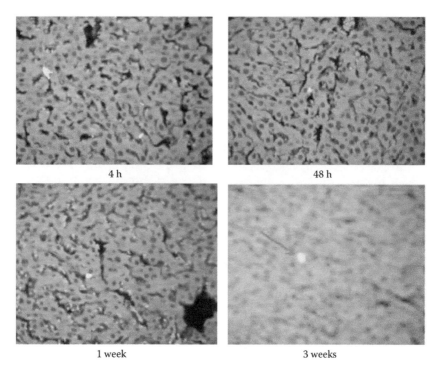

4 h   48 h

1 week   3 weeks

FIGURE 8.8   The distribution of ENP in liver tissues of IP-treated rats.

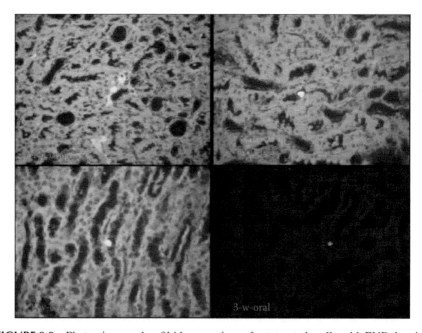

FIGURE 8.9   Photomicrographs of kidney sections of rats treated orally with ENP showing the ENP distribution in renal tissues.

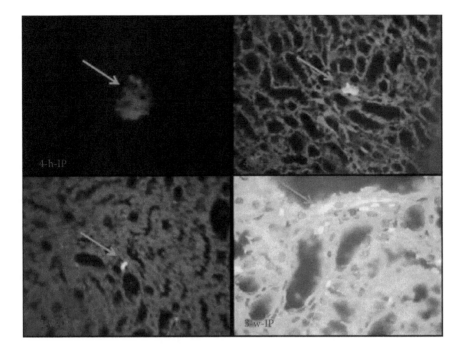

FIGURE 8.10 Photomicrographs of kidney sections of rats IP injected with ENP showing the ENP distribution in renal tissues.

selected dose of ENPs and the duration of exposure were based on our previous work (Abdel-Wahhab et al. 2014).

As mentioned in a previous work, the average size of the developed Eudragit® RL used in the current study was 300.0 ± 18.5 nm. Nanoparticle size is an important factor in gastrointestinal absorption, because only nanoparticles of the appropriate size can be absorbed significantly. Several mechanisms for gastrointestinal absorption of nanoparticles have been reported, that is, cell bypass channel transport, intestinal epithelial cells cross-cell uptake, and collection of lymph nodes in the *ileum* (Peyer's patches) of microfold cells (Hussain et al. 2001). Studies have shown a range of particle sizes to be suitable for gastrointestinal absorption (Florence et al. 1995), and that nanoparticles of around 100 nm are absorbed several times more efficiently than those of larger size (Win and Feng 2005). The nanoparticles prepared in the present experiment were 300 nm, could be absorbed well by the gastrointestinal tract, and thus would play a key role in their efficacy. In this concern, Keck and Müller (2013) reported that nanoparticles with a size below 100 nm can be taken up by macrophages. Moreover, many of them are difficult to access because they may be taken up by liver and spleen macrophages. Therefore, the smaller size NP has a higher toxicity risk and the 100 nm limit has also to be considered in the classification system.

The zeta potential values of the prepared ENPs were 57.5 ± 5.7 mV. It is well documented that the important factors for pharmaceutical nano-formulations are the increase in saturation solubility and the adhesiveness to surfaces/membranes. In the current study, the zeta potential value of the developed ENPs was higher than 30 mV, which may be due to the presence on the polymer backbone of quaternary ammonium groups with a positive zeta potential (Kim et al. 1997). Moreover, zeta potentials indicate the degree of repulsion between adjacent, similarly charged particles in dispersion and provide quantitative information on the stability of the particles more likely to remain dispersed if the absolute value of zeta potential is higher than 30 mV (Jiang et al. 2009). However, for molecules and particles that are small enough, a high zeta potential will confer the stability, that is, the solution or dispersion will resist aggregation (Martin et al. 1993).

The current results revealed that both oral treatment and IP injection of ENPs induced some disturbance in liver function tests AST, ALT, and ALP immediately after treatment; however, kidney function indices showed significant changes in urea after 4 hours and creatinine after 48 hours. After 1 week, all the tested parameters returned to the normal range. The activity of these biochemical parameters is normally used to evaluate the liver and kidney functions. Under normal circumstances, these parameters reside within the cells. The level is increased in cases of liver or kidney cell death resulting from factors such as shock, drug toxicity (Sally et al. 2001), and oxidative stress, inducing apoptosis (Rihn et al. 2000).

The present study also showed that MDA in the liver or kidney tissues was disturbed at all time periods of PO or IP administration but it was in the normal range by 3 weeks. However, TAC in serum, liver, or kidney tissue showed a significant increase in serum after 4 hours and 1 week, in the liver at all time points, and a significant decrease in kidney tissue at 4 hours, but was in the normal range thereafter. A previous study revealed that NPs may enter the circulation and produce adverse effects on different organs (Mohanan and Rathinam 1995), especially the liver, a major site where endogenous and exogenous substances accumulate. Free radicals are generated during the detoxification of reactive metabolites by cytochrome P-450 located in the smooth endoplasmic reticulum of hepatocytes and also by NADPH oxidase enzyme (Oesch et al. 1985) and also by NADPH oxidase enzyme (Eloisa et al. 1995) in the activated Kupffer cells (Wheeler et al. 2001). Reactive species, above a threshold, oxidize polyunsaturated fatty acids resulting in the onset of lipid peroxidation (Zacharias 2011), giving rise to peroxyl and alkoxyl radicals, the primary end products. Malondialdehyde is one of the toxic secondary products of lipid peroxidation which can diffuse and impairs cellular constituents such as lipids, nucleic acids, and proteins by their electrophilic nature, leading to cell death (Jain et al. 2008).

The current results indicated that serum inflammatory cytokine TNF-α was increased after 4 hours of oral administration or after 4 hours, 48 hours, and 1 week of IP injection, then it was in the normal range of the control at 1 and 3 weeks of oral administration and decreased at 3 weeks of IP injection. Moreover, IL-1α did not change significantly in orally treated rats but showed a significant increase in IP-treated rats at 48 hours. Pro-inflammatory cytokines are involved in the formation of toxic peroxynitrite by increasing the activity of the nitric oxide synthase (NOS) enzyme. Nitric oxide (NO) is a potent inflammatory mediator because of its strong reactivity with oxygen, superoxide, and iron-containing compounds. On the other hand, ENPs may be able to translocate from the gastrointestinal tract into the blood, resulting in systemic exposure of internal organs, although the extent of this may vary.

Moreover, several studies demonstrated the potential for nanomaterials to cause DNA mutation and induce major structural damage to mitochondria, even resulting in cell death. The main mechanism of nanoparticle toxicity is due to an increase of the production of reactive oxygen species (ROS). It results in oxidative stress; inflammatory cytokine production; and consequent damage to proteins, membranes, and DNA; and cell death (Nel et al. 2006). Similar to the current observation, Campbell et al. (2005) reported that inflammatory biomarkers such IL-1α and TNF-α were increased in the lungs of mice exposed to ambient air particulate matter compared to controls.

It is of interest to mention that exposure to ENPs resulted in a significant decrease in serum glucose level after 3 weeks of either PO or IP administration. These findings suggest a new function of ENPs in lowering blood glucose. Several studies indicated that insulin-loaded polycationic nonbiodegradable acrylic polymer (Eudragit® RS) has been used as a drug carrier for oral administration of a short-acting insulin analogue and suggested that Eudragit nanoparticles were able to preserve the biological activity of the insulin analogue and were effective in lowering blood glucose for about 24 hours (Damgé et al. 2009).

Histopathological examination of the liver and kidney tissues showed that no significant changes were observed in both tissues in animals receiving oral or IP injection of ENPs after different time periods, except the kidney of rats treated with ENPs both oral and IP after 48 hours and 1 week. These groups showed slight histological changes. Moreover, after 3 weeks of exposure, the liver and kidney tissue appeared normal. In this concern, Kim et al. (2015) reported that ENPs were efficiently retained in the knee joint up to 4 weeks and did not induce any side effect. Moreover, Morgen et al. (2013) suggested that Eudragit RL100 are biodegradable and form water-soluble products which can be cleared from the body through the kidneys with no significant effects. The observed histological alterations could be an indicator of slight injury of both hepatocytes and renal cells due to NPs which may be due to the metabolic and structural disturbances caused by these particles (Abdelhalim and Jarrar 2012).

Fluorescent microscopic examination of the liver and kidney tissues revealed that Nile Red–labeled ENPs were present in these tissues after 4 hours till 3 weeks after a single dose (either PO or IP). These results suggested that the retention of ENPs put them as a potential candidate for drug delivery for liver and kidney treatment. In this concern, Paul et al. (2013) reported that almost 50 percent and 85 percent of the drug was penetrating at 12 hours for nanoparticles of Eudragit RS 100 and RL 100 formulation, respectively. The authors concluded that penetration of the drug was higher in the case of the Eudragit RL 100 nanoparticle possibly due to higher permeation and zeta potential. Taken together, the current results supported our earlier findings (Abdel-Wahhab et al. 2014) and indicated the safe use of ENPs at a dose of 50 mg/kg bw for rats, which is equivalent to 8.1 mg/kg bw for humans (Reagan-Shaw et al. 2007).

8.5 CONCLUSION

ENPs prepared by the double emulsion/solvent evaporation technique having a size of 300.0 ± 18.5 nm and a zeta potential of 57.5 ± 5.5 mV were administrated to rats

PO or by IP injection. These nanoparticles did not induce any significant changes in serum biochemical parameters regarding liver and kidney functions as well as oxidative stress markers. Levels of both tested inflammatory cytokines, TNF-α and IL-1α, displayed transient changes, as well as the slight transient increase of MDA levels in the liver and kidney together with a decrease in TAC levels, reflecting a slight oxidative stress of NP-exposed rats. Moreover, the administration of ENPs resulted in a significant decrease in serum glucose level. The retention time of Eudragit® nanoparticles was long, as they were still found in the liver 3 weeks after their administration, inducing moderate portal fibrosis. Our results should prompt safety toxicologists to consider with caution the safety endpoints of the liver and kidney function before using nanoparticles, before using them as candidate for drug delivery for the treatment of liver diseases as was recently suggested for hepatitis virus infection (Lv et al. 2014).

ACKNOWLEDGMENTS

This work was supported by the National Research Centre, Dokki, Cairo, Egypt, project # S90402, and ANR "NanoSNO," Faculty of Pharmacy, Lorraine University, Nancy Cedex, France.

REFERENCES

Abdelhalim, M. A. K., and Jarrar, B. M. 2012. Histological alterations in the liver of rats induced by different gold nanoparticle sizes, doses and exposure duration. *J Nanobiotechnol* 10:5.

Abdel-Wahhab, M. A., Abdel-Wahhab, K. G., Mannaa, F. A., Hassan, N. S., Safar, R., Diab, R., Foliguet, B., and Rihn, B. H. 2014. Uptake of Eudragit® RL NP by human THP-1 cell line and its effects on hematology and erythrocyte damage in rats. *Materials* 7:1555–1572.

Bhardwaj, P., Chaurasia, H., Chaurasia, D., Prajapati, S. K., and Singh, S. 2010. Formulation and *in-vitro* evaluation of floating microballoons of indomethacin. *Acta Pol Pharm* 67(3):291–298.

Boczkowski, J., and Hoet, P. 2010. What's new in nanotoxicology? Implications for public health from a brief review of the 2008 literature. *Nanotoxicology* 4:1–14.

Buzea, C., Blandino, I. I. P., and Robbie, K. 2007. Nanomaterials and nanoparticles: Sources and toxicity. *Biointerphases* 2(4):MR17–MR172.

Campbell, A., Oldham, M., Beceria, A., Bondy, S. C., Meacher, D., Sioutas, C., Misra, C., Mendez, L. B., and Kleinman, M. 2005. Particulate matter in polluted air may increase biomarkers of inflammation in mouse brain. *Neurotoxicol* 26:133–140.

Dai, J., Nagai, T., Wang, X., Zhang, T., Meng, M., and Zhang, Q. 2004. Preparation of cyclosporine A pH sensitive nanoparticles and oral pharmacokinetics in rats. *Int J Pharm* 280:229–240.

Damgé, C., Socha, M., Ubrich, N., and Maincent, P. 2009. Poly (epsilon-caprolactone)/eudragit nanoparticles for oral delivery of aspart-insulin in the treatment of diabetes. *J Pharm Sci* 99(2):879–889.

Drury, R. A. V., and Wallington, E. A. 1980. *Carlton's Histological Techniques*, 5th ed. New York: Oxford University Press.

Eidi, H., Joubert, O., Attik, G., Duval, R. E., Bottin, M. C., Hamouia, A., Maincet, P., and Rihn, B. H. 2010. Cytotoxicity assessment of heparin nanoparticles in NR8383 macrophages. *Int J Pharm* 396(1–2):156–165.

Eidi, H., Joubert, O., Némos, C., Grandemange, S., Mograbi, B., Foliguet, B., Tournebize, J., Maincent, P., Le Faou, A., Aboukhamis, I., and Rihn, B. H. 2012. Drug delivery by polymeric nanoparticles induces autophagy in macrophages. *Int J Pharm* 422:495–503.

Eloisa, A., Manuel, C., Alberto, M., Francisco, S., and Consuelo, S. M. 1995. Decrease in free-radical production with age in rat peritoneal macrophages. *Biochem J* 312:555–560.

Florence, A. T., Hillery, A. M., Hussain, N., and Jani, P. U. 1995. Nanoparticles as carriers for oral peptide absorption: Studies on particle uptake and fate. *J Control Rel* 36:39–46.

Gargouri, M., Sapin, A., Bouli, S., Becuwe, P., Merlin, J. L., and Maincent, P. 2009. Optimization of a new non-viral vector for transfection: Eudragit NP for the delivery of a DNA plasmid. *Technol Cancer Res Treat* 8:433–444.

Hasovits, C., and Clarke, S. 2012. Pharmacokinetics and pharmacodynamics of intraperitoneal cancer chemotherapeutics. *Clin Pharmacokinet* 51(4):203–324.

Hoffart, V., Lamprecht, A., Maincent, P., Lecompte, T., Vigneron, C., and Ubrich, N. 2006. Oral bioavailability of a low molecular weight heparin using a polymeric delivery system. *J Control Release* 113:38–42.

Hussain, N., Jaitley, V., and Florence, A. T. 2001. Recent advances in the understanding of uptake of microparticulates across the gastrointestinal lymphatics. *Adv Drug Deliv Rev* 50:107–142.

Jain, D., Misra, R., Kumar, A., and Jaiswal, G. 2008. Levels of malondialdehyde and anti-oxidants in the blood of patients with vitiligo of age group 11–20 years. *Ind J Physiol Pharmacol* 52:297–301.

Jiang, J., Oberdörster, G., and Biswas, P. 2009. Characterization of size, surface charge, and agglomeration state of nanoparticle dispersions for toxicological studies. *J Nanopart Res* 11:77–89.

Jiao, Y., Ubrich, N., Marchand-Arvier, M., Vigneron, C., Hoffman, M., Lecompte, T., and Maincent, P. 2002. *In vitro* and *in vivo* evaluation of oral heparin-loaded polymeric NP in rabbits. *Circulation* 105:230–235.

Jose, S., Prema, M. T., Chacko, A. J., Thomas, A. C., and Souto, E. R. 2011. Colon specific chitosan microspheres for chronotherapy of chronic stable angina. *Colloids Surf B Biointerfaces* 83:277–283.

Keck, C. M., and Müller, R. H. 2013. Nanotoxicological classification system (NCS)—A guide for the risk-benefit assessment of nanoparticulate drug delivery systems. *Eur J Pharma Biopharm* 84:445–448.

Kim, B. Y., Rutka, J. T., and Chan, W. C. 2010. Nanomedicine. *New Engl J Med* 363:2434–2443.

Kim, S. R., Ho, M., Lee, E., Lee, J. W., Choi, Y. W., and Kang, L. J. 2015. Cationic PLGA/Eudragit RLnanoparticles for increasing retention time in synovial cavity after intra-articular injection in knee joint. *Int J Nanomed* 10:5263–5271.

Kim, Y., Fluckiger, L., Hoffman, M., Lartaud-Idjouadiene, I., Atkinson, J., and Maincen, P. 1997. The antihypertensive effect of PO administered nifedipine-loaded nanoparticles in spontaneously hypertensive rats. *Br J Pharmacol* 120:399–404.

Lv, S., Wang, J., Dou, S., Yang, X., Ni, X., Sun, R., Tian, Z., and Wei, H. 2014. Nanoparticles encapsulating hepatitis B virus cytosine-phosphate-guanosine induce therapeutic immunity against HBV infection. *Hepatology* 59(2):385–394.

Martin, A., Bustamante, P., and Chun, A. H. C. 1993. *Physical Pharmacy: Physical Chemical Principles in the Pharmaceutical Sciences*. Philadelphia, PA: Lea & Febiger.

Mohanan, P. V., and Rathinam, K. 1995. Biocompatibility studies on silicone rubber. *Proceed RC IEEE-EMBS and 14th BMESI* 4:11–12.

Morgen, M., Tung, D., Boras, B., Miller, W., Malfait, A., and Tortorella, M. 2013. Nanoparticles for improved local retention after intra-articular injection into the knee joint. *Pharm Res* 30:257–268.

Nel, A., Xia, T., Madler, L., and Li, N. 2006. Toxic potential of materials at the nanolevel. *Science* 311:622–627.

Oesch, F., Bentley, P., Gopalan, M., and Stassiecki, P. 1985. Benzopyrene metabolism in sub-cellular fractions. *Cancer Res* 45:4838–4843.

Oliveira, H. P., Tavares, G. F., Nogueiras, C., and Rieumont, J. 2009. Physico-chemical analysis of metronidazole encapsulation processes in Eudragit® copolymers and their blending with amphiphilic block copolymers. *Int J Pharm* 380:55–61.

Palena, M. C., Manzo, R. H., and Jimenez-Kairuz, A. F. 2012. Self-organized nanoparticles based on drug interpolyelectrolyte complexes as drug carriers. *J Nanopart Res* 14:867–878.

Paul, S. D., Mazumder, R., Bhattacharya, S., and Jha, A. K. 2013. An ex *vivo* study of amphotericin-B nanoparticle for ocular delivery. *Br Biomed Bull (BBB)* 1(2):119–125.

Pignatello, R., Bucolo, C., Ferrara, P., Maltese, A., Puleo, A., and Puglisi, G. 2002. Eudragit® RS100 nanosuspensions for the ophthalmic controlled delivery of ibuprofen. *Eur J Pharm Sci* 16:53–61.

Raula, J., Eerikäinen, H., and Kauppinen, E. I. 2004. Influence of the solvent composition on the aerosol synthesis of pharmaceutical polymer nanoparticles. *Int J Pharm* 284:13–21.

Ravikumar, C., Singh, S. K., and Bandyopadhyay, R. 2010. Formation of nanoparticles of water-soluble molecules: Experiments and mechanism. *J Phys Chem C* 114:8806–8813.

Reagan-Shaw, S., Nihal, M., and Ahmad, N. 2007. Dose translation from animal to human studies revisited. *FASEB J* 22:659–661.

Rihn, B. H., Bottin, M. C., Coulais, C., Rouget, R., Monhoven, N., Baranowski, W., Edorh, A., and Keith, G. 2000. Genotoxicity of 3-methylcholanthrene in liver of transgenic big Blue mice. *Environ Mol Mutagen* 36(4):266–273.

Sally, A., Tice, R. P. H., and Dean Parry, R. P. H. 2001. Medications that need hepatic monitoring. *Hospital Pharmacy* 36(4):456–464.

SAS Institute, Inc. 1982. SAS User's Guide Statistics. Cary, NC: SAS Institute.

Schaffazick, S. R., Siqueira, I. R., Badejo, A. S., Jornada, D. S., Pohlmann, A. R., Netto, C. A., and Guterres, S. S. 2008. Incorporation in polymeric nanocapsules improves the antioxidant effect of melatonin against liPid peroxidation in mice brain and liver. *Eur J Pharm Biopharm* 69:64–71.

Sze, A., Erickson, D., Ren, L., and Li, D. 2003. Zeta-potential measurement using the Smoluchowski equation and the slope of the current-time relationship in electroosmotic flow. *J Colloid Interface Sci* 261:402–410.

Tamizhrasi, S., Shukla, A., Shivkumar, T., Rathi, V., and Rathi, J. C. 2009. Formulation and evaluation of lamivudin loaded polymethacrylic acid nanoparticles. *Int J Pharm Tech Res* 1(3):411–415.

Wheeler, M. D., Kono, H., Yin, M., Nakagami, M., Uesugi, T., Arteel, G. E., Gäbele, E., Rusyn, I., Yamashina, S., Froh, M., Adachi, Y., Iimuro, Y., Bradford, B. U., Smutney, O. M., Connor, H. D., Mason, R. P., Goyert, S. M., Peters, J. M., Gonzalez, F. J., Samulski, R. J., and Thurman, R. G. 2001. The role of Kupffer cell oxidant production in early ethanol-induced liver disease. *Free Radic Biol Med* 31:1544–1549.

Win, K. Y., and Feng, S. S. 2005. Effects of particle size and surface coating on cellular uptake of polymeric nanoparticles for oral delivery of anticancer drugs. *Biomate* 26:2713–2722.

Zacharias, E. S. 2011. Liposomal antioxidants for protection against oxidant-induced damage. *J Toxicol* 152474.

Zhang, S., Kawakami, K., Yamamoto, M., Masaoka, Y., Kataoka, M., Yamashita, S., and Sakuma, S. 2011. Coaxial electrospray formulations for improving oral absorption of a poorly water-soluble drug. *Mol Pharm* 8(3):807–813.

9 In Vitro Exposure Systems to Assess the Toxicity of Airborne Substances

Tobias Krebs, Sonja Mülhopt,
Silvia Diabaté, Christoph Schlager,
Hanns-Rudolf Paur, and Marco Dilger

CONTENTS

9.1 BACKGROUND

There is an increasing need for toxicity testing of inhalable particulate matter: This is due to the number of adverse health effects caused by the PM10 emission (Pope et al. 2002; Dockery et al. 1993; Kappos et al. 2004), which will not significantly decrease in the coming years (Kiesewetter et al. 2015), on the one hand. On the other hand, an increasing need for material testing is linked with the use of submicron and nanosized particles in the industry, for example, in nanocomposites (Hussain 2006; Paul and Robeson 2008). Additionally, the regulation concerning the Registration, Evaluation, Authorisation, and Restriction of Chemicals (REACH) causes a long list of substances that must be tested (Hengstler et al. 2006; Scialli 2008).

9.1.1   ADVANTAGES OF *IN VITRO* TESTING USING
CELLS FROM THE RESPIRATORY TRACT

The use of human cell lines, primary cells, or 3D cell systems for the exposure to airborne substances offers a predictive value for human health hazards without the use of animals. There is a wide range of cells from different areas of the respiratory tract available as well as from donors with different health records. The use of *in vitro* tests allows for faster and less costly results than long-lasting animal tests (Gordon et al. 2015). Furthermore, a wide range of substances can be tested. The typical examples of atmospheres which are relevant to human health can be grouped into four major categories:

- Gases
- Liquid aerosols
  - E-cigarette vapors
  - Medical liquid aerosols
- Dry airborne particles
  - Nanomaterials
  - Pharmaceuticals
- Complex mixtures from gases and dry or liquid particles
  - Environmental atmospheres
  - Combustion-derived aerosols such as vehicle emissions and cigarette smoke

Most of the test atmospheres can be generated by using commercially available aerosol generators or can be sampled directly from the source, for example, the wood furnace, cigarette smoking machine, or an automotive engine.

More challenging is the sampling of environmental atmospheres. Some laboratories, especially when they are located in areas subject to heavy air pollution, have sampling lines to the outside of their environment. If tests need to be carried out in more remote areas, mobile test labs in a truck or container carry not only the *in vitro* exposure system, but also the required infrastructure, such as incubators and analyzers for the gas and particle phase of the test atmosphere.

9.1.2   SUBMERGED EXPOSURE CONDITIONS VERSUS
AIR–LIQUID INTERFACE (ALI) EXPOSURE

In the early phases of testing airborne materials *in vitro*, scientists had no other choice than to use a submerged exposure process. Here, the test substances were added to the cell culture media or for gaseous compounds the substances were bubbled through the media using impinger-like devices. Particles were extracted from filters or applied directly by suspension to the media.

When the first cell culture inserts became available, cells could be cultivated on porous membranes and then be exposed at the air–liquid interface—here the cells are not covered with culture media during exposure. The first developments were published in the 1970s by Aerts and Voisin (Voisin et al. 1977; Aerts and Voisin 1981) and later by Minuth et al. (1992) and Tippe et al. (2002). This procedure has the advantage that all constituents of the test atmosphere, thus the gas, semi-volatile, and particle phases can reach the cells directly and in their original composition. So the air–liquid interface enables the testing of substances without changing their original properties. Nutrition of the cell cultures is maintained at the same time through the pores of the membrane of the cell culture insert.

Figure 9.1 summarizes the advantages and disadvantages of the submerged exposure approach in comparison to the advantages and disadvantages of the air–liquid interface approach. Beside the fact that the exposure is not physiologically relevant when applying submerged exposures, one of the other major drawbacks is the undefined dose. In performing submerged exposures not only the gas and semi-volatiles phases of the test atmosphere are lost, but also the individual behavior of the particles when applied in the suspension influences the results and significance (Teeguarden et al. 2007). Particles show different floating properties according to (Figure 9.2) their sizes and nature. This results in size-dependent sedimentation times, buoyant behavior, or a combination of buoyant with upward diffusion. To overcome this

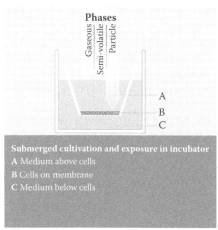
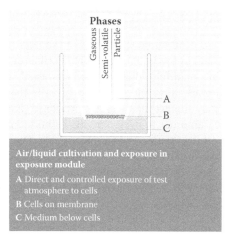

Submerged exposure

Advantages

+ Easy to perform
+ Low cost
+ Easy adaption to high throughput techniques

Disadvantages

- Changes in origin composition of test atmosphere
- Reaction of test components with culture media
- Physiologically not relevant
- No possibility testing gas phase and gas-particle interaction
- Low sensitivity
- Undefined dose

Air–liquid interface exposure

Advantages

+ No losses of original test atmosphere composition
+ No reaction of test components with culture media
+ Physiologically relevant
+ Complex cell systems with surfactant can be tested
+ High sensitivity of system
+ Defined dose

Disadvantages

- Complex technical solution
- Higher costs

FIGURE 9.1 Advantages and disadvantages of the submerged exposure approach in comparison to the advantages and disadvantages of the air–liquid interface approach.

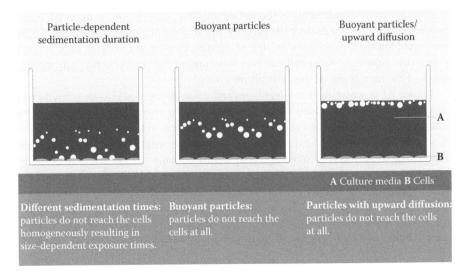

Particle-dependent   Buoyant particles   Buoyant particles/
sedimentation duration   upward diffusion

A Culture media B Cells

Different sedimentation times: Buoyant particles: Particles with upward diffusion:
particles do not reach the cells particles do not reach the particles do not reach the cells
homogeneously resulting in   cells at all.   at all.
size-dependent exposure times.

FIGURE 9.2   Different particle behavior in the suspension resulting in an unclear dose situation.

problem, numerical models have been developed to calculate the submerged dose, such as the ISDD model (Hinderliter et al. 2010). As the interactions in suspensions are manifold, different groups tested, for example, the influences of the medium composition and showed especially that the presence of fetal bovine serum (FBS) may supress the biological response (Panas et al. 2013).

In order to overcome these shortcomings, VITROCELL® offers exposure modules consisting of two major parts: The base module, which accommodates the cell culture inserts and the culture media and the aerosol exposure top. The latter has specially designed inlets that guide the aerosol in a controlled manner to the cell culture inserts. An integrated heating system by water circuit allows for exposure outside of an incubator (Figure 9.2).

9.2   EXPOSURE SYSTEMS

The complete *in vitro* exposure system consists of the following key components (Figure 9.3):

- Gas source or aerosol generator
- Distribution with optional dilution system
- Exposure modules
- Infrastructure equipment such as vacuum pumps, water bath, humidification systems

9.2.1   MANUAL EXPOSURE SYSTEMS

In vitro exposure systems have been traditionally configured according to the type of test substance, membrane insert diameters and throughput requirements. The

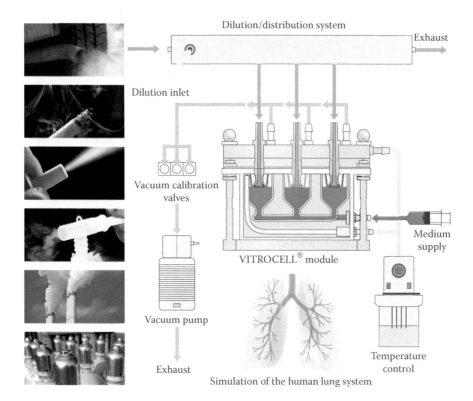

FIGURE 9.3 Typical system flow chart of an *in vitro* exposure system for *in vitro* inhalation toxicology testing.

required components are set up in the lab shown in Figure 9.4. The components are standalone, which must be handled manually in a clearly defined sequence by the lab technicians. This process is manageable but can be improved today by automation.

9.2.2 AUTOMATED EXPOSURE SYSTEM

The need for more automation emerged over the last few years. Automated systems have the advantage of a defined process for starting up and finishing an experiment and enabling at the same time a detailed monitoring of the process parameters, such as temperatures, aerosol flows, and humidity levels. Based on the experiences of many studies at KIT as reported by Diabaté et al. (2008), Comouth et al. (2013), Mülhopt et al. (2008), and Panas et al. (2014) the VITROCELL® automated exposure station as published by Mülhopt et al. (2016) was developed.

A VITROCELL® automated exposure station consists of the following key components (letters in parentheses correspond to Figure 9.5):

- Inlet with particle size selection (A)
- Clean air control system with control module (B)

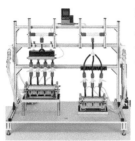

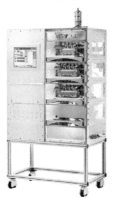

Manual exposure systems

Advantages	Disadvantages
+ Flexible and modular configuration	- Process parameters have to be set up manually
+ Lower cost	- No data logging of parameters
	- Risk that aerosol and exposure modules have different temperatures
	- Humidity control of entire system more difficult − No automated leak detection
	- GLP requirements difficult to implement

Automated exposure systems

Advantages	Disadvantages
+ User-friendly process	- Higher investment
+ Online monitoring of all relevant process parameters	
+ Integrated data logging	
+ Automatic leak detection	
+ Housed system with temperature and humidity control	

FIGURE 9.4 Different setup types of air–liquid interface systems suitable for different applications. The advantage and disadvantages are listed respectively.

- Aerosol exposure modules (C and D)
- Touch screen monitor and central computer system (E)
- Dose monitoring via Quartz Crystal Microbalances (F)
- Deposition enhancement function by electrical field (G)
- Integrated automatic leak testing function
- Central aerosol reactor with isokinetic sampling to exposure modules
- Humidification system
- Temperature control system
- Aerosol flow controllers
- Sampling ports for particle analyzers
- Vacuum pump

All items have their dedicated place in the entirely capsuled system. Depending on the research task and cell amount requirements, the stations can be equipped with two to four exposure modules with the choice of three to six compartments per module.

The system starts up with a fully automated heating cycle followed by an automated leak test for all positions of the exposure modules. The latter is very important to prevent streaming in of dry room air which will dry and kill the cells.

The inlet is equipped with a size-selective inlet and can be chosen according to the desired particle fraction of the aerosol in ranges of PM 1, 2.5, or 10.0. Most

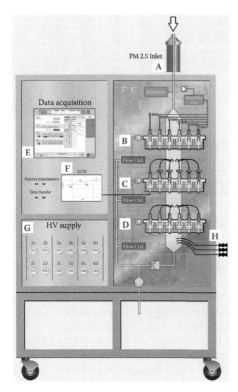

Flow chart of an exposure system with higher throughput

A   Inlet
B   Clean air exposure module (6 compartments)
C   Gas phase exposure module
D   Whole aerosol exposure module
E   Touch screen monitor
F   Microbalance online deposition monitoring
G   Deposition enhancement by electrical field
H   Sampling probes from central reactor to external aerosol measurements

FIGURE 9.5 Scheme of the automated exposure station showing the key components for the aerosol system, the exposure chambers and the automation.

frequently, the PM2.5 selector is used to reflect the typical size range of respirable airborne materials. The clean air module receives either synthetic air from a cylinder, from a compressor, or filtered room air. In order to maintain cell viability and to reflect the conditions in the human lung, the humidity of the test atmosphere is set to 85 percent. Due to a precise and sophisticated humidification system, this specification is reached with a precision of +/– 1 percent. The exposure modules receive the test substance from a central aerosol reactor with isokinetic sampling (Figure 9.6). The incoming aerosol is humidified to the same specifications of the clean air control module. The humidity levels at different positions as well as the aerosol flow through the reactor and the exposure positions are monitored and stored by the central computer. Easy-to-read graphs give the information at a glance.

9.2.3   DOSE MONITORING

One of the key advantages of the air–liquid interface is the possibility to integrate an online dose measurement and monitoring tools. A practical method is the use of quartz crystal microbalances (QCM), which can be placed in the exposure modules

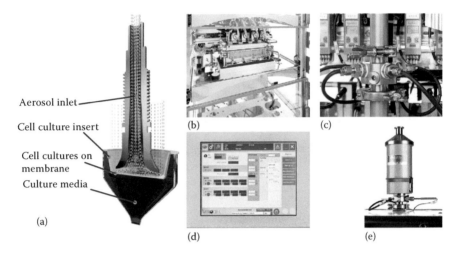

Aerosol inlet

Cell culture insert

Cell cultures on
membrane

Culture media

(a)

(b)

(c)

(d)

(e)

FIGURE 9.6 Close views to main components. (a) Principle of air–liquid interface exposure. (b) The exposure module shown has four compartments for exposure. Normally three positions are used to place cell culture inserts and the fourth position is used for dose monitoring via quartz crystal microbalance. (c) Isokinetic sampling with flow controllers. (d) Touch screen operation: All functions, such as aerosol and vacuum flows, temperature, humidity automatic leak test, charging, and start/end of the experiment can be edited using a large 15" touch-screen display. The central data management system provides valuable information on experimental parameters with user-friendly charts. The system can be networked and has a remote service module. (e) Size-selective central inlet.

(Mülhopt et al. 2009). The mass deposition rate per time at the measurement position can be displayed online with a resolution of 10 ng/(cm^2*h). A scheme of the QCM online monitoring chamber together with a typical measurement curve is shown in Figure 9.7b and d.

9.2.4 DEPOSITION ENHANCEMENT BY ELECTRICAL FIELD

When exposing cells to environmental atmospheres or nanomaterials with low initial particle concentrations there is an interest in observing the effects of increased particle deposition. An efficient way to increase deposition is to apply an electrical field below the cell cultures. In doing so, particles with a natural charge from the aerosolization process are forced to deposit on the membrane of the cell culture insert. There is the possibility to use a voltage of up to +/– 1.500V on the electrode placed in the media compartment as shown in Figure 9.7a.

The resulting increase in deposited mass varies aerosol-dependently with a factor of 5–10. Figure 9.7c shows the increase in deposition efficiency with and without electrostatic deposition among eleven positions of the exposure station in three independent experiments. To determine the deposited masses, the fluorescein sodium dosimetry according Mülhopt et al. (2016) was applied. The standard deviation

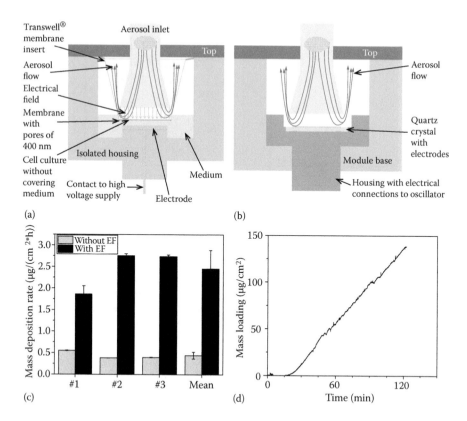

FIGURE 9.7 Increase of deposition efficiency by applying an electrical field. (a) Principle of deposition increase by integration of an electric potential below the cell culture to generate an electrical field. (b) Principle of online dose monitoring by integration of a Quartz Crystal Microbalance (QCM) sensor replacing the cell culture surface. (c) Deposition efficiency of fluorescein sodium nanoparticles for diffusional (without EF) and electrostatic (with EF) deposition. Results of 3 independent experiments (#1–#3) are shown; each bar represents the mean ± standard deviation of the deposited mass at four positions under diffusional and electrostatic conditions. (d) Typical sensor signal of the online dose measurement tool QCM exposed to an aerosol. It shows the dose increase per time in ng/cm².

among positions is remarkably low. It is important to note that the applied voltage has no effects on cell viability (Figure 9.8).

Several cell types representing different areas of the human lung are established at the air–liquid–interface: Cell lines as well as primary cells and 3D cell systems were used and analyzed for a set of biological responses as shown in Table 9.1.

9.2.5 Sampling Ports for Particle Analyzers

The system has sampling ports to connect particle and gas analyzers to the central reactor. In doing so, the aerosol can be characterized, for example, by taking filters for additional analytics as gravimetric or determination of the chemical composition.

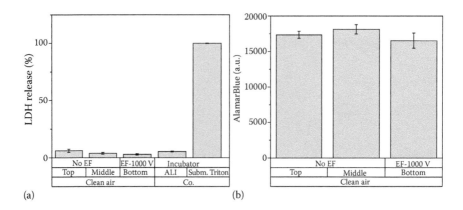

(a)   (b)

FIGURE 9.8 ALI exposure to clean air has no adverse effects. A549 cells were exposed to clean humidified air for 4 hours. (a) The LDH release was analyzed in the medium and shown as percentage of the positive control (Triton-lysed cells). (b) The AlamarBlue assay was performed and the results are shown as arbitrary units (au). Top = three positions in the upper row, middle = three positions in the middle row, bottom = three positions in the bottom row of the ALI system. No EF: no electrostatic field; EF: with electrostatic field (–1000 V). co. incub. ALI = stayed in the incubator but not covered with medium; co. incub. + Triton = control cells in the incubator lysed by Triton.

As shown in Figure 9.9b also the particle number size distribution could be determined using a scanning mobility particle sizer (SMPS). In this case, silica nanoparticles with a modal value of $x_{modal} = 25$ nm and a geometric standard deviation of $\sigma_g = 1.5$ were measured in the central aerosol reactor of the ALI exposure system. The same aerosol was collected on Formvar-coated copper grids, which were analyzed in a transmission electron microscope (Zeiss EM 109).

9.3 SUMMARY

The presented air–liquid interface systems are an appropriate method to assess the lung toxicity of inhalable toxins in gaseous and particulate form. There are several studies published with application of the ALI method to different aerosols: Oeder et al. and Sapcariu et al. investigated the influence of fuel type in a ship diesel engine on changes in the metabolism and proteome composition of cells (Sapcariu et al. 2016), to changes of the transcriptome composition and more (Oeder et al. 2015). More combustion-derived particles include diesel soot as tested by Cooney and Hickey (2011) and Kooter et al. (2013), tobacco smoke from cigarettes (Thorne et al. 2009; Kubatova et al. 2006; Nara et al. 2013) and recently also from e-cigarettes (Neilson et al. 2015; Thorne et al. 2016). A big topic is the testing of airborne manufactured nanomaterials: Cerium oxide nanoparticles were applied to a 3D cell model (Kooter et al. 2016), silica were tested by several groups as Panas et al. (2014). This only small excerpt on the possibilities and use of these methods underlies the statement Paur et al. published in 2011: the air–liquid interface exposure is the method of choice for the *in vitro* testing of inhalable aerosols.

TABLE 9.1

A List of Examples for Successfully Applied Cell Cultures and Observed Biological Effects

Cell Cultures				Biological Effects: Markers for			
Human Lung Epithelial Cells	Macrophages	Human Endothelial Cells	3D Cell System	Inflammatory Processes	Cytotoxicity	Oxidative Stress	Metabolism of Foreign Substances	Genotoxicity
A549, BEAS-2B, SK-MES-1	THP-1, RAW264.7	HUVEC	MucilAir EpiAirway	Release of IL-8, IL-6, MCP-1, expression of ICAM-1	Release of LDH, reduction of AlamarBlue, MTT assay	Expression of HMOX-1	Expression of CYP1A1	Expression of γ-H2AX
Co-cultures or triple-cultures of epithelial cells or macrophages or endothelial cells								

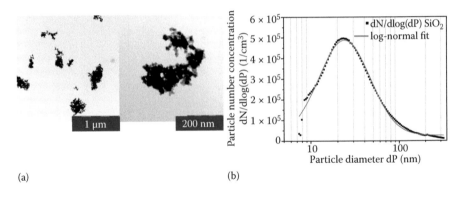

(a)   (b)

FIGURE 9.9 Aerosol measurement data. (a) Transmission electron microscopy image from silica nanoparticles. (b) Particle number size distribution dN/dlog(dP) in cm⁻³ of Silica nanoparticles determined by Scanning Mobility Particle Sizer (SMPS 3071, TSI GmbH Aachen, Germany). Shown are the mean +/– standard deviation in each channel of ten measurements.

ACKNOWLEDGMENTS

The authors acknowledge support from the European Commission's 7th Framework Programme within the project NanoMILE (Contract No. NMP4-LA-2013-310451) and the KIT Innovation Fund. We thank Sonja Schaaf, Marco Mackert, and Sivakumar Murugadoss for their technical support. Many thanks to Melanie Bucher for her help with the graphics.

REFERENCES

Aerts, C., and Voisin, C. 1981. In vitro toxicity of oxygen and oxygen-paraquat association on alveolar macrophages surviving in gas phase. *Clin Respir Physiol* 17(Suppl):145–151.

Comouth, A., Saathoff, H., Naumann, K.-H., Mülhopt, S., Paur, H.-R., and Leisner, T. 2013. Modelling and measurement of particle deposition for cell exposure at the air liquid interface. *J Aerosol Sci* 63:103–114.

Cooney, D. J., and Hickey, A. J. 2011. Cellular response to the deposition of diesel exhaust particle aerosols onto human lung cells grown at the air–liquid interface by inertial impaction. *Toxicol in Vitro* 25:1953–1965.

Diabaté, S., Mülhopt, S., Paur, H.-R., and Krug, H. F. 2008. The response of a co-culture lung model to fine and ultrafine particles of incinerator fly ash at the air liquid interface. *Altern Lab Anim* 36(3):285–298.

Dockery, D. W., Pope, III, C. A., Xu, X., Spengler, J. D., Ware, J. H., Fay, M. E., Ferris Jr., B. G., and Speizer, F. E. 1993. An association between air pollution and mortality in six U.S. cities. *New Engl J Med* 329(24):1753–1759. doi:10.1056/nejm199312093292401.

Gordon, S., Daneshian, M., Bouwstra, J., Caloni, F., Constant, S., Davies, D. E., Dandekar, G. et al. 2015. Non-animal models of epithelial barriers (skin, intestine and lung) in research, industrial applications and regulatory toxicology. *Altex* 32:327–378.

Hengstler, J. G., Foth, H., Kahl, R., Kramer, P. J., Lilienblum, W., Schulz, T., and Schweinfurth, H. 2006. The REACH concept and its impact on toxicological sciences. *Toxicology* 220(2–3):232–239.

Hinderliter, P. M., Minard, K. R., Orr, G., Chrisler, W. B., Thrall, B. D., Pounds, J. G., and Teeguarden, J. G. 2010. ISDD: A computational model of particle sedimentation, diffusion and target cell dosimetry for in vitro toxicity studies. *Part Fibre Toxicol* 7(1):36.

Hussain, F. 2006. Polymer-matrix nanocomposites, processing, manufacturing, and application: An overview. *Compos Mater* 40(17):1511–1575.

Kappos, A. D., Bruckmann, P., Eikmann, T., Englert, N., Heinrich, U., Hoppe, P., Koch, E. et al. 2004. Health effects of particles in ambient air. *Int J Hyg Environ Health* 207:399–407.

Kiesewetter, G., Borken-Kleefeld, J., Schöpp, W., Heyes, C., Thunis, P., Bessagnet, B., Terrenoire, E., Fagerli, H., Nyiri, A., and Amann, M. 2015. Modelling street level PM10 concentrations across Europe: Source apportionment and possible futures. *Atmos Chem Phys* 15(3):1539–1553.

Kooter, I. M., Alblas, M., Jedynska, A. D., Steenhof, M., Houtzager, M. M. G., and van Ras, M. 2013. Alveolar epithelial cells (A549) exposed at the air–liquid interface to diesel exhaust: First study in TNO's powertrain test centre. *Toxicol in Vitro* 27:2342–2349.

Kooter, I. M., Gröllers-Mulderij, M., Steenhof, M., Duistermaat, E., van Acker, F. A., Staal, Y. C., Tromp, P. C., Schoen, E., Kuper, C. F., and van Someren, E. 2016. Cellular effects in an in vitro human 3D cellular airway model and A549/BEAS-2B in vitro cell cultures following air exposure to cerium oxide particles at an air–liquid interface. *Appl In Vitro Toxicol* 2(1):56–66.

Kubatova, A., Dronen, L. C., Picklo, M. J., and Hawthorne, S. B. 2006. Midpolarity and nonpolar wood smoke particulate matter fractions deplete glutathione in RAW 264.7 macrophages. *Chem Res Toxicol* 19:255–261.

Minuth, W. W., Stöckl, G., Kloth, S., and Dermietzel, R. 1992. Construction of an apparatus for perfusion cell cultures which enables in vitro experiments under organotypic conditions. *Eur J Cell Biol* 57:132–137.

Mülhopt, S., Diabaté, S., Krebs, T., Weiss, C., and Paur, H.-R. 2009. Lung toxicity determination by in vitro exposure at the air liquid interface with an integrated online dose measurement. *J Phys Conf Ser* 170(1):012008.

Mülhopt, S., Dilger, M., Diabaté, S., Schlager, C., Krebs, T., Zimmermann, R., Buters, J. et al. 2016. Toxicity testing of combustion aerosols at the air–liquid interface with a self-contained and easy-to-use exposure system. *J Aerosol Sci* 96:18.

Mülhopt, S., Paur, H.-R., Diabaté, S., and Krug, H. F. 2008. In vitro testing of inhalable fly ash at the air liquid interface, in *Advanced Environmental Monitoring*, eds. Young J. Kim and Ulrich Platt, pp. 402–414. Dordrecht, the Netherlands: Springer.

Nara, H., Fukano, Y., Nishino, T., and Aufderheide, M. 2013. Detection of the cytotoxicity of water-insoluble fraction of cigarette smoke by direct exposure to cultured cells at an air–liquid interface. *Exp Toxicol Pathol* 65:683–688.

Neilson, L., Mankus, C., Thorne, D., Jackson, G., DeBay, J., and Meredith, C. 2015. Development of an in vitro cytotoxicity model for aerosol exposure using 3D reconstructed human airway tissue; application for assessment of e-cigarette aerosol. *Toxicol in Vitro* 29:1952–1962.

Oeder, S., Kanashova, T., Sippula, O., Sapcariu, S. C., Streibel, T., Arteaga-Salas, J. M., Passig, J. et al. 2015. Particulate matter from both heavy fuel oil and diesel fuel shipping emissions show strong biological effects on human lung cells at realistic and comparable in vitro exposure conditions. *PLOS ONE* 10(6):e0126536.

Panas, A., Comouth, A., Saathoff, H., Leisner, T., Al-Rawi, M., Simon, M., Seemann, G. et al. 2014. Silica nanoparticles are less toxic to human lung cells when deposited at the air–liquid interface compared to conventional submerged exposure. *Beilstein J Nanotechnol* 5:1590–1602.

Panas, A., Marquardt, C., Nalcaci, O., Bockhorn, H., Baumann, W., Paur, H.-R., Mülhopt, S., Diabaté, S., and Weiss, C. 2013. Screening of different metal oxide nanoparticles reveals selective toxicity and inflammatory potential of silica nanoparticles in lung epithelial cells and macrophages. *Nanotoxicology* 7(3):259–273.

Paul, D. R., and Robeson, L. M. 2008. Polymer nanotechnology: Nanocomposites. *Polymer* 49(15):3187–3204.

Paur, H.-R., Cassee, F. R., Teeguarden, J., Fissan, H., Diabate, S., Aufderheide, M., Kreyling, W. G. et al. 2011. In-vitro cell exposure studies for the assessment of nanoparticle toxicity in the lung-A dialog between aerosol science and biology. *J Aerosol Sci* 42:668–692.

Pope, C. A., Burnett, R. T., Thun, M. J., Calle, E. E., Krewski, D., Ito, K., and Thurston, G. D. 2002. Lung cancer, cardiopulmonary mortality, and long-term exposure to fine particulate air pollution. *J Am Med Assoc* 287:1132–1141.

Sapcariu, S. C., Kanashova, T., Dilger, M., Diabate, S., Oeder, S., Passig, J., Radischat, C. et al. 2016. Metabolic profiling as well as stable isotope assisted metabolic and proteomic analysis of RAW 264.7 Macrophages exposed to ship engine aerosol emissions: Different effects of heavy fuel oil and refined diesel fuel. *PLOS ONE* 11(6):e0157964.

Scialli, A. R. 2008. The challenge of reproductive and developmental toxicology under REACH. *Regul Toxicol Pharmacol* 51(2):244–50.

Teeguarden, J., Hinderliter, P. M., Orr, G., Thrall, B. D., and Pounds, J. G. 2007. Particokinetics in vitro: Dosimetry considerations for in vitro nanoparticle toxicity assessments. *Toxicol Sci* 95(2):300–312.

Thorne, D., Crooks, I., Hollings, M., Seymour, A., Meredith, C., and Gaca, M. 2016. The mutagenic assessment of an electronic-cigarette and reference cigarette smoke using the Ames assay in strains TA98 and TA100. *Mutat. Res.* 812:29–38.

Thorne, D., Wilson, J., Kumaravel, T. S., Massey, E. D., and McEwan M.. 2009. Measurement of oxidative DNA damage induced by mainstream cigarette smoke in cultured NCI-H292 human pulmonary carcinoma cells. *Mutat. Res.* 673:3–8.

Tippe, A., Heinzmann, U., and Roth, C. 2002. Deposition of fine and ultrafine aerosol particles during exposure at the air/cell interface. *J Aerosol Sci* 33(2):207–218.

Voisin, C., Aerts, C., Jakubczak, E., and Tonnel, A. B. 1977. A new experimental model for the in vitro study of alveolar macrophages. *Clin Respir Physiol* 13(1):69–82.

10 Nanoparticles as Nitroso-Glutathion Vehicles

Luc Ferrari, Roudayna Diab, Christophe Nemos, Ramia Safar, and Chloe Puisney

CONTENTS

10.1 INTRODUCTION

Eudragit RL is a nonbiodegradable copolymer of acrylic and methacrylic acid esters, which has been approved by regulatory agencies for oral delivery in polymeric form. This is in agreement with nanoparticles growth in the medical field, especially for drug delivery. Yet, for patient safety, before using such a formulation that seems to be promising in therapeutics, the absence of adverse effects and toxicity assessment must be ensured. But due to their dimensions, nanoparticles present new proprieties and conventional toxicology methods are no longer sufficient to completely characterize materials toxicity. Thus, we used a toxicogenomic approach to characterize it as it provides information on the whole transcriptome, which changes after a treatment, as suggested by national and international regulatory agencies (ANSM, NRC-US). This transcriptomic analysis was performed on Caco-2 cells following treatment by empty nanoparticles (NPs). This study is in addition to first viability and internalisation observations.

10.2 MATERIALS AND METHODS

10.2.1 CELL CULTURE

Caco-2 cells (ATCC, HTB-37™, Manassas, Virginia, United States; Pinto et al. 1983) were grown at 37°C under 5 percent CO_2 atmosphere in EMEM medium (Sigma Aldrich, Saint-Quentin Fallavier, France) supplemented with 20 percent fetal bovine serum (SVF, Eurobio, Les Ulis, France), 1 percent non-essential amino acids (Sigma Aldrich, Saint-Quentin Fallavier, France), 1 percent sodium pyruvate (Sigma Aldrich, Saint-Quentin Fallavier, France), and 1 percent antibiotics (100U/ mL of penicillin, 0.1 mg/mL streptomycin, Sigma Aldrich, Saint-Quentin Fallavier, France). Cells were trypsined once a week (Trypsin-EDTA, Sigma Aldrich, Saint-Quentin Fallavier, France). Passages 35 to 45 were used.

10.2.2 NANOPARTICLES PREPARATION

NP-ERL were prepared using a double emulsion—the solvent evaporation method from three phases as previously described (Wu et al. 2014). Briefly, a primary water–oil emulsion was prepared by sonication of the internal aqueous phase (0.5 mL of 0.1 percent aqueous solution of Pluronic F68 (w/v)) and the organic phase (10 percent solution (w/v) of Eudragit RL PO in 5 mL of DCM). After, a secondary emulsification was carried out by sonication after adding the external aqueous phase (20 mL of 0.1 percent Pluronic F68 aqueous solution) leading to a double water–oil–water emulsion. DCM was eliminated using a rotary evaporator (R-144, Büchi, Flawil, Switzerland). NP-ERL were collected by ultracentrifugation at 186000 g for 30 minutes. The pellet of NP-ERL was suspended in the medium used for experimentations by mechanical agitation.

10.2.3 NANOPARTICLES CHARACTERIZATION

The hydrodynamic diameter and size distribution of ENP, expressed as polydispersity index, were measured using dynamic light scattering (DLS, Zetasizer 3000E, Malvern Instruments Worcestershire, UK) and were calculated from the number distribution graph. Zeta potential was calculated using the Smoluchowski equation. (Sze et al. 2003). All measurements were performed in triplicate at 25°C.

10.2.4 CYTOTOXICITY ASSAY

Cells were seeded in 96-well plates with 5×10^4 cells/cm^2. After overnight incubation, the medium was removed by aspiration. Fresh medium with or without serum was added and cells were exposed with 0 to 2000 µg/mL Eudragit NP during 24 hours. Cell viability was examined by several assays as described below.

10.2.4.1 MTT Assay

MTT assay was performed according to Denizot's (Denizot and Lang 1989) recommendations. Briefly, after the nanoparticle exposure medium was removed and the cells were rinsed two times using HBSS. Cells were then incubated with 0.5 mg/mL MTT in medium solution during 4 hours. The working solution was removed. Cells were rinsed two times with HBSS and dimethylsulfoxide was added. Absorbance was measured at 570 nm.

10.2.4.2 WST-1 Assay

WST-1 assay was performed using Cell Proliferation Reagent WST-1 (Roche, Basel, CH) according to the manufacturer's protocol.

10.2.4.3 Neutral Red Assay

Neutral Red assay was performed according to Borenfreund's (Borenfreund and Puerner 1985) recommendations. Briefly, after the nanoparticle exposure medium was removed, cells were rinsed two times using HBSS. Cells were then incubated with 50 µg/mL Neutral Red in medium solution during 4 hours. The working solution was removed. Cells were rinsed two times with HBSS and lysis solution (50 percent water, 50 percent ethanol (v/v) + 1 percent acetic acid (v/v)) was added. Absorbance was measured at 540 nm.

10.2.5 UPTAKE STUDY

10.2.5.1 Transmission Electron Microscopy

Caco-2 cells were seeded in 6-well plates at a density of 5×10^4 cells/cm^2 and exposed after overnight incubation to 50 µg/mL of NP-ERL for 4 hours. Cells were fixed *in situ* with 2.5 percent glutaraldehyde in phosphate buffer (pH 7.4) for 60 minutes at 4°C. Cells were then postfixed with 2 percent osmium tetroxide and washed in cacodylate buffer containing 0.5 percent tannic acid. After extensive washes in 0.1 M Sorensen phosphate buffer (pH 7.2), they were dehydrated and embedded in epon (EMbed-812; Electron Microscopy Sciences). Ultra-thin sections were cut at a thickness of 50–90 nm and mounted on 300 mesh EM specimen supporting grids. Sections were then counterstained with uranyl acetate and lead citrate and examined with a JEM-ARF200 TEM (collaboration with C. Thevenot, UMR 7198 CNRS [NE2V Department], Jean Lamour Institute, University of Lorraine, Nancy, France).

10.2.5.2 Flow Cytometry

Cells were seeded in 24-well plates at a density of 5×10^4 cells/cm^2 and were exposed, after overnight preincubation, to 50 µg/mL of Nile Red–labeled NP in medium for 4 hours. The medium was removed and cells were dissociated with trypsin after an HBSS rinse step. Cells were then washed two times with HBSS and finally suspended in 1 percent (m/v) bovine serum albumin containing HBSS. Cell-associated fluorescence was detected by flow cytometry (FACSCalibur™, Becton Dickinson, BD Bioscience). Excitation and emission wavelengths were 488 and 585 nm, respectively. The results are reported as the mean of the fluorescence intensity distribution obtained by analyzing 10000 cells.

10.2.5.3 Confocal Study

Cells were seeded in Labtek plates at a density of 7×10^4 cells/cm^2 and were exposed, after overnight preincubation, to 50 µg/mL of Nile Red–labeled NP in medium (with or without serum) for 4 hours. Medium was removed and cells were washed two times with HBSS. Cells were then fixed with 4 percent (w/v) paraformaldehyde during 15 minutes at room temperature. After rinsing cells two times with HBSS, Hoechst (1 µg/mL in PBS) was used at room temperature during 15 minutes for nuclei staining.

10.2.5.4 Microarray Study

Total RNA was extracted using RNeasy Plus Mini Kit (Qiagen, Venlo, the Netherlands) according to the manufacturer's recommendations from cells exposed to 1.4 µM free GSNO, 50 µg/mL of NP-ERL, 50 µg/mL NP-GSNO. Unexposed cells were used as control. The quality of the extracted RNA was assessed by spectrophotometry and capillary electrophoresis as previously described (Safar et al. 2015). cDNA synthesis from RNA and Cy3-dye labeling as well as microarray hybridization were carried out with 100 ng of total RNA according to the manufacturer protocol (One-Color Microarray-Based Gene Expression Analysis, version 6.6). Microarray slides were scanned by Agilent DNA microarray scanner (SurePrint G3 Human GE v2 8x60K, Agilent Technologies). Acquisition of images and quantification of fluorescence signal as well as primary data analysis were performed using the Agilent Feature Extraction Software. Data were first normalized with Lowess's method and stringent filtering criteria were then used to identify genes whose expression level was significantly modified as compared to control. The means of at least three determinations for each condition were compared by the modified Student's t-test ($p \leq 0.001$). For a given gene, fold change (FC) of an expression ≥ 2.0 or ≤ 0.5 under one condition of exposure of cells in reference to the control was calculated. The analyzed genes displayed acceptable False Discovery Rate (< 20 percent) according to Benjamini et al. (2001). The selected genes were analyzed according to Gene Ontology (GO) terms and functions using (1) the Database for Annotation, Visualization, and Integrated Discovery (DAVID; http://david.abcc.ncifcrf.gov) and (2) the Genecard Database. Genes were grouped among clusters according to the functional pathways as defined in the DAVID database. The raw data of the microarrays are available on Gene Expression Omnibus database (GEO, http://www.ncbi.nlm.nih.gov/geo/), using the GSE 65911 accession number.

10.2.5.5 Statistical Analysis

Cell viability and cellular uptake data are presented as means ± standard error of the mean (SEM) of three biological replicates and six technical replicates. Statistical differences were determined by one-way analysis of variance (ANOVA) followed by Kruskall–Wallis test using the RLPlot software™.

10.3 RESULTS

10.3.1 CYTOTOXICITY STUDIES

Viability assays are presented in Figure 10.1 (without serum) and Figure 10.2 (with serum). Following exposure to nanoparticles in medium without or with serum,

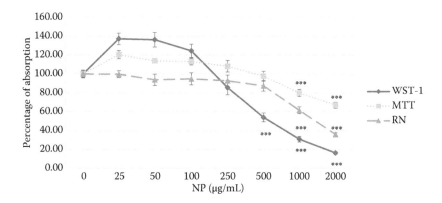

FIGURE 10.1 Viability assay of Caco-2 cell line after exposure to Eudragit nanoparticles in the absence of serum. Results are presented as mean ± SEM, n = 6, N = 3, * p < 0.05, ** p < 0.01, *** p < 0.001.

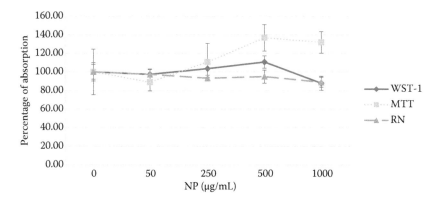

FIGURE 10.2 Viability assay of Caco-2 cell line after exposure to Eudragit nanoparticles in the presence of 20 percent of serum. Results are presented as mean ± SEM, n = 6, N = 3, * p < 0.05, ** p < 0.01, *** p < 0.001.

viability tests resultants shows an increase of mitochondrial activity at low concentrations (25 and 50 µg/mL) without toxicity in MTT and WST-1 tests, not recovered in Neutral Red test. In all tests, a dose dependent toxicity of Eudragit's empty nanoparticles can be noticed. It is clear that in presence of serum, the toxicity of Eudragit NPs is lowered (Figures 10.1 and 10.2).

10.3.2 FLOW CYTOMETRY ASSAY

Flow cytometry assay were realized on samples for which cells were exposed to nanoparticles with or without serum in the culture medium. Several controls were realized (Red Nile only, empty nanoparticles, cells only) and the results (data not shown) are congruent (absence of non-specific fluorescence).

Cells were first exposed to nanoparticles at usual temperature of 37°C. The results show a mean fluorescence of 98 for exposure to nanoparticles in medium containing serum (FBS: 20 percent) and a mean fluorescence of 360 for nanoparticles in medium without serum. Other cells were exposed to nanoparticles at 4°C. The results show a mean fluorescence of 84 for exposure to nanoparticles in medium containing serum (FBS: 20 percent) and a mean fluorescence of 92 for nanoparticles in medium without serum.

A significant difference ($p < 0.00001$) was recovery after exposure to nanoparticles dispersed in medium without serum between 37°C and 4°C. Exposure to nanoparticles at 4°C leading a blockage of energy-dependent internalization mechanisms, such a mechanism would be involved in nanoparticles internalization dispersed in medium without serum. Also, a significant difference was noticed between exposure with or without serum. However, we didn't find a significant difference between 4°C and 37°C for exposure to nanoparticles dispersed in medium with serum. This indicates an internalization of nanoparticles after exposure in medium without serum but leaves an ambiguity for exposure in medium with serum.

10.3.3 CONFOCAL LASER MICROSCOPY SCANNING

After exposure to Red Nile–labeled nanoparticles an increase of red fluorescence is noticed by observation of cells with confocal scanning microscopy. Increase of red fluorescence, attached to internalization of nanoparticles, is higher after exposure of cells to Eudragit's nanoparticles in medium without serum compared to exposure to nanoparticles in medium with 20 percent FBS. See Figure 10.3. These results are in agreement with flow cytometry assay. A higher internalization rate is noticed when cells are exposed to nanoparticles in medium without serum.

10.3.4 TRANSCRIPTOMIC STUDY

The analysis of transcriptomic data, obtained by DNA chips technology, permits to show differentially regulated genes groups: 191 genes are differentially regulated (up/down-regulation, FC > 2, $p < 0.05$) after exposure to 50 µg/mL of NP; 274 genes are differentially regulated after exposure to 50 µg/mL of NP-GSNO. For the exposure to active substance, GSNO at the concentration of 1.4 µM, 228 genes are differentially regulated.

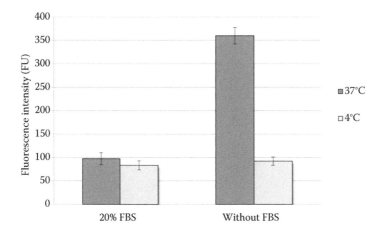

FIGURE 10.3 Internalization study after exposure of Caco-2 model to Red Nile–labeled Eudragit's nanoparticles by cytometry flow assay (n = 10 000, N = 3; without FBS, p < 0.001).

The most important network is linked to immune response and particularly "response to virus" (GO: 0009615), thanks to IFIT1, IFIT3, IFIT5, and MX1. The two other major clusters are linked to olfactory sensation (thanks to proteins which represent olfactory receptors: OR5F1, OR5M9, OR8U1, OR2AK2) and tight junction (CLDN18).

10.3.5 Clusters (PANTHER)

Genes differentially regulated after treatment (FC > 2, p < 0.05) were classified by groups (also called clusters) by using PANTHER™ (Thomas et al. 2003). Twelve major clusters are presented, corresponding to the first level of biological processes of the Gene Ontology database (Ashburner et al. 2000). Here, cellular process (GO: 009987) and metabolic process (GO: 0008152) clusters are the most affected. Indeed, these clusters are affected in a way that

- For "metabolic process" (GO: 008152) cluster: 55 genes are differentially regulated after exposure to empty Eudragit® RL PO's nanoparticles (NP).
- For "cellular process" (GO: 009987) cluster: 52 genes are differentially regulated after exposure to empty nanoparticles formed by Eudragit RL PO polymer (NP).

The type of response "Immune system process" was the subject of particular interest: 17 genes were differentially regulated after exposure to nanoparticles.

10.3.6 String

Figure 10.4 shows how interactions recover after nanoparticle exposure. This network represents protein–protein interactions of genes differentially regulated after exposure to empty and GSNO-loaded nanoparticles. We can identify two major interactions:

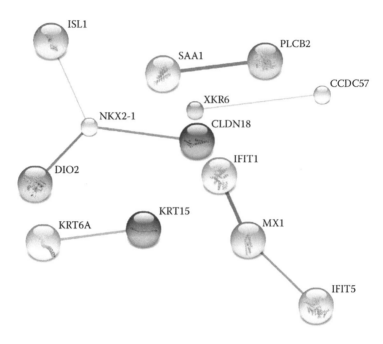

FIGURE 10.4   Protein–protein interactions identified after exposure to Eudragit's nanoparticles. DIO2: Deionidase; ISL1: ISL LIM homeobox; NKX2-1: NKZ homeobox; CLDN18: Claudin 18; SAA1: Serum Amyloid A1; PLCB2: Phospholipase C Beta 2; XKR6: Kell blood group complex subunit-related family; CCDC57: Coiled-coil domain containing 57; IFIT1: Interferon-induced protein with tetratricopeptide repeats 1; IFIT5: Interferon-induced protein with tetratricopeptide repeats 5; MX1: myxovirus (influenza virus) resistance 1 (interferon-inducible protein p78); KRT6A: Keratin 6A, KRT15: Keratin 15. Thickness of the link represents strength of interactions between them. (Done on http://string-db.org/.)

The first one is linked to tight junctions (CLDN18) and cytoskeleton (KRT6A, KRT15); the other to response to virus (IFIT1, MX1, IFIT5).

10.4   DISCUSSION

The cytotoxicity study of empty Eudragit® RL PO nanoparticles on Caco-2 model indicated a toxicity. For studies with serum, nanoparticles generally didn't present any toxicity. Differences between serum-free or with-serum studies suggest that a corona of protein is formed around our nanoparticles and this affects the behavior of cells in contact with them as suggested by several authors (see Rihn and Joubert 2015). However, in this study it seems important to note that mitochondrial activity increased during exposure at several doses of Eudragit RL PO nanoparticles in our cytotoxicity studies with or without serum. This mitochondrial activity burst has been noticed in previous works on different cell types (Hussien et al. 2013) after exposure to Eudragit's nanoparticles. This phenomenon is reported on other human cell types after exposure to the same nanoparticles as ours, THP-1 (Safar et al. 2015) or with Caco-2 cell lines, but with gold nanoparticles (Tarantini et al. 2015) or polymeric vectors, that is, insulin nanoparticles (Zhang et al. 2014).

Flow cytometry study showed an increase of fluorescence upon exposure of cells to nanoparticles in serum-free medium. When this experiment was reproduced at 4°C, fluorescence intensity decreased significantly, suggesting an energy-dependent mechanism. These results were confirmed by confocal microscopy study. The confocal results clearly showed a greater internalization of the nanoparticles in contact with cells in serum-free medium. Different results were obtained after exposure with and without serum, both in flow cytometry and in confocal microscopy. This is supporting the hypothesis of a corona formation. This interpretation is in agreement with the results of viability study. Aggregation of proteins on the surface of our nanoparticles change internalization behavior in cells and induce therefore a different cell reaction.

Our aim is to determine a very early adaptive response of cells after exposure to nanoparticles. However, conventional toxicological approach is not sufficient to characterize mechanistic toxicity. From our cytotoxicity study, we selected the concentration of 50 mg/ml. A transcriptomic approach was carried out after exposure to 50 µg/ml of nanoparticles dispersed in culture medium with serum to approximate physiological conditions (presence of proteins due the alimentary bolus). Validation of the transcriptomic study was performed following a discrimination of every transcript based on expression level. Dendrograms of samples enables realization of a supervised analysis (not shown). Transcriptomic analysis highlighted differentially regulated genes. Among these genes, some were found to be differentially regulated following different exposures. As a "vector" response, we can underline the identification of "response to a virus" cluster during exposure to nanoparticles which can be explained by the particle size (185 nm) about the size of a virus (Le Faou 2012).

Among the gene affected by the exposure to Eudragit NP, we found some genes which belong to the olfactory receptor cluster. These genes are usually supposed to be receptors for aromatic compounds present in the air. The presence and the regulation of these genes could be at first sight considered as a consequence of the carcinogenic status of the Caco-2 cell line. But a search in the literature indicates that several olfactory receptors are presents in various tissues (Kang and Koo 2012), including the colon (Flegel et al. 2013). Its regulation after exposure to chemicals remains to be understood.

We reanalyzed the data of Safar et al. (2016) following criteria selected for our study. Indeed, Safar et al. exposed the same nanoparticles as ours to a monocytes-macrophages model: THP-1. We then compared the differentially regulated gene groups following treatments. It appears that the response of THP-1 involved more genes than Caco-2 response. This difference could be explained by the fact that THP-1 cells are a model of monocytes–macrophages and thus represent the immune system of the body. Whereas Caco-2 cells represents the digestive system of the body less reactive than the immune system. Also, the signaling pathway mainly significantly affected by our conditions was the cytokine–cytokine receptor pathway in THP-1, but this route was not significantly affected on the Caco-2 model. This supports a specific cell response. While working with titanium dioxide nanoparticles,

Tilton et al. also demonstrated that THP-1 response differed from Caco-2 response model (Tilton et al. 2015). This suggests that study of the adaptive response following exposure to drug delivery nanoparticles should be performed on different cell models to predict various potentially harmful effects of these compounds.

In our study, we can assume interactions with cytoskeletal intermediate filaments via the identification of several types of keratin transcriptomic modulations. These interactions can lead to functional impairment of the intestinal epithelium, but also alterations in epithelial permeability linked to barrier function. Therefore, it would be useful to characterize transfer mechanisms of these nanoparticles at the intestinal epithelium. Indeed, only a few studies regarding nanoparticle transfer mechanisms have been done. However, if nanoparticles are transferred to the systemic circulation, other problems will come up. Finally, the functions of protection and repair of the epithelium may be affected by a change in transfer mechanisms.

In this study we presented some techniques useful to study the effects of nanoparticles on a cellular model. These studies could open a wide range of research and provide useful tools for the understanding of human interaction with a nanoparticular environment.

REFERENCES

Ashburner, M., Ball, C. A., Blake, J. A., Botstein, D., Butler, H., Cherry, J. M., Davis, A. P., Dolinski, K., Dwight, S. S., Eppig, J. T., Harris, M. A., Hill, D. P., Issel-Tarver, L., Kasarskis, A., Lewis, S., Matese, J. C., Richardson, J. E., Ringwald, M., Rubin, G. M., and Sherlock, G. 2000. Gene ontology: Tool for the unification of biology. The Gene Ontology Consortium. *Nat Genet* (1):25–29.

Benjamini, Y., Drai, D., Elmer, G., Kafkafi, N., and Golani, I. 2001. Controlling the false discovery rate in behavior genetics research. *Behav Brain Res* 125(1–2):279–284.

Borenfreund, E., and Puerner, J. A. 1985. Toxicity determined in vitro by morphological alterations and neutral red absorption. *Toxicol Lett* 24:119–124.

Denizot, F., and Lang, R. 1989. Rapid colorimetric assay for cell growth and survival— Modification to the tetrazolium dye procedure giving improved sensitivity and reliability. *J Immunol Methods* 89:271–277.

Flegel, C., Manteniotis, S., Osthold, S., Hatt, H., and Gisselmann, G. 2013. Expression profile of ectopic olfactory receptors determined by deep sequencing. *PLoS One* 8(2):e55368.

Hussien, R., Rihn, B. H., Eidi, H., Ronzani, C., Joubert, O., Ferrari, L., Vazquez, O., Kaufer, D., and Brooks, G. A. 2013. Unique growth pattern of human mammary epithelial cells induced by polymeric nanoparticles. *Physiol Rep* 1(4):e00027.

Kang, N., and Koo, J. 2012. Olfactory receptors in non-chemosensory tissues. *BMB Rep* 45(11):612–622.

Le Faou, A. 2012. *Virologie Humaine*. Rueil-Malmaison: Pradel Editions.

Pinto, M., Rabine-Leon, S., Appay, M. D., Kedinger, M., Triadou, N., Dussaulx, E., Lacroix, B., Simon-Assmann, P., Haffen, K., Fogh, J., and Zweibaum, A. 1983. Enterocyte-like differentiation and polarization of the human colon carcinoma cell line caco-2 in culture. *Biol Cell* 47:323–330.

Rihn, B. H., and Joubert, O. 2015. Comment on "Protein Corona Fingerprinting Predicts the Cellular Interaction of Gold and Silver Nanoparticles." *ACS Nano* 9(6):5634–5635.

Safar, R., Ronzani, C., Diab, R., Chevrier, J., Bensoussan, D., Grandemange, S., Le Faou, A., Rihn, B. H., and Joubert, O. 2015. Human monocyte response to s-nitrosoglutathione-loaded nanoparticles: Uptake, viability, and transcriptome. *Mol Pharm* 12(2):554–561.

Sze, A., Erickson, D., Ren, L., and Li, D. 2003. Zeta-potential measurement using the Smoluchowski equation and the slope of the current-time relationship in electroosmotic flow. *J Colloid Interface Sci* 261(2):402–410.

Tarantini, A., Lanceleur, R., Mourot, A., Lavault, M.-T., Casterou, G., Jarry, G., Hogeveen, K., and Fessard, V. 2015. Toxicity, genotoxicity and proinflammatory effects of amorphous nanosilica in the human intestinal Caco-2 cell line. *Toxicol In Vitro* 29:398–407.

Thomas, P. D., Campbell, M. J., Kejariwal, A., Mi, H., Karjak, B., Daverman, R., Diemer, K., Muruganujan, A., and Narechania, A. 2003. PANTHER: A library of protein families and subfamilies indexed by function. *Genome Res* 13:2129–2141.

Tilton, S. C., Karin, N. J., Tolic, A., Xie, Y., Lai, X., Hamilton, R. F. Jr., Waters, K., Holian, A., Witzmann, F. A., and Orr, G. 2014. Three human cell types respond to multi-walled carbon nanotubes and titanium dioxide nanobelts with cell-specific transcriptomic and proteomic expression patterns. *Nanotoxicol* 8(5):533–548.

Wu, W., Gaucher, C., Diab, R., Fries, I., Xiao, Y. L., Hu, X. M., Maincent, P., and Sapin-Minet, A. 2015. Time lasting S-nitrosoglutathione polymeric nanoparticles delay cellular protein S-nitrosation. *Eur J Pharm Biopharm* 89:1–8.

Zhang, Y., Du, X., Zhang, Y., Li, G., Cai, C., Xu, J., and Thang, X. 2014. Thiolated Eudragit-based nanoparticles for oral insulin delivery: Preparation, characterization, and evaluation using intestinal epithelial cells in vitro. *Macromol Biosci* 14:842–852.

Section IV

Medical Use

11 Transbarrier Trafficking of Nanoparticles

Perspectives for Cancer Therapeutics

*Lisa C. du Toit, Priyamvada Pradeep,
Thashree Marimuthu, Yahya E. Choonara,
Pradeep Kumar, and Viness Pillay*

CONTENTS

11.1 INTRODUCTION

Various internalization mechanisms are responsible for the cellular uptake of exogenous materials, including the drug–drug delivery system, such as phagocytosis, macropinocytosis, receptor-mediated endocytosis, clathrin-mediated endocytosis, caveolin-mediated endocytosis, and clathrin and caveolin-independent endocytosis as exemplified in Figure 11.1 (Soldati and Schliwa 2006; Sriraman et al. 2014). Endocytic pathways are most commonly followed by nanoparticulate drug delivery systems. Thereafter, trafficking of the internalized material to intracellular different locations occurs, dependant on cellular polarity, sorting and motor protein expression, protein–protein interactions, as well as cytoskeletal organization. Alterations to genes and phenotypes result in notable changes to intracellular transport mechanisms, and may be both the cause as well as result of certain disease states, such as cancer (Haglund et al. 2007).

Progression of cancer to the aggressive metastatic state emanates due to accumulation of genetic alterations, with malignant cells displaying substantial variation in cellular phenotype (e.g., intra- and extracellular protein expression, cell survival, and polarity). Non-malignant epithelial cells possess a polarized phenotype, which enables differing trafficking mechanisms apically and basolaterally. Malignant cells, however, generally display a loss in polarity, thus affecting intracellular sorting and

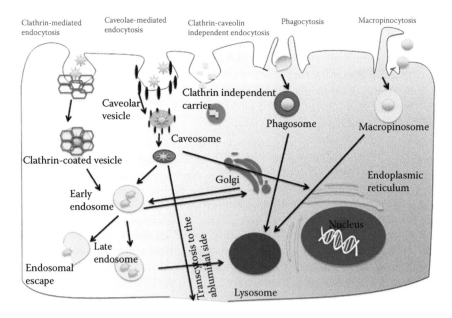

FIGURE 11.1 The various mechanisms of cellular internalization of nanoparticles via clathrin-mediated endocytosis, caveolin-mediated endocytosis, clathrin-caveolin independent endocytosis, phagocytosis and macropinocytosis and their subsequent intracellular trafficking. (Reproduced from Sriraman, S. K. et al., *Tissue Barriers*, 2, e29528-1–e29528-10, 2014. Landes Bioscience under Creative Commons Attribution—Non Commercial 3.0 Unported License.)

trafficking of the internalized material. Further, epithelial tumors have a heterogeneous nature, and phenotypic variations in cancer cells exert an important influence on material uptake, as well as intracellular sorting, trafficking, and localization (Barua and Rege 2009).

Nanoparticulate drug delivery systems (nanosystems) have a significant role as therapeutic, diagnostic, and imaging vehicles in cancer detection and treatment (Maier-Hauff et al. 2007). This is attributed to their (1) circulatory colloidal stability, which evades macrophage uptake; (2) multimodality—the potential to combine various properties in one object; and (3) capability for tumoral or diseased tissue concentration via the Enhanced Permeability and Retention (EPR) effect or through coupling with targeting biomolecules (Rima et al. 2013). Gaining knowledge of the pathways and fate of both targeted and untargeted nanosystems through tumor tissue and in cancer cells would enable the design and formulation of innovative targeted systems with enhanced efficacy and selectivity for the required intracellular site. The expression of specific receptors on cancer cells affects intracellular trafficking of targeted nanoparticles (NPs; Vasir and Labhasetwar 2007). Investigations have generally focused on conjugated NPs, which encompass polymers, cell-penetrating peptides, and serum proteins in untargeted (receptor-independent) cancer cell uptake and trafficking (Delehanty et al. 2006; Chithrani and Chan 2007; Ruan et al. 2007; Hauck et al. 2008) with a more recent and combinatory focus on NP size, shape, and surface properties (Barua and Rege 2009).

"Perfectly targeted" delivery of antineoplastic agents to the required intracellular site within the tumor cells of interest is the ultimate goal for achieving enhanced chemotherapeutic management of cancer. Attainment of this requires the successful trafficking of a number of tumoral barriers in order for the agent to reach its required intracellular site. We recently published a review on the "Parameters and Characteristics Governing Cellular Internalization and Trans-Barrier Trafficking of Nanostructures" (Murugan et al. 2015). In this chapter we specifically focus on elaboration of the tumor-specific barriers, the factors implicated in enhancing the transbarrier trafficking of nanosystems with specific regard to cancer chemotherapy, as well as progressive methods for quantifying the resultant NP uptake by cancer cells.

11.2 TUMOR MICROENVIRONMENTAL BARRIERS TO NANOPARTICLE TRAFFICKING

As emphasized, nanosystems inherently possess advantages over conventional therapeutics; however, only a limited fraction of the dose may reach the tumor site to elicit the required effect. This is mainly due to limited potential to reach the target site effectively as a result of physiological and cellular barriers (Agardan and Torchilin 2016). For effective delivery of the chemotherapeutic drug to the affected site, the nanosystem must be stable and undergo trafficking across various barriers. An understanding of the barriers encountered in achieving delivery to tumor sites is thus pertinent for designing optimal nanosystems (Agardan and Torchilin 2016).

The tumor microenvironment (TME) is characterized by malfunctioned vasculature with areas that are hypoxic, acidotic, and exposed to increased interstitial fluid pressure. Such features are exclusive to the TME, and are partly responsible for inefficiency of antineoplastic drug delivery. Targeted NPs can improve the bioavailability and intracellular drug concentration in cancer cells along with decreasing the toxicity to normal cells by employing both passive and active targeting strategies. Furthermore, because of their structural complexities, NPs bind to specific receptors and subsequently enter the cell; they are usually enclosed by endosomes via receptor-mediated endocytosis thus bypassing the recognition of P-glycoprotein which is one of the main drug-resistance mechanisms. The barriers to NP trafficking that must be overcome to reach and to penetrate the tumorous architecture can be broadly divided into (1) geometrical, (2) immunological, (3) hydraulic, (4) physicochemical, and (5) cellular barriers.

11.2.1 GEOMETRICAL BARRIER

The geometrical barrier refers to the abnormal and inconsistent distribution of vascular and avascular space ("vascular chaos") in the tumor which are often outlined and defined by the presence and absence of blood vessels (Ferrari 2005; Jain and Stylianopoulos 2010; Jain 2013). Tumor vasculature possesses structural abnormalities including an abnormal vessel wall, vessel architecture, and vascular density (Jain 2013). The tortuosity of the vascular system along with the nonuniform hierarchy of the blood vessels lead to division of the tumor into several varied dimensional avascular spaces, which may hinder the distribution and penetration of various nano-archetypes. The geometry of the tumorous vascular system is further complicated by the enlarged interendothelial junctions and pores as well as increased number of transendothelial channels and fenestrae as compared to normal tissue. The abnormally thick or thin basal membrane in the tumor vessels may also cause geometrical variance (Figure 11.2; Jain 1988; Heldin et al. 2004; Danhier et al. 2010; Jain and Stylianopoulos 2010). Furthermore, the continuous proliferation of the surrounding tumor tissue may exert pressure on the vasculature leading to rupture of blood vessels creating regions with under-perfusion or no-perfusion (Griffon-Etienne et al. 1999) These regions are often inaccessible to various therapeutic paradigms, including nanodelivery. Several researchers have exploited the irregular, saccular, convoluted, and leaky nature of tumor vessels (due to enlarged interendothelial junctions) for the delivery of bioactive payloads to tumor tissue (Heldin et al. 2004). NPs can undergo passive targeting via the enhanced permeability and retention (EPR) effect via extravasation into the tumor space via the enlarged pores with retention due to poor lymphatic drainage (Sriraman et al. 2014). However, absence or heterogeneity of permeability—by orders of magnitude—may jeopardize such an approach. The geometrical barrier in the form of varied vascular architecture may additionally affect the flow—rate as well as amount—of blood into the tumorous regions, making the therapeutic regimen ineffective and inaccessible (Groothuis 2000). The geometrical barrier may also constitute the pore size of the vessels perfusing the tumorous tissue. The pore size is dependent on the organ site ranging from ≈7 nm (brain) to ≈50–60 nm (breast and pancreas), hence making the "one-size-fits-all" paradigm of nanomedicine design ineffective (Hobbs et al. 1998; Chauhan et al. 2012; Chauhan and Jain 2013). Therefore, size selection in the case of nanomedicine for cancer therapeutics is very important. Small particles penetrate, and are cleared

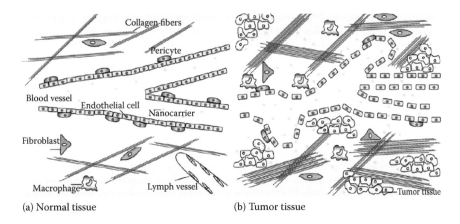

(a) Normal tissue   (b) Tumor tissue

FIGURE 11.2 Structural differences between normal and tumor tissues that affect interstitial fluid pressure. (a) Normal tissues contain linear blood vessels lined by a smooth layer of endothelial cells with pericytes maintaining the integrity of the vessel on its outside. The extracellular matrix consists of a loose network of collagen and other fibers, and contains a few fibroblasts and macrophages. Lymph vessels are also present in normal tissues. (b) Tumor tissues contain defective blood vessels that are leaky and irregularly shaped, with many sac-like formations, dead-ends, and highly activated endothelia. Blood flow is therefore inefficient. These blood vessels are also covered by fewer pericytes than in normal tissues, resulting in decreased vessel stability. Furthermore, many tumors lack lymph vessels, thus interstitial fluid and soluble proteins are inefficiently removed. The extracellular matrix of tumors contains a much denser network of collagen fibers, which are thicker than in normal tissues. Therefore, the tumor tissue is more rigid than normal loose connective tissue. Tumors also contain an increased number of fibroblasts, which bind to the collagen fibers in an integrin-dependent manner and exert an increased tension between the fibers, as well as an increased number of macrophages and other inflammatory cells; these cells release cytokines and growth factors that act on cells of blood vessels and stroma fibroblasts to increase interstitial fluid pressure. (Reproduced with permission from Heldin, C. H. et al., *Nat Rev Cancer*, 4, 806–813, 2004. Nature Publishing Group ©2004; Danhier, F. et al., *J Control Release*, 148, 135–146, 2010. Elsevier B.V. Ltd. ©2010.)

from tumors easily as compared to their large counterparts requiring a precise balance between the upper and lower limits of particle size. Interestingly, rod- and disc-shaped particles penetrate much more efficiently than their spherical equivalents but they are only applicable in vessels with a small pore size (Chauhan and Jain 2013).

11.2.2 Hydraulic Barrier

The hydraulic barrier in the TME refers to high interstitial fluid pressure (IFP), which can reach as high as 60 mm Hg in tumor tissue (such as in breast carcinoma, metastatic melanoma, head and neck carcinoma, and colorectal carcinoma) as compared to 0 mm Hg in the case of normal tissue. The inherent cause of such an increase in pressure has been attributed to leakage from the vascular system and the vascular–lymphatic imbalance (Boucher et al. 1990; Heldin et al. 2004; Ferrari 2005; Alexis 2008;

Jain and Stylianopoulos 2010). Heldin and coworkers provided a very detailed account of factors responsible for high IFP as

- Release of vascular endothelial cell growth factor (VEGF) ≈ ↑ vascular permeability ≈ ↑ protein and biomolecules outflow ≈ ↑ interstitial colloid osmotic pressure
- Non-functional lymphatic vessels ≈ ↓ fluid and biomolecules drainage
- Proliferation of stromal fibroblasts ≈ ↑ fibrosis of the interstitial tissue ≈ ↑ density of connective-tissue ≈ ↑ contraction and compression of tumor tissue ≈ ↑ IFP (Heldin et al. 2004)

In the tumor tissue, the IFP may become equal to the microvascular pressure (MVP) while at the tumor periphery, the IFP may drop down to normal levels leading to the formation of a pressure gradient. Additionally, a further increase in IFP (higher than MVP) may cause extravasation of the NPs from the tumor vascular system to surrounding healthy tissue. A higher IFP may render the therapeutic paradigm inefficient as both the convection (high molecular weight bioactives) and diffusion (low molecular weight bioactives) based drug transport is affected (Heldin et al. 2004; Owens and Peppas 2006; Ferrari 2010; Chauhan and Jain 2013).

11.2.3 PHYSICOCHEMICAL BARRIER

Following extravasation, NPs encounter the tumor interstitium, which differs extensively from normal tissue. It combines cancerous and noncancerous cells and their dynamic microenvironment, created by the tumor and controlled by tumor-induced interactions (Whiteside 2008). Non-specific binding of NPs with intracellular or extracellular macromolecules in the tumorous tissues can lead to decreased diffusional penetration into tumor cells. Thus, high NP concentration in the tumor is not an indicator of uniform distribution of the same throughout the tumor, but may rather indicate higher binding at the periphery and low drug concentration deep into the tumorous mass. This leads to increased variability in drug exposure in the tumor cells. The physicochemical barrier refers to the resistance provided by the interstitial space and the TME lined by collagen fibers and intertwined with proteo- and glycosamino-glycans. The TME is much denser (pore size ≈10 nm) than the normal tissue microenvironment and only allows diffusion of small chemotherapeutics agents and NPs with sizes smaller than ~50 nm (Danhier 2010). Large and charged NPs and high molecular weight biomolecules profoundly interact (hydrodynamically and electrostatically) with the TME and hence can only exert local action after extravasation from vessels to the interstitial fluid (Danhier 2010). The diffusion of nanomedicines is further hindered by an increase in the viscosity of the microenvironment due to long and elongated fibers of sulfated glycosaminoglycan—a negatively charged material capable of forming strong aggregated with cationic NPs. The physicochemical barrier additionally affects the formation of a geometrical barrier wherein the tumor space is divided into viscous (collagen rich) and non-viscous regions causing heterogeneity in the nanomedicine distribution (Curti 1993; Netti et al. 2000). Jacobson and coworkers (2003) proposed that transforming growth factor-β (TGFβ) may be the inherent cause of an increase in collagen content of the tumors, which in turn leads to an increased fibrosis and IFP. Additionally, activation of fibroblasts and macrophages may affect the growth of the highly contractile extracellular matrix which further stalls the movement of NPs across the tumorous region due to high density and hence low diffusion (Cairns 2006; Stylianopoulos et al. 2012).

11.2.4 Immunological Barrier

Immunogenicity towards the administered nanomedicine can be termed as a *nano-induced barrier*. Opsonization, or removal of drug-loaded NPs from the systemic circulation by the mononuclear phagocytic system (MPS), also known as the reticuloendothelial system (RES), acts as a major sequestering mechanism for the administered NPs affecting tumor targeting as well as the circulatory half-life of the nano-entities. Several complement proteins such as C3, C4, and C5, laminin, fibronectin, C-reactive protein, type I collagen, and immunoglobulins may bind to the NPs within a few seconds after their introduction into the bloodstream via van der Waals forces, electrostatic, ionic, or hydrophobic/hydrophilic attractions, thus rendering them more visible to phagocytosis mechanism through cells like macrophages, which are typically Kupffer cells, or macrophages of the liver. These macrophages do not have the ability to directly identify NPs rather they recognize specific opsonin proteins attached to the surface of the NPs and result in consumption and final removal of the NPs from the systemic circulation. In the systemic circulation, drug-loaded NPs are typically taken up by the liver, spleen, and other parts of the RES, rendering fewer NPs able to reach their target and thus posing as hindrance to efficient cancer drug therapy. Based on characteristics of conventional surface non-modified NPs, they are taken up by RES, depending on their size and surface features (Cho et al. 2008). NPs with surface hydrophobicity demonstrate preferential uptake by the liver, then by the spleen and lungs. Conversely, NPs with surface hydrophilicity have displayed <1 percent spleen and liver uptake. Although various researchers have proposed that coating the NPs with polyethylene glycol may circumvent the problem, the RES is still a major hurdle in cancer nanomedicine (Li and Huang 2009; Guo and Huang 2011). The new generation nanoarchetypes, such as fullerenes, dendrimers, and carbon nanotubes, may induce an antibody-mediated immunogenic response, which is even more noticeable in case of polymer-dendrimer conjugates (Ferrari 2005). Another crucial immunogenic aspect relates to targeted NP therapeutics wherein antibodies (or their fragments) are employed for targeting the tumor environment (Alexis et al. 2008). Monoclonal antibodies (mAb) provide two binding sites per antibody and provide better binding avidity than the fragmented counterparts. However, if the F_c portion of the antibody binds to the F_c portion of normal cell, a macrophage-like reaction occurs, causing uptake of the mAb-bound NPs via liver or spleen and thereby compromising the nano-therapy (Peer et al. 2007). The stimulation of such an immune response can lead to release or activation of various cytokines (such as TGFβ) and angiogenic factors which in turn interact with various cell types causing a cascade of biochemical reactions leading to an increased IFP (Heldin et al. 2004). Although there are strategies to counter the immunological barrier; complete avoidance of the RES is difficult (Nie 2010). NP physicochemical characteristics including shape, size, charge, and surface chemistry affect their ulti-mate opsonization and clearance (Albanese et al. 2012).

11.2.5 CELLULAR BARRIERS

Once the nanosystem reaches the tumor interstitium, it needs to traverse the cell membrane barrier, which is essentially impermeable to water soluble molecules, to reach the cytoplasm with subsequent delivery of the therapeutic payload to vari-ous subcellular compartments (e.g., nucleus, mitochondrion, or lysosomes). Most NPs undergo internalization via specific endocytosis (clathrin-mediated, caveolae-mediated, and clathrin- and caveolae-independent endocytosis, or micropinocyto-sis) and release the loaded drug intracellularly (Hillaireau and Couvreur 2008). For efficient intracellular delivery, NP size, shape, surface characteristics (lipo-philicity), and charge require optimization. Cationic NPs display a stronger affin-ity for the anionic cell membrane. Further, cellular uptake of polymeric NPs has demonstrated cell-line dependence, which is also affected by NP composition (He et al. 2010; Agardan and Torchilin 2016). Following cell internalization, the NP may need to reach an intracellular target for drug content delivery, which is achieved by endosomal vesicles. An additional barrier the nanosystem thus faces is lysosomal degradation. However, certain cationic polymers and lipids can evade transportation to the lysosomal compartment and be recycled back to the cell surface (Biswas and Torchilin 2014).

11.3   STRATEGIES TO OVERCOME TUMOR BARRIERS

From the above discussion, it is clear that one of the primary hurdles to nanothera-peutics in cancer is the heterogeneity of the TME and strategies to overcome the tumor barriers must look into its normalization (Figure 11.3). Among these, cor-recting the vascular angiogenesis, reducing the IFP, and intruding the complex col-lagenous network are of particular interest. Below is a list of potential nano- and biostrategies to enhance the transbarrier trafficking of cancer therapeutics:

1. In several reports, Jain (2001) proposed the administration of anti-angiogenic factors to arrest the overexpression of proangiogenic factors such as VEGF, basic fibroblast growth factor, and platelet-derived growth factor (PDGF). In addition to preventing the excessive and heterogeneous spread of blood vessels in the tumor, this strategy can contribute towards the lowering of the IFP by reducing vessel diameter and hence may render better control and distribution of bioactives across the TME (Jain 2001; Datta et al. 2015).
2. Pharmacologically active monoclonal antibodies such as trastuzumab and bevacizumab can exert an indirect anti-angiogenic effect and instigate tumor normalization by reducing the tumor diameter, density, and perme-ability with a reduction in IFP by ~70 percent (Izumi et al. 2002; Batchelor et al. 2007).

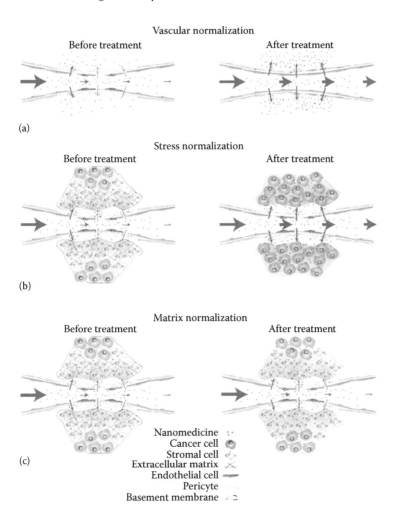

FIGURE 11.3 Normalizing the tumor microenvironment to improve drug delivery and efficacy. Drug-delivery barriers resulting from tumor pathophysiology cannot all be overcome by nanomedicine design. Nanomedicines can be combined with therapies that normalize these physiological abnormalities for enhanced anti-tumor efficacy. (a) Vascular normalization repairs blood vessels, rendering them more mature, more homogenous and less leaky. This lowers interstitial fluid pressure which restores a transvascular fluid pressure difference that results in improved blood flow and convective NP penetration in tumors. (b) Stress normalization reduces solid stress, the mechanical stress that compresses tumor blood vessels to restore perfusion throughout tumors. This increases the supply of drugs, such as nanomedicines, throughout tumors. (c) Matrix normalization modulates the structure of matrix molecules such as collagen, reducing their hindrance to nanomedicine distribution. This results in a more uniform distribution of nanomedicines in tumors. Depending on the extent of matrix depletion and reorganization, matrix normalization can potentially also normalize solid stress and lead to increased perfusion in addition to improved matrix penetration. (Reproduced with permission from Chauhan, V. P., and Jain, R. K., *Nat Mater*, 12, 958–962, 2013. Nature Publishing Group ©2013.)

3. Another approach is evading the binding-site barrier induced by targeting nanomedicines towards mutant receptors instead of merely targeting over-expressing receptors on the tumor surface. Additionally, programming the release of drugs "deep into the tumor tissue" away from blood vessels can also provide better therapeutic outcomes as the pH and enzymatic profile of the TME can be explored here as the trigger (Helmlinger et al. 1997; Schmidt and Wittrup 2009).

4. Eikenes and coworkers (2004, 2005) in two separate studies demonstrated that the administration of enzymes such as collagenase and hyaluronidase may modulate the TME by disentangling the collagen-based tumor net-work, thereby reducing the interstitial and microvascular pressure. This may eventually lead to achievement of enhanced transvascular filtration and interstitial transport of macromolecules such as monoclonal antibodies (Eikenes et al. 2004, 2005).

The fate of the injected NP should be controlled by fine-tuning their size and surface features. Table 11.1 provides a summary of various strategies which can be implemented to overcome the barriers discussed for achieving enhanced cancer nanotherapy. The subsequent section will focus on specific nanostrategies for enhancing transbarrier trafficking for enhanced cancer therapy.

TABLE 11.1
Summary of Strategies to Overcome Various Barriers to Cancer Nanomedicine

Barrier to Nanomedicine Delivery and Performance	Strategies to Overcome the Barrier
Geometrical barrier	• Adjustment in particle size to obtain mesoscopic range • Customized size according to location/organ of tumor and by taking pore-size heterogeneity into consideration • Rod- or disc-shaped NPs as compared to spherical particles
Hydraulic barrier	• Inhibition of cytokines such as TGFβ, VEGF, PDGF, and other angiogenic factors
Physicochemical barrier	• Permeation enhancers such as zonula-occludens toxin • Co-administration of bradykinin antagonist • Employing macromolecules with linear, semi-flexible configurations • Neutralization of NP charge to circumvent matrix interactions
Immunological barrier	• NP size below 35 nm diameter • Rendering the NP surface hydrophilic by coating with polymers such as polyethylene glycol and N-(2-hydroxypropyl) methacrylamide • Steric stabilization • Forming conjugates with protein such as albumin

Source: Alexis et al. 2008; Cho et al. 2008; Ferrari 2010; Nie 2010; Chauhan et al. 2012; Chauhan and Jain 2013.

11.4 SPECIFIC NANO-STRATEGIES FOR ENHANCING CANCER CELL UPTAKE AND INTRACELLULAR TRAFFICKING

Endocytic pathways differ in the proteins involved, vesicle size, and located cell type. Following engulfment, the nanosystem's intracellular fate depends on the endocytic pathway followed. As NPs become more advanced, there is an increased concern with their intracellular pathway, as this becomes critical to their biomedical application (Kou et al. 2013; Bai et al. 2015). Nanosystems have presented with limitations related to their toxicity in the body inherent to their minute size. Reductions in potential toxicity are achievable through close examination of the endocytic pathway mechanisms (in addition to the ensuing exocytosis and NP clearance). A low-targeting efficiency of the NP emanates in excessive toxicity of chemotherapeutic nanosystems (Oh and Park 2014). In this regard, the physicochemical properties of the NP as a drug delivery vehicle are a pertinent consideration in controlling the biological response elicited. NP size, surface chemistry, and charge, and morphology (shape) in concert with various intracellular components of the specific cell type all impact on the endocytic pathway (Wang et al. 2011; Xiang et al. 2012; Oh and Park 2014). Important to note is that no single factor has been isolated for predicting intracellular transport (Kou et al. 2013). The past decade has seen a heightened focus on the physical, chemical, and biological interactions at the NP–biological barrier interface, which improves the knowledge of the manner in which the nano-architecture impacts nanosystem cellular uptake. However, it is clear that no generalizations can be applied in terms of NP attributes and a number of facets still yet to be further investigated owing to the complexity of the process (Bai et al. 2015). The ensuing discussion will delve into each NP characteristic as well as various examples in order to identify trends, or dispute the fact that trends exist in accordance with a specific physicochemical property.

11.4.1 NANOPARTICLE SIZE

Vesicle size following NP endocytosis depends on the pathway employed. NP size may be considered to have a degree of influence in determining the transport pathway. For vesicular entry, the size should be sufficiently small, with a range preferably of 10–500 nm but less than 5 μm, with a potentially more rapid rate of cell entry for smaller particles (Zhang et al. 2008; Kou et al. 2013). Macropinocytosis is the mechanism of choice for large particles. Additionally, as highlighted, the RES, which consists of sinusoid in the spleen, and fenestra of the Kupffer cells in the liver, presents with openings from 150 nm to 200 nm. Furthermore, the size of gap junction between the endothelial cells of the leaky vasculature of tumor tissues varies from 100 nm to 600 nm. Thus the size of NPs should not exceed 100 nm to effectively reach tumor tissues via these specific vascular structures. Further, the size of NPs should be optimized to prevent their leakage into blood capillaries. Numerous critical *in vivo* NP attributes, for example, circulation time, targeting, internalization, and clearance, are size dependent (Oh and Park 2014). Vesicles of ~100 nm participate in clathrin-mediated endocytosis. Caveolae-mediated endocytosis is followed by vesicles of 60–80 nm (Kou et al. 2013). There is, however, evidence that size may not be of utmost significance relative to other factors in the selection of a NP entry pathway (Huang et al. 2002).

Investigations have been undertaken in attempts to explore the size-dependent internalization of NPs in cancer cells. Unconjugated gold NPs of various sizes were investigated for uptake in human cervical cancer (HeLa) cells (Chithrani et al. 2006; Chithrani and Chan 2007; Jiang et al. 2008). Size was demonstrated to influence the uptake mechanism and saturation concentration. Gold NPs having a size of 50 nm demonstrated the most efficient cellular uptake comparatively, within the 14–100 nm range. It was proposed that serum-containing protein absorption of the anionic surface promoted non-specific uptake by cancer cells (Chithrani and Chan 2007). Herceptin-conjugated gold NPs having a size of 25–50 nm exhibited the best uptake in SK-BR-3 breast cancer cells when a size range of 2–100 nm was examined (Jiang et al. 2008).

Uptake of polymeric particles <25 nm has been demonstrated to be via non-degradative, cholesterol-independent, and non-clathrin and non–caveolae-dependent endocytosis, emanating in their conveyance as punctate structures in the HeLa cell perinuclear region. This was not exhibited for larger NPs >40 nm (Lai et al. 2007; Barua and Rege 2009). Various sizes of polystyrene NP uptake were evaluated in a human colon adenocarcinoma cell line (Win and Feng 2005). The uptake of particles of size 100 nm was enhanced compared to 50, 200, 500 and 1000 nm NPs, with the internalization efficiency of 50 nm particles being the lowest. It is thus evident that often in concert with size, the NP material also has a pertinent effect on cellular uptake.

11.4.2   NANOPARTICLE COMPOSITION AND STIMULUS-RESPONSIVENESS

When evaluating the effect of NP composition on cellular uptake, Oh and Park (2014) proposed that particle stiffness may be responsible for this phenomenon, as there is more rapid endocytosis if there is a tighter interaction, which would occur between stiffer particles and the cell membrane, for example, inorganic NPs vs. polymeric NPs. The therapeutic use of inorganic and semiconductor NPs has grown due to the interaction potential of inorganic NPs with light or magnetic fields, thus having application in imaging of cancer sites via fluorescence or magnetic resonance imaging, X-ray imaging, or Raman imaging, as well for chemotherapeutic drug delivery via external stimulus-triggered release. Gold NPs have demonstrated certain advantages above other inorganic NPs owing to simple synthetic approaches achieving controlled sizes and shapes and good biocompatibility due to their inertness, with various studies on their cellular uptake into mammalian cells (Kobayashi et al. 2014).

The composition of NPs can also be tailored to be responsive to external stimuli (e.g., ultrasound, light, heat) or internal stimuli (e.g., change in pH, redox potential, enzymes) with resultant drug release. The NPs maintain a stealth nature until triggered to transform or degrade to elaborate drug release with subsequent enhanced intracellular delivery in the presence of an environmental or focused applied stimulus. Ultrasound has been commonly employed to illicit drug release to solid tumors from NPs, as reported by Rapoport and coworkers (2009, 2010, 2011). The mild hyperthermia induced following ultrasound-mediated delivery of micelles enhances their extravasation into the tumor, while the mechanical action of ultrasound causes drug release. In their recent investigation (Rapoport et al. 2011), they employed a core-forming compound of perfluoro-15-crown-5-ether (PFCE) in their perfluoro-carbon nanoemulsions, displaying both ultrasound and fluorine (^{19}F) MR contrast properties.

NPs composed of photo-sensitive polymers can be light-triggered for employment in targeted cancer therapy. Cell uptake and liberation of the payload may be by photo-driven isomerization and activation, de-crosslinking, surface plasmon absorption and photochemical effects, hydrophobicity changes, and polymer backbone fragmentation (Biswas and Torchilin 2004). For example, You et al. (2010) developed dual-functional hollow gold nanospheres (HAuNS) transporting doxorubicin (DOX), which were ~40 nm in diameter and enabled both photothermal ablation of MDA-MB-231 breast cancer cells and drug release with near-infrared (NIR) light irradiation. HAuNS with the DOX were internalized by the MDA-MB-231 cells via phagocytosis and distributed to the endolysosomal compartments with distribution to cell nuclei 1hr after incubation. This investigation highlights the potential for controlling intracellular DOX release from HAuNS by NIR laser irradiation. The specific composition of iron oxide NPs also allows them to be driven by an external magnetic field promoting cancer cell uptake (El-Dakdouki et al. 2012; Kaaki et al. 2012; Huang et al. 2013). Huang and coworkers (2013) developed pH-responsive superparamagnetic iron oxide NP (SPION)-micelles including β-lapachone (β-lap), an innovative anticancer agent demonstrating notable cancer specificity through selective enhancement of reactive oxygen species (ROS) stress in tumor cells. The synergism between SPION and β-lap was exploited for enhanced chemotherapy. Following four hours of incubation, localization of most of the SPION-micelles (>80 percent) occurred in late endosomes and lysosomes, with the acidic microenvironment eliciting iron ion release.

Internal stimuli, including pH, temperature, redox potential, overexpressed proteolytic enzymes of the TME can also activate and promote the uptake of NPs, where specific moieties become exposed revealing the required functionality. In polymeric and co-polymeric micelles and dendritic structures, an integrated stimulus-responsive moiety as part of the fabricated composition enables triggered spatial or temporal bioactive release. For polymeric and copolymeric micelles and dendritic structures, such a moiety could be a fundamental component of the structural polymer. pH-tunable moieties, for example, carboxyl or tertiary amino groups, are incorporated into pH-sensitive self-assembled polymeric NPs, functioning as pH sensors due to alteration of their hydrophobicity on protonation and deprotonation (Schmaljohann 2006; Bawa et al. 2009). Polymers employed to achieve this include poly(acrylic acid) (PAA) and its derivatives, which swell or collapse with pH variation. pH-sensitive linkages may also be employed, including hydrazine, hydrazide, or acetal. The chemotherapeutic agent may be conjugated to a dendritic scaffold's functional group (Lee et al. 2006); the low pH of the TME triggers drug release, with the alteration in hydrophobicity following cleavage of the pH-sensitive bonds potentially inducing the dendrimer to undergo a conformational change. Liposomal structures may incorporate a pH-responsive component as an inherent segment of the composing lipid or may be included via chemical modification, resulting in carriers only undergoing cleavage at a lower pH, avoiding premature and non-specific drug release. Thus cleavage generally occurs intracellularly, with more options for enhanced cellular uptake via endocytic pathways (Fleige et al. 2012).

NP composition may also be exploited to promote endosomal escape. Liposomes and micelles may be composed of lipids possessing the ability to fuse with endosomal membranes, thus destabilizing the nanosystem, with subsequent drug release. Dioleoyl phosphatidylethanolamine (DOPE) is a lipid existing in both lamellar and hexagonal phases, and has been employed as a fusogenic lipid (Farhood et al. 1995; Kogure et al. 2007). At the low endosomal pH, it transforms from lamellar to inverted hexagonal, thus promoting fusion of the nanosystem and endosomal membrane, with payload release (Hafez and Cullis 2001; Biswas and Torchilin 2014).

11.4.3 NANOPARTICLE SURFACE CHARGE

The zeta (ζ) potential represents the electrostatic potential at the NP shear plane, relating both to surface charge and the local milieu of the NP. It is a pertinent parameter in colloid science for explicating electrostatic interactions and is employed in cell biology for investigation of cell adhesion, activation, and agglutination centered on cell–surface charge properties (Zhang et al. 2009). The impact of zeta potential on cellular interaction could be significant (Altankov et al. 2003).

The cytomembrane is negatively charged (Coulman et al. 2009); it thus follows that there would be a strong electrostatic interaction with cationic NP, facilitating rapid entry. There may be escape of positively charged particles from endosomes following internalization with the "proton sponge effect," eliciting perinuclear localization (Kou et al. 2013). Neutral NPs could undergo cell interaction via hydrophobic and hydrogen bond interactions (Vandamme and Brobeck 2005). Coating of these particles with hydrophilic polymers could prevent interaction with the cytomembrane, thus limiting absorption. Endocytosis of anionic NPs could be via interactions with positive sites of membrane proteins; extensive capturing is possible due to repulsive interactions with the negatively charged cell surface (Yeung et al. 2008). The choice of pathway depending on surface charge is not clear: The majority of cationic NPs enter via clathrin-mediated endocytosis; however, micropinocytosis or caveolae- or clathrin-independent endocytosis may occur (Harush-Frenkel et al. 2008; Perumal et al. 2008; Kovács et al. 2009). Caveolae-mediated endocytosis is more common for anionic NPs, with some exception (Vina-Vilaseca et al. 2011). Neutral NPs show no specific pathway preference (Kou et al. 2013).

Specific investigations on the impact of charge density and charge type (i.e., positive, negative, or neutral) in nonphagocytic cells highlighted that charged polystyrene and iron oxide NPs showed enhanced uptake compared to their unionized counterparts (Thorek and Tsourkas 2008; Villanueva et al. 2009; Jiang et al. 2011). Further, cationic NPs demonstrated enhanced uptake compared to anionic NPs. Fröhlich et al. (2012) summarized that it has been specifically shown in various investigations that there was higher ingestion of cationic gold and silver, superparamagnetic iron oxide, hydroxyapatite, silicon dioxide, lipid, and polymer (e.g., poly(lactic acid), chitosan, polystyrene) NPs than their anionic complements (Miller et al. 1998; Cho and Caruso 2005; Lorenz et al. 2006; Harush-Frenkel 2008; Ge et al. 2009;

Mailander and Landfester 2009; Brandenberger et al. 2010; Chen et al. 2011; Marquis et al. 2011; Yue et al. 2011).

As examples of the manner in which modified surface charge affects the trafficking of polymeric NPs, Lorenz et al. (2006) surmised that surface charge affected cellular uptake in the absence of transfection agents. The surface charge of the fluorescent-labeled polymeric NPs was varied through adjustment of the amount of copolymerized monomer–bearing amino groups for investigation of the cellular uptake and intracellular trafficking in correlation to the zeta potential in three cancer cell lines (HeLa and leukemic cell lines, Jurkat, and KG1a), as visualized in Figure 11.4. It was concluded that surface charge mainly affects the first step of attachment of the NPs to the cell membrane, whereas the differences in the intracellular localization among various cell lines is attributed to endocytotic/pinocytotic specific properties of each cell line. Chung and coworkers (2010) demonstrated similar results for poly (lactide-co-glycolide) (PLGA)–based NPs coated with either heparin-Pluronic (negative) or chitosan-Pluronic (positive) conjugate, for potentially enhancing the tumor-targeting efficacy compared to pure Pluronic-coated PLGA NPs (control) in the SCC7 tumor-bearing athymic mouse model. Yue et al. (2011) investigated the uptake and intracellular trafficking of polymeric NPs possessing varying surface charges in various cell lines, including a human lung cancer cell line (A549).

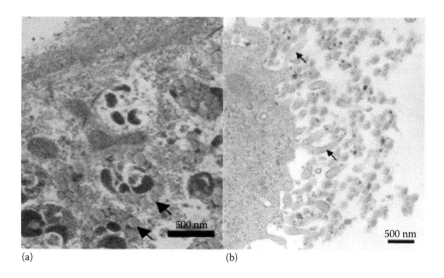

(a) (b)

FIGURE 11.4 (a) Surface functionalization with cationic groups enhanced the uptake of the NPs in the absence of transfection agents compared to neutral NPs into HeLa cells, and intracellular uptake into endosomal compartments was visualized. HeLa cells incubated with NPs (arrows) for 24 hours show their localization inside organelles. (b) In KG1a there was clustered attachment of the NPs to the cell membrane with surrounding microvilli. TEM analysis of KG1a cells incubated for 24 hours with NPs showed adhesion of NP clusters on the cell membrane. Microvilli (arrows) extend between the particle clusters and the particles are bridged by electron dense material (arrowhead). A similar observation was made with Jurkat cells. (Reproduced with permission from Lorenz, M. R. et al., *Biomaterials*, 27 2820–2828, 2006. Elsevier B.V. Ltd. ©2006.)

They reported that rate and amount of cellular uptake have a positive correlation with the surface charge in all cell lines investigated. In the ensuing intracellular trafficking there was escape of some positively charged chitosan NPs from the lysosome with perinuclear localization, whereas the negatively and neutrally charged NPs displayed preferential colocalization with the lysosome, as depicted in Figure 11.5.

In a smart approach to tumor-targeted NP delivery, Hung and coworkers (2016) formulated PLGA NPs coated with pH-responsive N-acetyl histidine modified D-α-tocopheryl polyethylene glycol succinate (NAcHis-TPGS), for enhancing chemotherapeutic agent uptake and penetration. The resultant nanocarriers possessed responsiveness to tumor extracellular acidity (pH$_e$) via switching of their surface charge, and delivered the photothermal agent, indocyanine green (ICG), and the chemotherapeutic drug doxorubicin (DOX). There was enhanced *in vitro* cancer cell and macrophage uptake of the ICG/DOX NPs in a weak acidic environment owing to increased NAcHis (imidazole) moiety protonation causing attraction to the negatively-charged cell membrane surface. Ex vivo and *in vivo* biodistribution studies highlighted notable accumulation of the theranostic NPs in the TRAMP-C1 solid tumor mouse model following intravenous injection. The NPs achieved active permeation into deep hypoxic tumor sites owing to their small size, neutral surface induced by the pH$_e$, as well as hitchhiking transport via tumor-associated macrophages. Following tumor accumulation, image-guided photothermal therapy by the ICG/DOX NPs caused extensive tumor/vessel ablation, further enhancing NP extravasation and permeation of tumors by DOX. This photothermal/chemo dual-modality therapy is promising for cancer theranosis (Hung et al. 2016).

With specific reference to uptake of metal-based NPs by cancer cells, the internalization and biocompatibility of iron oxide NPs displaying functionalization of their surfaces by four carbohydrates possessing various charges (dextran, amino-dextran, heparin, and dimercaptosuccinic) was evaluated by Villanueva et al. (2009) in the HeLa cell line. Neutral NPs demonstrated no detectable uptake. The behavior of anionic NPs differed with regard to the chemical makeup of the coating: dimercaptosuccinic-coating resulted in low cellular uptake with non-toxic effects, while heparin-coating of NPs required high NP concentrations for cellular uptake,

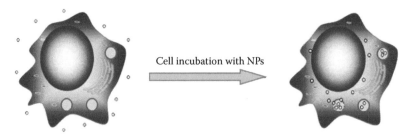

Cell incubation with NPs

○ Positively charged NPs   ◔ Neutrally charged NPs   ○ Negatively charged NPs   ◯ Lysosome

FIGURE 11.5 Cellular uptake and intracellular distribution of NPs with different surface charge. (Reproduced with permission from Yue, Z. G. et al., *Biomacromolecules*, 12, 2440–2446, 2011. American Chemical Society ©2011.)

with induction of abnormal mitotic spindle configurations. In contrast, cationic magnetic NPs entered the cells with high efficacy with endosomal localization, were readily detectable within cells by optical microscopy, were retained for comparatively longer time periods, and did not induce cytotoxicity. Thus, the cationic NPs demonstrated favorable properties for potential *in vivo* biomedical applications including cell tracking by magnetic resonance imaging (MRI), as well as hyperthermic cancer treatment (Villanueva et al. 2009). Employing cerium oxide NPs ("nanoceria") Asati et al. (2010) investigated the previously poorly understood interaction of polymer-coated nanoceria with normal and cancer cells lines, their mechanism of uptake, subcellular localization, and whether there was a correlation between cytotoxicity and localization in lysosomes. Positive and neutral nanoceria entered most cell lines investigated, while negative nanoceria mostly internalized within the cancer cell lines, as demonstrated in Figure 11.6. The anionic NPs underwent lysosomal uptake,

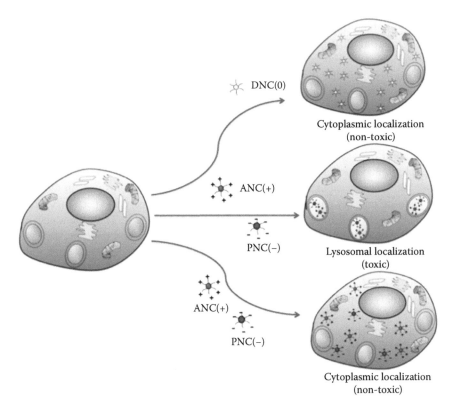

FIGURE 11.6 Polymer-coated nanoceria cell internalization, localization and proposed toxicity mechanism. Neutral DNC(0) internalized and localized mostly into the cytoplasm of cells; therefore not cytotoxic. ANC(+) and PNC(−) can localize either into the cytoplasm or the lysosomes, depending on cell type. With localization of nanoceria to the lysosome, the low organelle pH activates the NP oxidase-like activity, exhibiting toxicity. ANC(−) or PNC(+) that localized into the cytoplasm displayed no cytotoxicity. (Reproduced with permission from Asati, A. et al., *ACS Nano*, 4, 5321–5331, 2010. American Chemical Society ©2010.)

subsequently instigating significant cell death; whereas there was localization in the cytoplasm of viable tumor cells when cationic nanoceria were employed, with minimal toxicity. Nanoceria internalization and subcellular localization thus depended on the surface charge, exhibiting a pertinent role on the cytotoxicity profile.

11.4.4 Nanoparticle Shape

The NP shape could have a notable impact on the biological behavior of NPs such as blood circulation, margination ability, and binding affinity (Oh and Park 2014). It thus follows that NP shape has notable effects on the tumor deposition rate and the drug cargo's therapeutic efficacy. The role of particle shape on drug delivery has been explored; however, the main focus has been on phagocytosis rather than the actual pathway selected on uptake of the NPs (Champion and Mitragotri 2009; Lu et al. 2010). NPs with the correct aspect ratio may be more rapidly internalized (Gratton et al. 2008; Mitragotri and Lahann 2009; Meng et al. 2011). Investigations have highlighted the varied effects of NP shape on cellular uptake (Chithrani et al. 2006; Qiu et al. 2010). The highest uptake in HeLa is demonstrated by nanoscale rods, followed by spheres, cylinders, and cubes. The aspect ratio notably affects the uptake of cylindrically shaped NPs. However, an increase in the aspect ratio of gold nanorods significantly decreased their receptor-mediated endocytosis (Oh and Park 2014).

As evidenced, NPs size pertinently influences intratumoral deposition via the EPR effect. Investigations have indicated that an optimal diameter of 100 nm is required for tumoral deposition of spherical NPs (which also depends on the vascular pore size, pharmacokinetics and potential to surmount high interstitial pressures; Mayer et al. 1989; Nagayasu et al. 1994). Tumor microvascular systems vary in the size of the endothelial gaps, interstitial pressure, microvessel density and geometry; further various tumor types have differing vascular wall pore shapes. Thus, the aspect ratio of a NP would also uniquely influence extravasation rates and patterns, depending on the tumor type, which was aptly demonstrated in the study of Smith et al. (2012). They exposed three tumor types: human glioblastoma (U87MG), ovarian adenocarcinoma (SKOV-3), and colon adenocarcinoma (LS174T) to two widely applied but contrastingly shaped NPs: Quantum dots (QDs) and single-walled carbon nanotubes (SWNT). QDs and SWNTs possess notable variation in their physical properties, such as shape and size, but display a similar surface area despite their geometrical differences. Intravital micrsocopy (IVM) was employed, which enables detailed microscopic imaging of phenomena in living subjects for elucidation of the manner in which NPs target cancer sites. Results demonstrated that both NPs displayed almost no extravasation in SKOV-3 tumors; however, there was fourfold greater extravasation of QDs compared to SWNTs of the same surface area in a LS174T tumor; whereas when it came to an U87MG tumor, only the nanotubes extravasated. This differential extravasation is detailed in Figure 11.7. Data may highlight that slightly smaller U87MG pores could enable notably more SWNTs to diffuse than QDs, while the somewhat larger size of LS174T pores could favor diffusion of QDs. However, other factors could also contribute to extravasational variations observed, for example, U87MG tumors possess a fenestrated endothelium which creates gaps

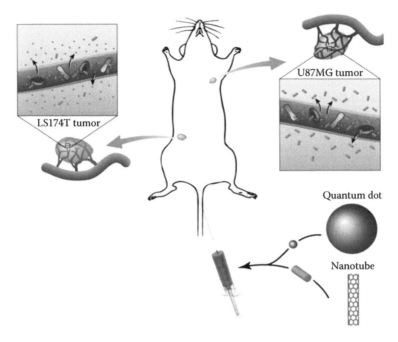

FIGURE 11.7 Schematic of NP extravasation in murine tumor models highlighting QD extravasation from LS174T tumor but not U87MG tumor, and SWNTs extravasation from U87MG tumor with minimal trafficking from LS174T tumor. (Reproduced with permission from Smith, B. R. et al., *Nano Lett*, 12, 3369–3377, 2012. American Chemical Society ©2012.)

~5.5 nm. U87MG tumors possessed the lowest pore cut-off size as demonstrated by the spherical particle challenge; however, they had the highest permeability to albumin. This indicates the presence of very small pores through which SWNTs could traffick via Brownian motion; however, movement of QDs was sterically restricted. This study does highlight that having a knowledge of the physical parameters of a patient's tumor would be essential in providing personalized oncological care, as a specific NP architecture (shape and size) could be fabricated for the apt tumor conditions (Smith et al. 2012). This study also highlights the interplay between the physicochemical properties of the NPs as well as the tumor/cell type.

Peiris and coworkers (2012) undertook investigations highlighting the enhanced delivery of NPs with a greater aspect ratio (in their case nanochains were exploited) to overexpressed vascular targets in tumors. The vascular targeting system comprised an $\alpha v \beta 3$ integrin-targeted nanochain particle which consisted of four chemically linked iron oxide nanospheres as a linear assemblage. The chain-shaped NPs enabled enhanced recognition of the vascular bed tumor-associated remodeling for more specific targeting of metastatic tumors. *In vivo* evaluation via multimodal *in vivo* imaging (Fluorescence Molecular Tomography and MRI) in an orthotopic 4T1 mammary adenocarcinoma mouse model revealed two times enhanced targeting of $\alpha_v \beta_3$ integrin at the tumor site by the nanochains compared to spherical NPs after 45 minutes due to geometrically enhanced multivalent docking. In the investigation of Karaman et al. (2012), the effect of various NP properties in addition to the shape on cellular internalization was realized. Both spherical and rod-shaped porous silica NPs were prepared and their cellular uptake efficiency examined in the HeLa and Caco-2 (human epithelial colorectal adenocarcinoma) cell lines. HeLa cells readily internalized both rod-shaped and spherical NPs, having slight shape and charge-associated differences; however, rod-shaped NPs demonstrated more efficient internalization in Caco-2 cells compared to their spherical counterparts. Thus, in addition to NP shape and surface functionalization, the cell origin and its features also has an effect on NP trafficking. NP shape appears to have a cell-dependent influence and can be exploited as such (Karaman et al. 2012). Barua et al. (2013) have demonstrated that an oblate shape enhances binding and cellular membrane trafficking of antibody-displaying NPs compared to a nanospherical geometry. A fivefold greater inhibition of BT-474 breast cell growth was attained for their trastuzumab-coated nanorods in comparison to nanospheres carrying the same dose.

An important point to note as that beyond the shape and the size, composition, surface charge and polymeric coating, non-spherical NPs possess unique properties to their spherical counterparts, for example, their enhanced response to a magnetic field or photothermal triggered therapy (Toy et al. 2014), which further affects mechanisms of transbarrier trafficking. PRINT, a top-down particle fabrication technique, has been employed in NP preparation to acquire the desired size, shape, and surface chemistry (Gratton et al. 2008; DeSimone 2009; Kou et al. 2013).

11.4.5 NANOPARTICLE SURFACE CHEMISTRY/HYDROPHOBICITY AND SURFACE MODIFICATION

Efficacious chemotherapy and side effect reduction requires that drug delivery to the tumor site should be controlled and tumor cell-specific—this is the ultimate goal of nanosystem-based chemotherapy. This has emanated on various investigations being undertaken on the relationship between the NP surface characteristics, the site of accumulation, and localization of NPs within the organ, and cell specificity (Kobayashi et al. 2014). The lack of precise control over the chemistry of the NP surface is an important factor that limits mechanistic studies of cellular uptake, as there is difficulty in preparing model NPs where there is systematic variation of a single structural parameter. Metal NPs, silica NPs, and QDs are more commonly investigated and display surface homogeneity, with modifications limited to surface deposition and ligand exchange reactions. Single-molecule polymeric organic NPs (ONPs), including dendrimers, intramolecularly crosslinked polymers and hyperbranched polymers, have a bottom-up synthetic approach, and could provide enhanced flexibility for surface functionalization through presentation of a precise number of specific functional groups, ordered internal architecture, and a narrow size distribution. Bai et al. (2015) described a novel approach for formulating water-soluble, biocompatible ONPs via consecutive ring-opening metathesis polymerization and ring-closing metathesis (ROMP-RCM) process for facile incorporation of a wide range of functional groups, synthetic scalability, and enhanced size control. They demonstrated that the monomer employed in the linear polymerization had a significant effect on the lipophilicity and thus degree of cell internalization in HeLa cells, and the resultant ONP could serve as platform (with ready incorporation of fluorophores) for a systematic study of NP–cell interactions with regard to surface properties and size (Figure 11.8). The cell internalization rate was enhanced with an increase in repeating unit lipophilicity as well as by decreasing ONP size. They demonstrated the concept of "masked" vs. "unmasked" ONPs employing a thiol-bearing ONP that underwent predictable changes in cellular uptake with maleimide conjugation (Bai et al. 2015).

The affinity for the cell membrane, and therefore cell uptake kinetics and amount, is enhanced with increasing NP hydrophobicity, which depends on the NP chemical composition. Modification of NPs with hydrophilic polymers, for example, polyethylene glycol (PEG; Lankveld et al. 2011), poly (N-vinyl-2-pyrrolidone; PVP; Kaneda et al. 2004), poly(amino acids; Riche et al. 2004) and dextran (Moore et al. 2000), can form a suppressive cloud that limits NP–lipid bilayer interaction. However, circulation lifetime is enhanced allowing more time to reach the target site. The endocytic pathway employed could depend on the polymeric composition of the NP (Kou et al. 2013).

It must further be borne in mind that the attainment of a balance of the NP hydrophobicity and hydrophilicity is pertinent in order to maintain dispersibility in serum, as well as enable basic cellular uptake. On penetration of hydrophobic NPs within the cell membrane into the cytosol, a switch to hydrophilicity is required for facile permeation. A stimulus-responsive switch between the hydrophobicity and hydrophilicity of the NP would accelerate cellular permeation (Kobayashi et al. 2014). Such stimuli, which have successfully altered the surface properties, include light (Han et al. 2006; Shao et al. 2010; Subramani et al. 2011; Tong et al. 2012; Jonsson et al. 2013) and temperature (Zhu et al. 2004; Liu et al. 2012). Several groups (Han et al. 2006; Shao et al. 2010; Jonsson et al. 2013) have demonstrated hydrophilic/hydrophobic photoswitching on spiropyrane-immobilized NP surfaces. Han et al. (2006) employed this reversal of surface charge on exposure to ultraviolet irradiation for the intracellular delivery of genes, which could have application in cancer

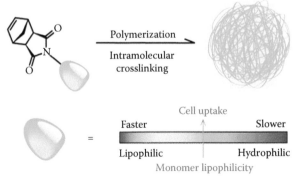

FIGURE 11.8 Schematic representation demonstrating institution of surface functional groups to control the cellular uptake of polymeric ONPs. (Reproduced with permission from Bai, Y. et al., *ACS Nano*, 9, 10227–10236, 2015. American Chemical Society ©2015).

therapy. Gold NPs with a PEG-derivative thiol ligand possessing *o*-nitrobenzaldehyde were developed possessing a cationic group at the end. The initially cationic particles are converted to anionically charged NPs through cleavage of *o*-nitrobenzaldehyde via ultraviolet irradiation, as depicted in Figure 11.9. Similarly, coating of NPs with thermoresponsive polymers will enable temperature control of the state of aggregation (Kobayashi et al. 2014).

A significant challenge in the design of targeted NPs for enhanced cancer therapy is the identification of targeting ligands enabling differential binding and internalization by the targeted cancer cells (Cho et al. 2008; Xiao et al. 2012). Targeting ligands/agents can be employed to achieve cell-specific delivery, especially as tumor cells characteristically overexpress certain receptors or molecules which normal cells do not (You et al. 2013). An example is binding of a folate-targeted conjugate to the surface folate receptor. The plasma membrane invaginates to envelop the receptor–ligand complex, thus forming an endosome, which subsequently undergoes trafficking to target organelles. The interior of the endosome progressively becomes more acidic, resulting in activation of lysozymes, thereby releasing the drug from the conjugate enabling cytoplasmic entry with subsequent trafficking by the target organelle. Significantly, the physicochemical properties of the drug will also affect its potential for partitioning across the endosomal membrane. The released folate receptor returns to the cell membrane for participation in further transportation (Cho et al. 2008). Further, the breast cancer cell line, SK-BR-3, overexpresses the Herceptin receptor, HER-2 (human epidermal growth factor receptor 2). Conjugation of Herceptin as a targeting agent to NPs thus enables their selective internalization by the SK-BR-3 cell line (Baselga et al. 1998; You et al. 2013). Rathinaraj et al. (2014) described the precise interaction and internalization of gold NPs on which the Herceptin monoclonal antibody was immobilized (GNP–HER) into SK-BR3

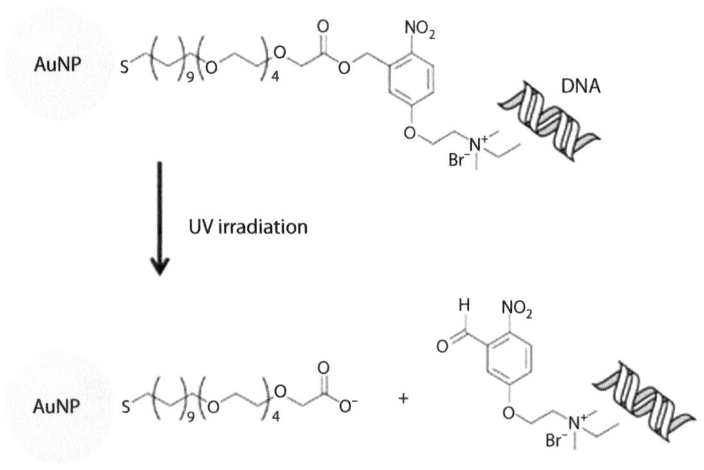

FIGURE 11.9 Charge reversal surface ligands upon UV irradiation with associated intracellular DNA release. (Reproduced with permission from Kobayashi, K. et al., *Polymer Journal*, 46, 460–468, 2014. Nature Publishing Group ©2014.)

cells (confirmed by confocal laser scanning microscopy, CLSM, as demonstrated in Figure 11.10). The GNPs possessed a mean size of 29 nm, which increased to 82 nm following herceptin attachment. Fluorescence images in Figure 11.10 thus highlight there was initiation of interaction of SK-BR3 with GNP-HER following one hour of incubation which accelerated and saturated by six hours, highlighting effective attainment of NP-mediated delivery of monoclonal antibodies, with resultant cell death. The internalization mechanism implicated endocytosis, with consequential release of the GNP-HER into the cytoplasm. The specific binding of herceptin to the receptor on SK-BR3 membrane withdraws the growth signal to SK-BR3 cells with consequent cell death (Rathinaraj et al. 2014). Xiao et al. (2012) focused on prostate cancer (PCa), and conceptualized a cell-uptake selection strategy for isolation of PCa-specific internalizing 2'-O-methyl RNA aptamers (Apts) to incorporate onto NPs. Pertinently their strategy focused on enriching cancer cell-specific internalizing Apts rather than isolating high-affinity Apts (Xiao et al. 2012).

There is also overexpression of certain sugar receptors by tumor cells. NPs functionalized with galactose selectively enter human liver hepatocellular carcinoma (HepG2) cells as a result of receptor-mediated endocytosis, rather than HeLa cells (Lai et al. 2010; Lee et al. 2012). This was demonstrated by Lai et al. (2010), who synthesized fluorescent galactosyl–conjugated magnetic NPs (MNPs) as potential biomedical probes. These MNPs interacted with the extracellular asialoglycoprotein

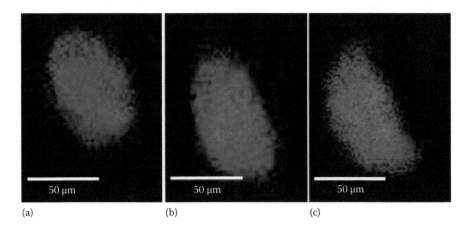

(a)　　　　　　　　　(b)　　　　　　　　　(c)

FIGURE 11.10 Fluorescence images of SK-BR3 cells highlighting specific HER-2 interaction with herceptin (using the blue dye, 4,6-diamidino-2-phenylindole dihydrochloride, DAPI) and the internalized GNP–Her (red). Images were obtained from the culture of SK-BR3 cells for (a) 1 hour, (b) 3 hours, and (c) 6 hours in the presence of DAPI. After 1 hour, there was visualization of weak GNP–Her conjugates in the fluorescence image (red color) after 1 hour (a), with a slight increase in intensity at 3 hours (b) and intense fluorescence at 6 hours (c). Conversely, at 1 hour, there was strong blue fluorescence due to nuclei staining with DAPI which decreased as incubation time increased and was almost not visible after 6 hours of incubation. (Reproduced from Rathinaraj, P. et al., *Breast Canc Targets Ther*, 7, 51–58, 2014. Dove Medical Press Ltd., under Creative Commons Attribution—Non Commercial [unported, v3.0 License].)

receptor (ASGP-R) on the cell surface, triggering internalization via receptor-mediated endocytosis. The group also highlighted that the spatial orientations of the multivalent galactosyl-conjugated ligands had an effect on the ingestion ability of the liver cells, with the tri-antennary galactosyl-conjugated MNP demonstrating the highest efficacy.

Following cellular uptake, certain surface modifications can control nanoparticulate localization within cells. An additional selective barrier to nuclear import includes the nuclear pores located on the nuclear envelope. The nuclear import of maltotriose(Glc_3)-displaying QDs through the pores of digitonin-treated HeLa cells was increased due to enhanced affinity between the nuclear pore and surface QD sugar pendant, whereas mono- and disaccharide QDs failed to be transported, as confirmed by Sekiguchi et al. (2012) and represented in Figure 11.11. It was thus demonstrated that the nuclear pores–carbohydrate interaction propelled the nuclear import of maltooligo-QDs. Functionalization of QDs with various sugars for intracellular localization was also investigated by Benito-Alifonso and team (2014), demonstrated in a HeLa cell line, where they highlighted the effect of the type of sugar employed on cellular uptake of QDs. Lactose functionalization elicited a Trojan horse effect for enabling the cellular uptake of QDs possessing additional noninternalizable moieties (e.g., mannose and maltotriose). The organelle-defined uptake is provided in Figure 11.12.

An issue associated with a number of the currently employed tumor targeting probes is the poor permeability of tumors to bloodborne compounds, specifically in solid tumors, having a particularly high IFP (Ruoslahti et al. 2012). Drug penetration is limited to 3–5 cell diameters from the blood vessel, thus deeper tumor cells

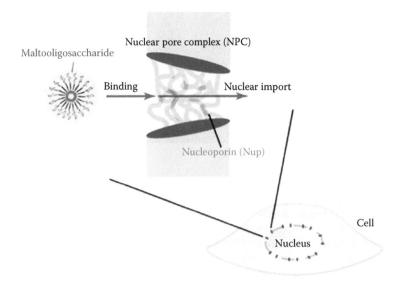

FIGURE 11.11 Schematic illustration of nuclear import through the nuclear pore. (Reproduced with permission from Sekiguchi, S. et al., *RSC Advances*, 2, 1656–1662, 2012. Royal Society of Chemistry ©2011.)

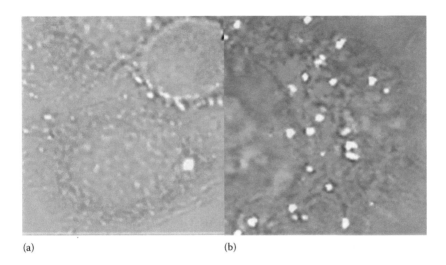

(a)   (b)

FIGURE 11.12   Representative confocal microscopy images showing internalization after 2 hours incubation of (a) galactose-QD in the Golgi of HeLa cells; (b) lactose-QD in the Golgi of HeLa cells; QD shown in green, organelle tracker in red, and overlap in yellow. (Reproduced with permission from Benito-Alifonso, D. et al., *Angew Chem Int Ed*, 53, 810–814, 2014. John Wiley and Sons ©2013.)

may not receive sufficient drug exposure leading to the development of resistance (Hambley and Hait 2009). Ruoslathi et al. (2012) highlighted their laboratory work on a tissue–cell penetration system that stimulates both homing to the target tissue and, as well as tissue penetration. A tissue penetration motif (R/KXXR/K) is contained by the peptide, which requires exposure at the C terminus of the peptide or protein for activity as per the C-end rule (CendR). A tumor-homing CendR peptide incorporates a tumor-specific homing sequence as well as a cryptic (not C terminal) CendR sequence. The homing sequence transports the peptide to the target tissue vascular endothelium; proteolytic processing of the CendR motif transforming it to the active C terminal. This subsequently binds to the neuropilin-1 receptor, enabling the C-terminally truncated peptide to be extravasated, undergo tissue penetration and ultimate cell entry, together with any payload transported with it (Sugahara et al. 2009; Ruoslahti et al. 2012). In other attempts to achieve tumor specificity, Jiang and coworkers (2004) investigated a cationic cell-penetrating peptide to which a negatively charged sequence is attached, thus blocking cell penetration until cleavage via a tumor protease, achieving tumor-homing that was enhanced three-times (Ruoslahti et al. 2012).

11.5   CANCER CELL TYPE AS A SELECTIVE BARRIER TO NP TRAFFICKING

The effect of cancer cell types has been highlighted in each of the above discussions on NP properties, as there is an inextricable link. There is tumor cell-specific expression of different endocytic pathways which affects the amount and velocity of NP uptake (Fröhlich et al. 2012). Certain cells may lack the necessary proteins for a specific endocytic pathway, for example, HepG2 cells do not possess endogenous caveolin thus endocytosis via this pathway is not possible (Fujimoto et al. 2000). Cellular growth conditions (e.g., cell density and hormones) could affect the cell phenotype and thus the endocytic pathway. Pertinently, this is evident in the variation between normal and tumor cells, thus rendering the different endocytic pathway of tumor cells as an apt target (Sahay et al. 2010). The connection between cell origin and the resultant endocytic pathway is not well-defined and requires further research (Kou et al. 2013).

11.6 QUANTIFICATION OF NANOPARTICLE CANCER CELL UPTAKE AND INTRACELLULAR TRAFFICKING

As highlighted in this chapter, NP–cancer cell interactions involve a number of cellular uptake steps followed by active and kinetic intracellular trafficking. Additionally, the heterogeneity of the TME may lead to small deviations in cellular uptake which requires large sample sizes to obtain statistically meaningful results (Turnbull et al. 2015). Therefore, advanced state-of-the-art instrumental techniques are carried out to accurately, precisely, and efficiently characterize these processes at a single cell level (Vanhecke et al. 2014). *In vitro* assays generally employ methods based on quantification techniques such as (1) laser scanning microscopy (LSM; fluorescent NPs), (2) flow cytometry (fluorescence labeling), (3) Inductively Coupled Plasma Techniques (metallic NPs), and (4) Transmission Electron Images (TEM; electron density; Vanhecke et al. 2014). The selection of either the microscopy or spectroscopy techniques and stereology will depend on the characteristics of the NPs with regards to organic, inorganic, or hybrid-based nanocarriers and the environment of the targeted cancer cells (Ekkapongpisit et al. 2012). To this end, these methods will be briefly discussed to highlight their suitability and limitations to NPs cellular uptake and distribution at single cancer cell environments.

11.6.1 Laser Scanning Microscopy

Traditional fluorescence microscope imaging with the use of fluorescent biomarkers and dyes has been effectively used to show cellular uptake. Moreover trafficking studies have been reported, for instance Ekkapongpisit (2012) observed that trafficking depends on both the physiochemical of NPs and the biochemical composition of the cell membrane of the targeted cancer cell. However, this method lacks the axial (z-axis) resolution to precisely detect the locations of intracellular NPs (Ichimura et al. 2014). This limitation is overcome by employing confocal microscopy, which lends itself to two methods, namely confocal laser scanning microscopy (CLSM) and spinning disk confocal laser microscopy (SDCLM). The former method requires relative longer acquisition time but provides better axial resolution and signal-to-noise ratio. Furthermore, it is possible to view the intracellular compartments such as the membrane, cytoplasm, mitochondria, and nucleus by independently labeling

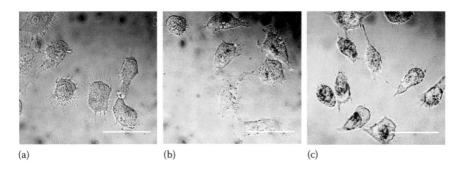

(a)   (b)   (c)

FIGURE 11.13   Two-color confocal laser scanning microscopy imaging of HeLa cells after incubation time of 3 hours with 2 nm (200 nM), 4 nm (100 nM), and 6 nm (30 nM) NPs, respectively. Scale bar is 50 mm. (Images in panels a–c were reproduced from Kim, C. S. et al., *Methods X*, 2, 306–315, 2015. Elsevier B.V. Ltd. under Creative Commons Attribution License.)

with different color-emitting fluorescent tags, which upon absorption of selected laser wavelengths will result in viewing of the different cell structures (Tsai et al. 2008). This method is also quite applicable to investigate the uptake of metal-based NPs, for example AuNPs due to their inherent scattering and reflecting of laser light in the presence of fluorescence-dyed cellular compartments (Tsai et al. 2008). Kim et al. (2015) investigated the effect of concentration and size of NPs on their cellular uptake in HeLa cells using CLSM imaging (Figure 11.13; Kim et al. 2015). In another study the use of SDCLM provided dynamic results of NP uptake in live HeLa cells (Yang et al. 2013).

Moreover, the detection of intracellular/nuclear localization of DOX released from AuNPs AuNPs-DOX has also been demonstrated using LSM methods (Madhusudhan et al. 2014; Figure 11.14). Overall LSM methods require practical sample preparation time (hours), it can be used to distinguish between extracellular and intracellular NP events, and merged images for observation of colocalization with cellular components are possible. However, the resolution obtained is still limited to 200 nm laterally and 500–900 nm axially, which is below the standards of high resolution microscopy techniques (Schermelleh et al. 2010).

11.6.2   FLOW CYTOMETRY

Flow cytometry is an established method that is used for high throughout rapid measurements that furnish semi-quantitative analysis of high statistical standards (Picot et al. 2012). Consequently, this method is used to determine the proportion of cells that have internalized fluorescently labelled or NPs that inherently display light scattering phenomena. However, flow cytometry is characterized by low resolution and cannot be used alone to study membrane bound and internalized cellular NP localization. Image flow cytometry affords rapid imaging of large amount of cells in flow by using the high sensitivity fluorescence quantification with the added benefits

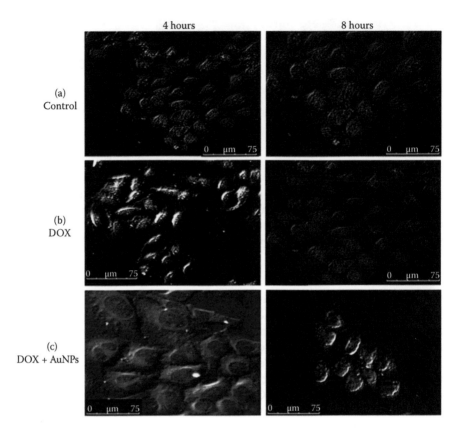

FIGURE 11.14 Confocal laser scanning microscopy images showed intracellular/nuclear localization of DOX released from AuNPs in HeLa cells previously treated with 10 ppm DOX and DOX loaded AuNPs after 4 and 8 hours, respectively. Scale bar is 75 mm. (Images in panels a–c were reproduced from Madhusudhan, A. et al., *Int J Mol Sci*, 15, 8216–8234, 2014. MDPI under Creative Commons Attribution License.)

of microscopy. The computationally assisted method involves creating a whole cell mask eroded by 3 µm to remove the fluorescence intensity emitted by adsorbed NPs and subsequently images were taken with ImageStreamX platform (Vranic et al. 2013). Nevertheless, the method cannot account for extracellular NPs, and NPs bound within the mask would also be quantified as intracellular particles.

To this end, a recent imaging flow cytometry procedure for distinguishing between membrane bound and internalized particles by eukaryotic cells was proposed by Smirnov and coworkers (2015). A spot counting algorithm procedure was developed to measure the number of extracellular and intracellular particles per cell (Smirnov et al. 2015). The procedure was reported to be suitable to any cell type and any particle provided it can be identified using antibodies or other reagents (Smirnov et al. 2015). Nonetheless, more research is needed to show that this method can be applicable to all cancer cell types and particles of the nano-range.

11.6.3 INDUCTIVELY COUPLED PLASMA TECHNIQUES

Inductively Coupled Plasma (ICP) techniques combined with mass spectrometry (ICP-MS) or optical emission spectrometry (ICP-OES) are the current gold standard to determine average elemental concentrations of total metal NPs within the cell (Rashkow et al. 2014; Albanese et al. 2013). Notably, ICP methods do not give information regarding NPs distribution within the cell, or cell heterogeneity, and cannot be used for detection of non-metal–based NPs. Moreover, harsh acid-promoted digestion of metal NPs is required (Fabricius et al. 2014). Nonetheless, accurate and precise results of multiple elements with detection limits of <1 ppb are unprecedented. A potential to harness the superior quantitative power of ICP with another method to quantify intracellular NPs has resulted in the implementation of multimodal spectroscopies such as LA-ICP-MS to visualize the distribution of NPs (Mueller et al. 2014). A further hyphenation of LA-ICP-MS with micro-mapping with Raman microspectroscopy offers both quantification of NPs in single cells and following of the NP pathway from endocytotic uptake and intracellular processing (Büchner et al. 2014). The future is promising for emerging ICP-MS techniques (Mueller et al. 2014); nonetheless, the complexity of the cancer cell environment requires complementary analysis to ICP methods to fully understand the fate of NPs.

11.6.4 TRANSMISSION ELECTRON MICROSCOPY

Transmission electron microscopy provides essential qualitative and quantitative information with regard to the exact intra- and extracellular location of NPs, and the number of internalized NPs within different cellular components without the use of fluorescence tagging (Vanhecke et al. 2014). Reasonable resolution higher than SEM in the nanometer range is possible and high-resolution transmission electron microscopy (HRTEM) provides unsurpassed resolved NPs interactions at the 10 nm level (Dam et al. 2012). However, TEM methods requires samples to be freeze-dried with a preferable sample thickness between 50 and 200 nm, which limits the application towards the study of NP uptake in living cells. An example of the successful integration of TEM, ICP-MS, confocal microscopy, and Western blot was reported by Zhang and co-workers (2013), who studied and proposed the trafficking mechanism of AuNPs in breast cancer incubated and chased at different intervals, as shown in Figure 11.15. Additionally, the impact of the impact of cell division on the NP load within cells was studied.

Despite the successful application, TEM for the detection of electron-dense NPs such as inorganic metal NPs, the analysis of organic components in hybrid organic structures and core–shell type NPs is not easily achievable. To this end, there are emerging platforms such as high-angle annular dark-field scanning TEM (HAADF STEM) and ADF-STEM (Sentosun et al. 2015) that have shown promising application. A more recent advent is the use of Two-color Stochastic Optical Reconstruction Microscopy (STORM), which combines high resolution with confocal and electron microscopy to study the intracellular drug delivery by NPs

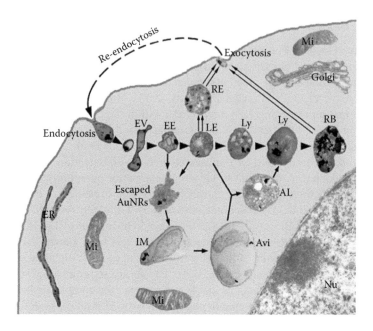

FIGURE 11.15 Collation transmission electron microscopy (TEM) images to study trafficking of AuNPs in breast cancer cells. (Reproduced with permission from Zhang, W. et al., *ACS App Mat Interfaces*, 5, 9856–9865, 2013. American Chemical Society ©2013.)

(van der Zwaag et al. 2016). However, the full potential and efficiency of this method has to be demonstrated in future investigations.

11.7 FUTURE PERSPECTIVES AND CONCLUDING REMARKS

Nanotechnology is a strategic rational design tool to enable transbarrier trafficking to access the intracellular environment of the cancer cell. With the growing benefits of nanoscience being realized, investigations into approaches for enhancing transbarrier trafficking of NPs across cancer barriers are gaining impetus. An increasing number of studies are employing "smart," including dual-pronged approaches combining antibody conjugation and as well stimulus-responsive targeting, for the delivery of the anti-tumor drug to its ultimate intracellular destination. Furthermore, there is increasing attention on the actual mechanisms implicated in transbarrier trafficking into the tumor cell in order to understand the manner in which NP properties enhance transbarrier trafficking, as well as the investigation into progressive techniques for characterization of the efficacy of mechanisms employed to achieve enhanced tumoral delivery. This is pertinent for the conceptualization of innovative targeted systems with enhanced efficacy and selectivity for the required intracellular site. From these discussions it is evident that various NP factors work together in determining the selected uptake pathway and ultimate cellular destination. A summative representation of the diverse approaches discussed for enhancing the uptake and trafficking of nanosystems is provided in Figure 11.16 and could be considered

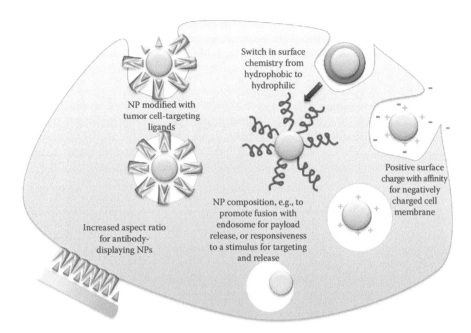

FIGURE 11.16 Nanosystem architectural strategies: Including surface charge and lipophilicity, targeting ligand, shape, and NP composition, for enhancing uptake and intracellular trafficking in cancer cells. Once internalized, the pH value in the interior of the endosome becomes acidic; the drug is released from the NPs and enters the cytoplasm. Drug-loaded NPs bypass the P-glycoprotein efflux pump, leading to high intracellular concentration.

in designing the desired nanosystem for the required chemotherapeutic application. A deep understanding of NP architecture and cell biology coupled with predictive computer-aided tools must also be considered to develop a system that meets all requirements for selective release of drug-to-tumor sites. Future efforts may even witness triple-pronged approaches for further improving tumor barrier trafficking. Therefore there is enormous potential for the development of the next generation of nano-engineered chemotherapeutic delivery systems with more potential for translation into clinical applications.

REFERENCES

Agardan, B. M., and Torchilin, V. P. 2016. Engineering of stimulus-repsonsive nanopreparations to overcome physiological barriers and cancer multidrug resistance, in *Engineering of Nanobiomaterials: Applications of Nanobiomaterials*, ed. A. Grumezescu. Norwich, NY: William Andrew.

Albanese, A., Tang, P. S., and Chan, W. C. W. 2012. The effect of nanoparticle size, shape, and surface chemistry on biological systems. *Annu Rev Eng* 14:1–16.

Albanese, A., Tsoi, K. M., and Chan, W. C. W. 2013. Simultaneous quantification of cells and nanomaterials by inductive-coupled plasma techniques. *J Lab Automation* 18:99–104.

Alexis, F., Pridgen, E., Molnar, L. K., and Farokhzad, O. C. 2008. Factors affecting the clearance and biodistribution of polymeric nanoparticles. *Mol Pharmaceutics* 5:505–515.

Altankov, G., Richau, K., and Groth, T. 2003. The role of zeta potential and substratum chemistry for resulation of dermal fibroblasts interaction. *Materialwiss Werkst* 34:1120–1128.

Asati, A., Santra, S., Kaittanis, C., and Perez, J. M. 2010. Surface-charge-dependent cell localization and cytotoxicity of cerium oxide nanoparticles. *ACS Nano* 4:5321–5331.

Bai, Y., Xing, H., Wu, P., Feng, X., Hwang, K., Lee, J. M. et al. 2015. Chemical control over cellular uptake of organic nanoparticles by fine tuning surface functional groups. *ACS Nano* 9:10227–10236.

Barua, S., and Rege, K. 2009. Cancer-cell-phenotype-dependent differential intracellular trafficking of unconjugated quantum dots. *Small* 5:370–376.

Barua, S., Yoo, J. W., Kolhar, P., Wakankar, A., Gokarn, Y. R., and Mitragotri, S. 2013. Particle shape enhances specificity of antibody-displaying nanoparticles. *Proc Natl Acad Sci USA* 110:3270–3275.

Baselga, J., Norton, L., Albanell, J., Kim, Y.-M., and Mendelsohn, J. 1998. Recombinant humanized anti-HER2 antibody (Herceptin) enhances the antitumor activity of paclitaxel and doxorubicin against HER2/neuoverexpressing human breast cancer xenografts. *Cancer Res* 58:2825–2831.

Batchelor, T. T., Sorensen, A. G., di Tomaso, E., Zhang, W.-T., Duda, D. G., Cohen, K. S. et al. 2007. AZD2171, a pan-VEGF receptor tyrosine kinase inhibitor, normalizes tumor vasculature and alleviates edema in glioblastoma patients. *Cancer Cell* 11:83–95.

Bawa, P., Pillay, V., Choonara, Y. E., and du Toit, L. C. 2009. Stimuli-responsive polymers and their applications in drug delivery. *Biomed Mater* 4:022001.

Benito-Alifonso, D., Tremel, S., Hou, B., Lockyear, H., Mantell, J., Fermin, D. J. et al. 2014. Lactose as a "Trojan horse" for quantum dot cell transport. *Angew Chem Int Ed* 53:810–814.

Biswas, S., and Torchilin, V. P. 2014. Nanopreparations for organelle-specific delivery in cancer. *Adv Drug Deliv Rev* 66:26–41.

Boucher, Y., Baxter, L. T., and Jain, R. K. 1990. Interstitial pressure gradients in tissue-isolated and subcutaneous tumors: Implications for therapy. *Cancer Res* 50:4478–4484.

Brandenberger, C., Rothen-Rutishauser, B., Mühlfeld, C., Schmid, O., Ferron, G. A., Maier, K. L. et al. 2010. Effects and uptake of gold nanoparticles deposited at the air-liquid interface of a human epithelial airway model. *Toxicol Appl Pharmacol* 242:56–65.

Büchner, T., Drescher, D., Traub, H., Schrade, P., Bachmann, S., Jakubowski, N. et al. 2014. Relating surface-enhanced Raman scattering signals of cells to gold nanoparticle aggregation as determined by LA-ICP-MS micromapping. *Analyt Bioanalyt Chem* 406:7003–7014.

Cairns, R., Papandreou, I., and Denko, N. 2006. Overcoming physiologic barriers to cancer treatment by molecularly targeting the tumor microenvironment. *Mol Cancer Res* 4:61–70.

Champion, J. A., and Mitragotri, S. 2009. Shape induced inhibition of phagocytosis of polymer particles. *Pharm Res* 26:244–249.

Chauhan, V. P., and Jain, R. K. 2013. Strategies for advancing cancer nanomedicine. *Nat Mater* 12:958–962.

Chauhan, V. P., Stylianopoulos, T., Martin, J. D., Popovic, Z., Chen, O., Kamoun, W. S. et al. 2012. Normalization of tumour blood vessels improves the delivery of nanomedicines in a size-dependent manner. *Nat Nanotech* 7:383–388.

Chen, L., McCrate, J. M., Lee, J. C., and Li, H. 2011. The role of surface charge on the uptake and biocompatibility of hydroxyapatite nanoparticles with osteoblast cells. *Nanotechnology* 22:105708.

Chithrani, B. D., and Chan, W. C. 2007. Elucidating the mechanism of cellular uptake and removal of protein-coated gold nanoparticles of different sizes and shapes. *Nano Lett* 7:1542–1550.

Chithrani, B. D., Ghazani, A. A., and Chan, W. C. 2006. Determining the size and shape dependence of gold nanoparticle uptake into mammalian cells. *Nano Lett* 6:662–668.

Cho, J., and Caruso, F. 2005. Investigation of the interactions between ligand-stabilized gold nanoparticles and polyelectrolyte multilayer films. *Chem Mater* 17:4547–4553.

Cho, K., Wang, X., Nie, S., Chen, Z. G., and Shin, D. M. 2008. Therapeutic nanoparticles for drug delivery in cancer. *Clin Cancer Res* 14:1310–1316.

Chung, Y. I., Kim, J. C., Kim, Y. H., Tae, G., Lee, S.-Y., Kim, K. et al. 2010. The effect of surface functionalization of PLGA nanoparticles by heparin- or chitosan-conjugated Pluronic on tumor targeting. *J Control Release* 143:374–382.

Coulman, S. A., Anstey, A., Gateley, C., Morrissey, A., Mcloughlin, P., Allender, C. et al. 2009. Microneedle mediated delivery of nanoparticles into human skin. *Int J Pharm* 366:190–200.

Curti, B. D. 1993. Physical barriers to drug delivery in tumors. *Crit Rev Oncol Hematol* 14:29–39.

Dam, D. H. M., Lee, J. H., Sisco, P. N., Co, D. T., Zhang, M., Wasielewski, M. R. et al. 2012. Direct observation of nanoparticle–cancer cell nucleus interactions. *ACS Nano* 6:3318–3326.

Danhier, F., Feron, O., and Préat, V. 2010. To exploit the tumor microenvironment: Passive and active tumor targeting of nanocarriers for anti-cancer drug delivery. *J Control Release* 148:135–146.

Datta, M., Via, L. E., Kamoun, W. S., Liu, C., Chen, W., Seano, G. et al. 2015. Anti-vascular endothelial growth factor treatment normalizes tuberculosis granuloma vasculature and improves small molecule delivery. *PNAS* 112:1827–1832.

Delehanty, J. B., Medintz, I. L., Pons, T., Brunel, F. M., Dawson, P. E., and Mattoussi, H. 2006. Self-assembled quantum dot-peptide bioconjugates for selective intracellular delivery. *Bioconjugate Chem* 17:920–927.

DeSimone, J. 2009. Engineered colloids having particles of controlled size, shape, and chemistry. *BAPS* 54.

Eikenes, L., Bruland, O. S., Brekken, C., and de Lange Davies, C. 2004. Collagenase increases the transcapillary pressure gradient and improves the uptake and distribution of monoclonal antibodies in human osteosarcoma xenografts. *Cancer Res* 64:4768–4773.

Eikenes, L., Tari, M., Tufto, I., Bruland, O. S., and de Lange Davies, C. 2005. Hyaluronidase induces a transcapillary pressure gradient and improves the distribution and uptake of liposomal doxorubicin (Caelyx) in human osteosarcoma xenografts. *Br J Cancer* 93:81–88.

Ekkapongpisit, M., Giovia, A., Follo, C., Caputo, G., and Isidoro, C. 2012. Biocompatibility, endocytosis, and intracellular trafficking of mesoporous silica and polystyrene nanoparticles in ovarian cancer cells: Effects of size and surface charge groups. *Int J Nanomed* 7:4147–4158.

El-Dakdouki, M. H., Zhu, D. C., El-Boubbou, K., Kamat, M., Chen, J., Li, W. et al. 2012. Development of multifunctional hyaluronan-coated nanoparticles for imaging and drug delivery to cancer cells. *Biomacromolecules* 13:1144–1151.

Fabricius, A.-L., Duester, L., Meermann, B., and Ternes, T. A. 2014. ICP-MS-based characterization of inorganic nanoparticles—Sample preparation and off-line fractionation strategies. *Analyt Bioanalyt Chem* 406:467–479.

Farhood, H., Serbina, N., and Huang, L. 1995. The role of dioleoyl phosphatidylethanolamine in cationic liposome mediated gene transfer. *Biochim Biophys Acta* 1235:289–295.

Ferrari, F. 2010. Frontiers in cancer nanomedicine: Directing mass transport through biological barriers. *Trends Biotechnol* 28:181–188.

Ferrari, M. 2005. Cancer nanotechnology: Opportunities and challenges. *Nat Rev Cancer* 5:161–171.

Fleige, E., Quadir, M. A., and Haag, R. 2012. Stimuli-responsive polymeric nanocarriers for the controlled transport of active compounds: Concepts and applications. *Adv Drug Deliv Rev* 64:866–884.

Fröhlich, E. 2012. The role of surface charge in cellular uptake and cytotoxicity of medical nanoparticles. *Int J Nanomedicine* 7:5577–5591.

Fujimoto, T., Kogo, H., Nomura, R., and Une, T. 2000. Isoforms of caveolin-1 and caveolar structure. *J Cell Sci* 113:3509–3517.

Ge, Y., Zhang, Y., Xia, J., Ma, M., He, S., Nie, F. et al. 2009. Effect of surface charge and agglomerate degree of magnetic iron oxide nanoparticles on KB cellular uptake in vitro. *Colloids Surf B Biointerfaces* 73:294–301.

Gratton, S. E., Ropp, P. A., Pohlhaus, P. D., Luft, J. C., Madden, V. J., Napier, M. E. et al. 2008. The effect of particle design on cellular internalization pathways. *Proc Natl Acad Sci* 105:11613–11618.

Griffon-Etienne, G., Boucher, Y., Brekken, C., Suit, H. D., and Jain, R. K. 1999. Taxane-induced apoptosis decompresses blood vessels and lowers interstitial fluid pressure in solid tumors: Clinical implications. *Cancer Res* 59:3776–3782.

Groothuis, D. R. 2000. The blood–brain and blood–tumor barriers: A review of strategies for increasing drug delivery. *Neuro-Oncology* 2:45–59.

Guo, S., and Huang, L. 2011. Nanoparticles escaping RES and endosome: Challenges for siRNA delivery for cancer therapy. *J Nanomater* 2011:742895. doi:10.1155/2011/742895.

Hafez, I. M., and Cullis, P. R. 2001. Roles of lipid polymorphism in intracellular delivery. *Adv Drug Deliv Rev* 47:139–148.

Haglund, K., Rusten, T. E., and Stenmark, H. 2007. Aberrant receptor signaling and trafficking as mechanisms in oncogenesis. *Crit Rev Oncog* 13:39–74.

Hambley, T. W., and Hait, W. N. 2009. Is anticancer drug development heading in the right direction? *Cancer Res* 69:1259–1262.

Han, G., You, C.-C., Kim, B.-J., Turingan, R. S., Forbes, N. S., Martin, C. T. et al. 2006. Light-regulated release of DNA and its delivery to nuclei by means of photolabile gold nanoparticles. *Angew Chem Int Ed* 45:3165–3169.

Harush-Frenkel, O., Rozentur, E., Benita, S., and Altschuler, Y. 2008. Surface charge of nanoparticles determines their endocytic and transcytotic pathway in polarized MDCK cells. *Biomacromolecules* 9:435–443.

Hauck, T. S., Ghazani, A. A., and Chan, W. C. 2008. Assessing the effect of surface chemistry on gold nanorod uptake, toxicity, and gene expression in mammalian cells. *Small* 4:153–159.

He, C., Hua, Y., Yin, L., Tang, C., and Yin, C. 2010. Effects of particle size and surface charge on cellular uptake and biodistribution of polymeric nanoparticles. *Biomaterials* 31:3657–3666.

Heldin, C. H., Rubin, K., Pietras, K., and Östman, A. 2004. High interstitial fluid pressure—An obstacle in cancer therapy. *Nat Rev Cancer* 4:806–813.

Helmlinger, G., Yuan, F., Dellian, M., and Jain, R. K. 1997. Interstitial pH and pO2 gradients in solid tumors in vivo: High-resolution measurements reveal a lack of correlation. *Nat Med* 3:177–182.

Hillaireau, H., and Couvreur, P. 2009. Nanocarriers entry into the cell: Relevance to drug delivery. *Cell Mol Life Sci* 66:2873–2896.

Hobbs, S. K., Monsky, W. L., Yuan, F., Roberts, W. G., Griffith, L., Torchilin, V. P. et al. 1998. Regulation of transport pathways in tumor vessels: Role of tumor type and microenvironment. *PNAS* 95:4607–4612.

Huang, G., Chen, H., Dong, Y., Luo, X., Yu, H., Moore, Z. et al. 2013. Superparamagnetic iron oxide nanoparticles: Amplifying ROS stress to improve anticancer drug efficacy. *Theranostics* 3:116–126.

Huang, M., Ma, Z., Khor, E., and Lim, L. Y. 2002. Uptake of FITC-chitosan nanoparticles by A549 cells. *Pharm Res* 19:1488–1494.

Hung, C. C., Huang, W. C., Lin, Y. W., Yu, T. W., Chen, H. H., Lin, S.-C. et al. 2016. Active tumor permeation and uptake of surface charge-switchable theranostic nanoparticles for imaging-guided photothermal/chemo combinatorial therapy. *Theranostics* 6:302–317.

Ichimura, T., Jin, T., Fujita, H., Higuchi, H., and Watanabe, T. M. 2014. Nano-scale measurement of biomolecules by optical microscopy and semiconductor nanoparticles. *Front Physiol* 5:273. doi:10.3389/fphys.2014.00273.

Izumi, Y., Xu, L., di Tomaso, E., Fukumura, D., and Jain, R. K. 2002. Tumour biology: Herceptin acts as an anti-angiogenic cocktail. *Nature* 416:279–280.

Jacobson, A., Salnikov, A., Lammerts, E., Roswall, P., Sundberg, C., Heldin, P. et al. 2003. Hyaluronan content in experimental carcinoma is not correlated to interstitial fluid pressure. *Biochem Biophys Res Commun* 305:1017–1023.

Jain, R. K. 1988. Determinants of tumor blood flow: A review. *Cancer Res* 48:2641–2658.

Jain, R. K. 2001. Normalizing tumor vasculature with anti-angiogenic therapy: A new paradigm for combination therapy. *Nat Med* 7:987–989.

Jain, R. K. 2013. Normalizing tumor microenvironment to treat cancer: Bench to bedside to biomarkers. *J Clin Oncol* 31:2205–2218.

Jain, R. K., and Stylianopoulos T. 2010. Delivering nanomedicine to solid tumors. *Nat Rev Clin Oncol* 11:653–664.

Jiang, T., Olson, E. S., Nguyen, Q. T., Roy, M., Jennings, P. A., and Tsien, R. Y. 2004. Tumor imaging by means of proteolytic activation of cell-penetrating peptides. *Proc Natl Acad Sci USA* 101:17867–17872.

Jiang, W., Kim, B. Y., Rutka, J. T., and Chan, W. C. 2008. Nanoparticle-mediated cellular response is size-dependent. *Nat Nanotechnol* 3:145–150.

Jiang, X., Musyanovych, A., Rocker, C., Landfester, K., Mailander, V., and Nienhaus, G. U. 2011. Specific effects of surface carboxyl groups on anionic polystyrene particles in their interactions with mesenchymal stem cells. *Nanoscale* 3:2028–2035.

Jonsson, F., Beke-Somfai, T., Andréasson, J., and Nordén, B. 2013. Interactions of a photochromic spiropyran with liposome model membranes. *Langmuir* 29:2099–2103.

Kaaki, K., Herve-Aubert, K., Chiper, M., Shkilnyy, A., Sourcé M., Benoit, R. et al. 2012. Magnetic nanocarriers of doxorubicin coated with poly(ethylene glycol) and folic acid: Relation between coating structure, surface properties, colloidal stability, and cancer cell targeting. *Langmuir* 28:1496–1505.

Kaneda, Y., Tsutsumi, Y., Yoshioka, Y., Kamada, H., Yamamoto, Y., Kodaira, H. et al. 2004. The use of PVP as a polymeric carrier to improve the plasma half-life of drugs. *Biomaterials* 25:3259–3266.

Karaman, D. S., Desai, D., Senthilkumar, R., Johansson, E. M., Ratts, N., Odén, M. et al. 2012. Shape engineering vs organic modification of inorganic nanoparticles as a tool for enhancing cellular internalization. *Nanoscale Res Lett* 7:358.

Kim, C. S., Li, X., Jiang, Y., Yan, B., Tonga, G. Y., Ray, M. et al. 2015. Cellular imaging of endosome entrapped small gold nanoparticles. *Methods X* 2:306–315.

Kobayashi, K., Wei, J., Iida, R., Ijiro, K., and Niikura, K. 2014. Surface engineering of nanoparticles for therapeutic applications. *Polym J* 46:460–468.

Kogure, K., Akita, H., and Harashima, H. 2007. Multifunctional envelope-type nano device for non-viral gene delivery: Concept and application of Programmed Packaging. *J Control Release* 122:246–251.

Kou, L., Sun, J., Zhai, Y., and He, Z. 2013. The endocytosis and intracellular fate of nanomedicines: Implication for rational design. *Asian J Pharm Sci* 8:1–10.

Kovács, T., Kárász, A., Szöllosi, J., and Nagy, P. 2009. The density of GM1-enriched lipid rafts correlates inversely with the efficiency of transfection mediated by cationic liposomes. *Cytometry A* 75:650–657.

Lai, C.-H., Lin, C.-Y., Wu, H.-T., Chan, H.-S., Chuang, Y.-J., Chen, C.-T. et al. 2010. Galactose encapsulated multifunctional nanoparticle for HepG2 cell internalization. *Adv Funct Mater* 20:3948–3958.

Lai, K., Hida, K., Man, S. T., Chen, C., Machamer, C., Schroer, T. A. et al. 2007. Privileged delivery of polymer nanoparticles to the perinuclear region of live cells via a non-clathrin, non-degradative pathway. *Biomaterials* 28:2876–2884.

Lankveld, D. P., Rayavarapu, R. G., Krystek, P. Oomen, A. G., Verharen, H. W., van Leeuwen, T. G. et al. 2011. Blood clearance and tissue distribution of PEGylated and non-PEGylated gold nanorods after intravenous administration in rats. *Nanomedicine* 6:339–349.

Lee, C. C., Gillies, E. R., Fox, M. E., Guillaudeu, S. J., Fréchet, J. M. J., Dy, E. E. et al. 2006. A single dose of doxorubicin-functionalized bow-tie dendrimer cures mice bearing C-26 colon carcinomas. *PNAS* 103:16649–16654.

Lee, M. H., Han, J. H., Kwon, P.-S., Bhuniya, S., Kim, J. Y., Sessler, J. L. et al. 2012. Hepatocyte-targeting single galactose-appended naphthalimide: A tool for intracellular thiol imaging *in vivo*. *J Am Chem Soc* 134:1316–1322.

Li, S. D., and Huang, L. 2009. Nanoparticles evading the reticuloendothelial system: Role of the supported bilayer. *Biochim Biophys Acta* 1788:2259–2266.

Liu, Y., Han, X., He, L., and Yin, Y. 2012. Thermoresponsive assembly of charged gold nanoparticles and their reversible tuning of plasmon coupling. *Angew Chem Int Ed* 51:6373–6377.

Lorenz, M. R., Holzapfel, V., Musyanovych, A., Nothelfer, K., Walther, P., Frank, H. et al. 2006. Uptake of functionalized, fluorescent-labeled polymeric particles in different cell lines and stem cells. *Biomaterials* 27:2820–2828.

Lu, Z., Qiao, X., Zheng, X. T., Chan-Park, M. B., and Li, C. M. 2010. Effect of particle shape on phagocytosis of CdTe quantum dot–cystine composites. *Med Chem Commun* 1:84–86.

Madhusudhan, A., Reddy, G. B., Venkatesham, M., Veerabhadram, G., Kumar, D. A., Natarajan, S. et al. 2014. Efficient pH dependent drug delivery to target cancer cells by gold nanoparticles capped with carboxymethyl chitosan. *Int J Mol Sci* 15:8216–8234.

Maier-Hauff, K., Rothe, R., Scholz, R., Gneveckow, U., Wust, P., Thiesen, B. et al. 2007. Intracranial thermotherapy using magnetic nanoparticles combined with external beam radiotherapy: Results of a feasibility study on patients with glioblastoma multiforme. *J Neurooncol* 81:53–60.

Mailander, V., and Landfester, K. 2009. Interaction of nanoparticles with cells. *Biomacromolecules* 10:2379–2400.

Marquis, B. J., Liu, Z., Braun, K. L., and Haynes, C. L. 2011. Investigation of noble metal nanoparticle ζ-potential effects on single-cell exocytosis function in vitro with carbon-fiber microelectrode amperometry. *Analyst* 136:3478–3486.

Mayer, L. D., Tai, L. C., Ko, D. S., Masin, D., Ginsberg, R. S., Cullis, P. R. et al. 1989. Influence of vesicle size, lipid composition, and drug-to-lipid ratio on the biological activity of liposomal doxorubicin in mice. *Cancer Res* 49:5922–5930.

Meng, H., Yang, S., Li, Z., Xia, T., Chen, J., Ji, Z. et al. 2011. Aspect ratio determines the quantity of mesoporous silica nanoparticle uptake by a small GTPase-dependent macropinocytosis mechanism. *ACS Nano* 5:4434–4447.

Miller, C. R., Bondurant, B., McLean, S. D., McGovern, K. A., and O'Brien, D. F. 1998. Liposome-cell interactions in vitro: Effect of liposome surface charge on the binding and endocytosis of conventional and sterically stabilized liposomes. *Biochemistry* 37:12875–12883.

Mitragotri, S., and Lahann, J. 2009. Physical approaches to biomaterial design. *Nat Mater* 8:15–23.

Moore, A., Marecos, E., Bogdanov, A., and Weissleder, R. 2000. Tumoral distribution of long-circulating dextran-coated iron oxide nanoparticles in a rodent model. *Radiology* 214:568–574.

Mueller, L., Traub, H., Jakubowski, N., Drescher, D., Baranov, V. I., and Kneipp, J. 2014. Trends in single-cell analysis by use of ICP-MS. *Analyt Bioanalyt Chem* 406:6963–6977.

Murugan, K., Choonara, Y. E., Kumar, P., du Toit, L. C., and Pillay, V. 2015. Parameters and characteristics governing cellular internalization and trans-barrier trafficking of nanostructures. *Int J Nanomedicine* 10:2191–2206.

Nagayasu, A., Shimooka, T., Kinouchi, Y., Uchiyama, K., Takeichi, Y., and Kiwada, H. 1994. Effects of fluidity and vesicle size on antitumor activity and myelosuppressive activity of liposomes loaded with daunorubicin. *Biol Pharm Bull* 17:935–939.

Netti, P. A., Berk, D. A., Swartz, M. A., Grodzinsky, A. J., and Jain, R. K. 2000. Role of extracellular matrix assembly in interstitial transport in solid tumors. *Cancer Res* 60:2497–2503.

Nie, S. 2010. Understanding and overcoming major barriers in cancer nanomedicine. *Nanomedicine* 5:523–528.

Oh, N., and Park, J.-H. 2014. Endocytosis and exocytosis of nanoparticles in mammalian cells. *Int J Nanomedicine* 9(Suppl 1):51–63.

Owens, D. E., and Peppas, N. A. 2006. Opsonization, biodistribution, and pharmacokinetics of polymeric nanoparticles. *Int J Pharm* 307:93–103.

Peer, D., Karp, J., Hong, S., Farokhzad, O., Margalit, R., and Langer, R. 2007. Nanocarriers as an emerging platform for cancer therapy. *Nat Nanotechnol* 2:751–760.

Peiris, P. M., Toy, R., Doolittle, E. Pansky, J., Abramowski, A., Tam, M. et al. 2012. Imaging metastasis using an integrin-targeting chain-shaped nanoparticle. *ACS Nano* 6:8783–8795.

Perumal, O. P., Inapagolla, R., Kannan, S., and Kannan, R. M. 2008. The effect of surface functionality on cellular trafficking of dendrimers. *Biomaterials* 29:3469–3476.

Picot, J., Guerin, C. L., Le Van Kim, C., and Boulanger, C. M. 2012. Flow cytometry: Retrospective, fundamentals and recent instrumentation. *Cytotechnology* 64:109–130.

Qiu, Y., Lu, Y., Wang, L., Xu, L., Bai, R., Ji, Y. et al. 2010. Surface chemistry and aspect ratio mediated cellular uptake of Au nanorods. *Biomaterials* 31:7606–7619.

Rapoport, N. Y., Kennedy, A. M., Shea, J. E., Scaife, C. L., and Nam K. H. 2009. Controlled and targeted tumor chemotherapy by ultrasound-activated nanoemulsions/microbubbles. *J Control Release* 138:268–276.

Rapoport, N., Kennedy, A. M., Shea, J. E., Scaife, C. L., and Nam, K. H. 2010. Ultrasonic nanotherapy of pancreatic cancer: Lessons from ultrasound imaging. *Mol Pharm* 7:22–31.

Rapoport, N., Nam, K.-H., Gupta, R., Gao, Z., Mohan, P., Payne, A. et al. 2011. Ultrasound-mediated tumor imaging and nanotherapy using drug loaded, block copolymer stabilized perfluorocarbon nanoemulsions. *J Control Release* 153:4–15.

Rashkow, J. T., Patel, S. C., Tappero, R., and Sitharaman, B. 2014. Quantification of single-cell nanoparticle concentrations and the distribution of these concentrations in cell population. *J Royal Soc Interface* 11:94.

Rathinaraj, P., Al-Jumaily, A. M., and Sung Huh, D. 2015. Internalization: Acute apoptosis of breast cancer cells using herceptin-immobilized gold nanoparticles. *Breast Canc Targets Ther* 7:51–58.

Riche, E. L., Erickson, B. W., and Cho, M. J. 2004. Novel long-circulating liposomes containing peptide library-lipid conjugates: Synthesis and *in vivo* behavior. *J Drug Target* 12:355–361.

Rima, W., Sancey, L., Aloy, M.-T., Armand, E., Alcantara, G. B., Epicier, T. et al. 2013. Internalization pathways into cancer cells of gadolinium-based radiosensitizing nanoparticles. *Biomaterials* 34:181–195.

Ruan, G., Agrawal, A. A., Marcus, I., and Nie, S. 2007. Imaging and tracking of tat peptide-conjugated quantum dots in living cells: New insights into nanoparticle uptake, intracellular transport, and vesicle shedding. *J Am Chem Soc* 129:14759–14766.

Ruoslathi, E., Bhatia, S. N., Sailor, M. J. 2010. Targeting of drugs and nanoparticles to tumors. *JCB* 188:759.

Sahay, G., Kim, J. O., Kabanov, A. V., and Bronich, T. K. 2010. The exploitation of differential endocytic pathways in normal and tumor cells in the selective targeting of nanoparticulate chemotherapeutic agents. *Biomaterials* 31:923–933.

Schermelleh, L., Heintzmann, R., and Leonhardt, H. 2010. A guide to super-resolution fluorescence microscopy. *J Cell Biol* 190:165–175.

Schmaljohann, D. 2006. Thermo- and pH-responsive polymers in drug delivery. *Adv Drug Deliv Rev* 58:1655–1670.

Schmidt, M. M., and Wittrup, K. D. 2009. A modeling analysis of the effects of molecular size and binding affinity on tumor targeting. *Mol Cancer Ther* 8:2861–2871.

Sekiguchi, S., Niikura, K., Matsuo, Y., Yoshimura, S. H., and Ijiro, K. 2012. Nuclear transport facilitated by the interaction between nuclear pores and carbohydrates. *RSC Advances* 2:1656–1662.

Sentosun, K., Sanz Ortiz, M. N., Batenburg, K. J., Liz-Marzán, L. M., and Bals, S. 2015. Combination of HAADF-STEM and ADF-STEM tomography for core–shell hybrid materials. *Part & Part Systems Charact* 32:1063–1067.

Shao, N., Jin, J., Wang, H., Zheng, J., Yang, R., Chan, W. et al. 2010. Design of bis-spiropyran ligands as dipolar molecule receptors and application to *in vivo* glutathione fluorescent probes. *J Am Chem Soc* 132:725–736.

Smirnov, A., Solga, M. D., Lannigan, J., and Criss, A. K. 2015. An improved method for differentiating cell-bound from internalized particles by imaging flow cytometry. *J Immunol Methods* 423:60–69.

Smith, B. R., Kempen, P., Bouley, D., Xu, A., Liu, Z., Melosh, N. et al. 2012. Shape matters: Intravital microscopy reveals surprising geometrical dependence for nanoparticles in tumor models of extravasation. *Nano Lett* 12:3369–3377.

Soldati, T., and Schliwa, M. 2006. Powering membrane traffic in endocytosis and recycling. *Nat Rev* 7:897–908.

Sriraman, S. K., Aryasomayajula, B., and Torchilin, V. P. 2014. Barriers to drug delivery in solid tumors. *Tissue Barriers* 2:e29528-1–e29528-10.

Stylianopoulos, T., Martin, J. D., Chauhan, V. P., Jain, S. R., Diop-Frimpong, B., Bardeesy, N. et al. 2012. Causes, consequences, and remedies for growth-induced solid stress in murine and human tumors. *PNAS* 109:15101–15108.

Subramani, C., Yu, X., Agasti, S. S., Duncan, B., Eymur, S., Tonga, M. et al. 2011. Direct photopatterning of light-activated gold nanoparticles. *J Mater Chem* 21:14156–14158.

Sugahara, K. N., Teesalu, T., Karmali, P. P., Kotamraju, V. R., Agemy, L., Girard, O. M. et al. 2009. Tissue-penetrating delivery of compounds and nanoparticles into tumors. *Cancer Cell* 16:510–520.

Thorek, D. L., and Tsourkas, A. 2008. Size, charge and concentration dependent uptake of iron oxide particles by non-phagocytic cells. *Biomaterials* 29:3583–3590.

Tong, R., Hemmati, H. D., Langer, R., and Kohane, D. S. 2012. Photoswitchable nanoparticles for triggered tissue penetration and drug delivery. *J Am Chem Soc* 134:8848–8855.

Toy, R., Peiris, P. M., Ghaghada, K. B., and Karathanasis, E. 2014. Shaping cancer nanomedicine: The effect of particle shape on the *in vivo* journey of nanoparticles. *Nanomed (Lond)* 9:121–134.

Tsai, S.-W., Chen, Y.-Y., and Liaw, J.-W. 2008. Compound cellular Imaging of laser scanning confocal microscopy by using gold nanoparticles and dyes. *Sensors (Basel, Switzerland)* 8:2306–2316.

Turnbull, T., Douglass, M., Paterson, D., Bezak, E., Thierry, B., and Kempson, I. 2015. Relating intercellular variability in nanoparticle uptake with biological consequence: A quantitative x-ray fluorescence study for radiosensitization of cells. *Analyt Chem* 87:10693–10697.

Vandamme, T. F., and Brobeck, L. 2005. Poly (amidoamine) dendrimers as ophthalmic vehicles for ocular delivery of pilocarpine nitrate and tropicamide. *J Control Release* 102:23–38.

Van der Zwaag, D., Vanparijs, N., Wijnands, S., De Rycke, R., De Geest, B. G., and Albertazzi, L. 2016. Super resolution imaging of nanoparticles cellular uptake and trafficking. *ACS App Mat Interfaces* 8:6391–6399. doi:10.1021/acsami.6b00811.

Vanhecke, D., Rodriguez-Lorenzo, L., Clift, M. J. D., Blank, F., Petri-Fink, A., and Rothen-Rutishauser, B. 2014. Quantification of nanoparticles at the single-cell level: An overview about state-of-the-art techniques and their limitations. *Nanomedicine* 9:1885–1900.

Vasir, J. K., and Labhasetwar, V. 2007. Biodegradable nanoparticles for cytosolic delivery of therapeutics. *Adv Drug Delivery Rev* 59:718–728.

Villanueva, A., Canete, M., Roca, A. G., Calero, M., Veintemillas-Verdaguer, S., Serna, C. J. et al. 2009. The influence of surface functionalization on the enhanced internalization of magnetic nanoparticles in cancer cells. *Nanotechnology* 20:115103.

Vina-Vilaseca, A., Bender-Sigel, J., Sorkina, T., Closs, E., and Sorkin, A. 2011. Protein kinase C-dependent ubiquitination and clathrin-mediated endocytosis of the cationic amino acid transporter CAT-1. *J Biol Chem* 286:8697–8706.

Vranic, S., Boggetto, N., Contremoulins, V. Mornet, S., Reinhardt, N., Marano, F. et al. 2013. Deciphering the mechanisms of cellular uptake of engineered nanoparticles by accurate evaluation of internalization using imaging flow cytometry. *Part Fibre Toxicol* 10:2.

Wang, J., Byrne, J. D., Napier, M. E., and DeSimone, J. M. 2011. More effective nanomedicines through particle design. *Small* 7:1919–1931.

Whiteside, T. L. 2008. The tumor microenvironment and its role in promoting tumor growth. *Oncogene* 27:5904–5912.

Win, K. Y., and Feng, S. S. 2005. Effects of particle size and surface coating on cellular uptake of polymeric nanoparticles for oral delivery of anticancer drugs. *Biomaterials* 26:2713–2722.

Xiang, S., Tong, H., Shi, Q., Fernandez, J. C. Jin, T., Dai, K. et al. 2012. Uptake mechanisms of non-viral gene delivery. *J Control Release* 158:371–378.

Xiao, Z., Levy-Nissenbaum, E., Alexis, F. Lupták, A., Teply, B. A., Chan, J. M. et al. 2012. Engineering of targeted nanoparticles for cancer therapy using internalizing aptamers isolated by cell-uptake selection. *ACS Nano* 6:696–704.

Yang, L., Shang, L., and Nienhaus, G. U. 2013. Mechanistic aspects of fluorescent gold nanocluster internalization by live HeLa cells. *Nanoscale* 5:1537–1543.

Yeung, T., Gilbert, G. E., Shi, J., Silvius, J., Kapus, A., and Grinstein, S. 2008. Membrane phosphatidylserine regulates surface charge and protein localization. *Science* 319:210–213.

You, J., Zhang, G., and Li, C. 2010. Exceptionally high payload of doxorubicin in hollow gold nanospheres for near-infrared light-triggered drug release. *ACS Nano* 4:1033–1041.

You, J.-O., Guo, P., and Auguste, D. T. 2013. A drug-delivery vehicle combining the targeting and thermal ablation of HER2+ breast-cancer cells with triggered drug release. *Angew Chem Int Ed* 52:4141–4146.

Yue, Z. G., Wei, W., Lv. P. P., Yue, H., Wang, L.-Y., Su, M. J. et al. 2011. Surface charge affects cellular uptake and intracellular trafficking of chitosan-based nanoparticles. *Biomacromolecules* 12:2440–2446.

Zhang, S., Li, J., Lykotrafitis, G., Bao, G., and Suresh, S. 2008. Size-dependent endocytosis of nanoparticles. *Adv Mater* 21:419–424.

Zhang, W., Ji, Y., Wu, X., and Xu, H. 2013. Trafficking of gold nanorods in breast cancer cells: Uptake, lysosome maturation, and elimination. *ACS App Mat Interfaces* 5:9856–9865.

Zhang, Y., Yang, M., Park, J. H., Singelyn, J., Ma, H., Sailor, M. J. et al. 2009. A surface-charge study on cellular-uptake behavior of F3-peptide-conjugated iron oxide nanoparticles. *Small* 5:1990–1996.

Zhu, M.-Q., Wang, L.-Q., Exarhos, G. J., and Li, A. D. Q. 2004. Thermosensitive gold nanoparticles. *J Am Chem Soc* 126:2656–2657.

12 Polymeric Nanoparticles as a Vehicle for Delivery of Antioxidants in the Brain
Potential Application in Neurodegenerative Diseases

Jean-Michel Rabanel, Ghislain Djiokeng-Paka, and Charles Ramassamy

CONTENTS

12.1 INTRODUCTION

The deleterious effect of oxidative stress in some neurodegenerative disorders (NDDs) such as Alzheimer's disease (AD) or Parkinson's diseases (PD) is well established. For instance, lipid peroxidation, protein oxidation, and nucleic acid oxidation damage markers were found to be elevated while antioxidant levels decreased in vulnerable region of the brain from patients with NDDs (Scheff et al. 2016). In AD, these oxidative alterations were evidenced before the onset of the disease, in patients with mild cognitive impairment (MCI), a preclinical stage of AD (Arce-Varas et al. 2016; Scheff et al. 2016; Di Domenico et al. 2016). So, these alterations could contribute to the etiology of AD and may play a detrimental role in the pathogenesis of this disease and suggest that antioxidants intake should be beneficial for the prevention of AD. Major efforts have been made to determine whether antioxidant supplementation could be an efficient way of preventing or even treating AD. However, the beneficial effects of antioxidants such as vitamin C, E, or some polyphenols (e.g., curcumin, catechin, quercetin, resveratrol, anthocyanins, rutin, and many others as presented in Figure 12.1) in NDDs is still not consistent (see the critical reviews Ramassamy 2006; Devore et al. 2010; Vina et al. 2011; Harrison 2012).

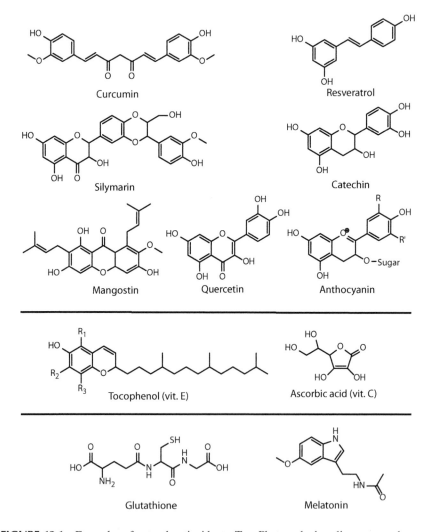

FIGURE 12.1 Examples of natural antioxidants. Top: Phyto-polyphenolic compounds structures with antioxidant activity. Middle: Vitamins. Bottom: Structure of glutathione and melatonin.

Curcumin, the phytochemical agent in the spice turmeric is one of the most recognized *in vitro* and *in vivo* antioxidant with neuroprotective potential (Barnham et al. 2004; Cuajungco et al. 2000; Belkacemi and Ramassamy 2012; Swomley and Butterfield 2015; Singh et al. 2008; Ramassamy 2006). It has even been cited as the best antioxidants and inhibitors of Amyloid-β (Aβ) fibril formation among 214 other natural antioxidant compounds (Kim et al. 2005). However, curcumin brain bioavailability is low due to its low stability in solution (Wang et al. 1997) and its poor permeability across the blood–brain barrier (BBB; see reviews by Belkacemi et al. 2011; Begum et al. 2008). For instance, clinical trials conducted in California (United States), where patients receiving 2–10 mg curcumin for 6 months showed no significant improvement in cognitive function (Ringman et al. 2012).

Chemical stability is an issue shared by all natural antioxidants. Thus, the issue of whether antioxidant treatment could be used in AD or other NDDs such as PD (Blesa et al. 2015) or multiple sclerosis (Gilgun-Sherki et al. 2004) remain a great challenge likely due to their limited bioavailability and their very low cerebral permeability in addition to the property of the BBB.

12.1.1 SOME PROPERTIES OF THE BLOOD–BRAIN BARRIER

The BBB is well-known as a gatekeeper in regards to exogenous substances. The BBB is composed by endothelial cells, pericytes, astrocytes, and basal membrane (Celia et al. 2011). In comparison with peripheral capillaries, the brain capillaries do not have fenestrations and microvessel endothelial cells (MECs) are recovered by pericytes and which confer a more tightly structure. The BBB is characterized by the presence of tight junctions (TJs) between MECs which induce a high transendothelial electrical restriction. TJs are the most important element in the junctional complex which is formed by transmembranar proteins such as claudins, a protein associated to the regulation of the microenvironment and in the control of cell proliferation (Kniesel and Wolburg 2000; Huber et al. 2001). Astrocyte projections surrounding the MECs of the BBB are providing biochemical support to those cells and are involved in the production of growth factors and inflammatory compounds. Pericytes and basal membrane are involved in the physical stability of the BBB. Physicochemical properties of drugs, such as lipophilicity and molecular weight, are key components in paving drug BBB permeability. So, drugs or compounds that are lipophilic, non-ionized at physiological pH, and with low molecular weight (<500 Da) can cross the BBB by diffusion mechanisms. Other essential compounds, such as amino acids, neuropeptides, and hexoses, normally need specific carriers to permeate into the brain (Rapoport 1996), while peptides and proteins can cross the BBB by saturable transport systems (Banks et al. 1991). To overcome the limited access of drugs to the brain, different strategies have been investigated including the osmotic BBB opening using compounds such as arabinose and mannitol (Rapoport 1996), the use of biologically active agents such as histamine, serotonin, substance P, metalloproteinases, and so on (Abbott and Revest 1991), and finally, the development of the so-called drug carriers such as liposomes and nanoparticles (NPs).

12.1.2 GENERAL ASPECTS OF NANOPARTICLES

The definition of polymer NPs depends on the organization but they are generally defined as solid, colloidal particles in the range of 10 to 1000 nm. In most assays, NPs used in biological assays are in the range of 10 to 200 nm for diverse biological reasons. NPs can be a nanosphere, that is, a matrix particle with a solid core or a nanocapsule, that is, a vesicular system with an aqueous or oily liquid core containing the drug surrounded by a solid polymer wall. The reason why these NPs are attractive for medical use is based on their important and unique features, such as their high surface to mass ratio, their quantum properties, and their ability to adsorb and carry compounds, drugs, proteins, or dyes. It is hypothesized that NPs encapsulation can increase, for example, the dispersion of poorly soluble compounds, increase their chemical stability, and enhance their adsorption through endothelial barriers and cell membranes. Several types of polymeric NPs have been proposed (Figure 12.2): A first generation, best described as a simple polymeric matrix to provide protection and controlled release; a second generation, which corresponds to NPs with surface modifications for a better biocompatibility and increased time of residence in circulation; and finally, a third generation with ligand-receptor targeting capabilities such as toward the BBB, the neuronal cells, or both. A fourth generation corresponding to NPs systems having stimuli responsive element for specific drug release will be discussed briefly in a following section.

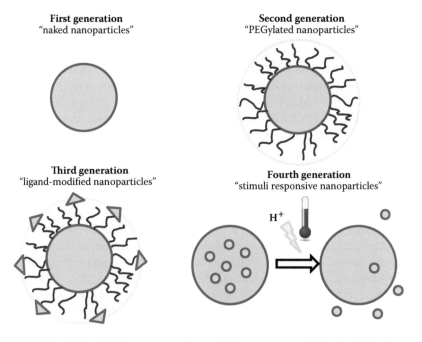

FIGURE 12.2 NPs of different generations. (1) First-generation NPs, "naked" polymeric matrix type NPs. (2) Second-generation NPs, "PEG-coated surface" NPs. (3) Third-generation NPs, "ligand-modified surface" NPs. (4) Fourth-generation NPs, "stimuli responsive" NPs: Upon external inducers such as pH, temperature, or redox potential, drug release is triggered.

12.2 POLYMERS AND NANOPARTICLES PREPARATION

12.2.1 POLYMERS USED FOR BIOMEDICAL APPLICATIONS

Several polymers have been used for the preparation of biomedical particles: Natural polymers such as chitosan, albumin, gelatin, and sodium alginate; or synthetic polymers such as poly(lactic-co-glycolic) (PLGA), poly(lactic) (PLA), poly(alkylcyanoacrylate) (PACA), and many others (Soppimath et al. 2001; Kamaly et al. 2016). Due to its biocompatibility and low toxicity, PLGA has been approved for human use by the U.S. Food Drug Administration (Makadia and Siegel 2011; Anderson and Shive 1997). PLGA is the most clinically used polymer (Nair and Laurencin 2007). PLGA is a copolymer composed of repeating units of lactic acid (LA) and glycolic acid (GA) according to a variable arrangement based on preferred intrinsic properties and the applications. The ratio between LA and GA defines in part the hydrophilicity of the matrix. A PLGA 50:50, means 50 percent of monomer is LA, and 50 percent is GA. A PLGA 50:50 constitutes a more hydrophilic matrix than a PLGA 75:25. This ratio determines the affinity of the matrix for hydrophobic compounds, the rate of hydration in aqueous suspension, and kinetic of hydrolytic degradation. Degradation is initiated by the hydrolytic rupture of ester bonds resulting in the formation of two monomers: LA and GA (Ramchandani and Robinson 1998). LA and GA formed enter the Krebs cycle where they are metabolized to CO_2 and H_2O (Athanasiou et al. 1996). PLGA is used in many areas, but the main application remains in the biomedical industry, where it plays the role of pharmaceutical excipient for slow release depot system, scaffold for tissue regeneration, sutures, and surgical plates. Therefore, in this chapter, more emphasis will be put on PLGA-derived NPs.

12.2.2 PREPARATION OF NANOPARTICLES

PLGA NPs are mainly prepared by two techniques: (1) emulsion/evaporation technique or (2) nanoprecipitations. Emulsion/evaporation consists in dissolving the polymer along with the drug in a water-insoluble organic phase and transferring the mixture into an aqueous phase to form an emulsion stabilized by a surfactant. After solvent removal, particles are washed by different techniques to remove the surfactant and free drugs. Nanoprecipitation (or solvent displacement technique) consists in the dissolution of the polymer along with the drug in a water-soluble phase (typically acetone). The injection of the organic phase in an aqueous phase under stirring (or other rapid phase-mixing technique such as microfluidic or flash nanoprecipitation), results in the formation of NPs, which are collected after purification to remove residual organic solvent and free drug. Both techniques suffer from drawbacks: The use of organic solvent and their convenience limited to the encapsulation of relatively hydrophobic drugs.

12.3 FIRST GENERATION NANOPARTICLE SYSTEM

The first generation of NP system can be defined as the naked polymer matrix type NP (Figure 12.2). The active molecules are entrapped inside the matrix, the core or adsorbed on the surface. The NPs in biological medium are providing a dispersion of nanoreservoirs containing the active molecules. The rationale behind the development of this type of particle is based on the modification of the pharmacokinetic (PK) parameters of an active compound, offered by its entrapment in a polymer matrix. The influenced PK parameters are t_{max} and C_{max} with the modified release, that is, with modification of the dissolution rate, the chemical stability (elimination), and the bioavailability at the pathological site. The issues relevant to these NPs are (1) the quantity of active molecule encapsulated; (2) the controlled and sustained release compared to other conventional drug administration devices. This approach can lead to significant improvement of treatments by decreasing administration frequency and insure a constant level of the active compounds like antioxidant at the desired site (Kamaly et al. 2016).

Our early attempt to encapsulate curcumin in PLGA NPs shows the potential of polymer NPs to protect neuronal cell lines from induced oxidative stress (Doggui et al. 2012). The PLGA NPs were prepared by emulsion/evaporation method using DMAB as a stabilizer and ethyl acetate as the organic phase. We were able to efficaciously entrapped curcumin (about 15 percent drug loading) and to show an increase of the antioxidant activity in comparison with free curcumin *in vitro*. This increased of antioxidant activity was related to curcumin entry into cells as monitored by fluorescence microscopy, to a decrease of intracellular ROS level, to a prevention of the decrease level of intracellular glutathione (GSH) following H_2O_2 oxidative stress induction and suppression of Nrf2 activation. Very interestingly, the antioxidant activity of curcumin was found to be preserved up to 6 months when encapsulated (Doggui et al. 2012), while free curcumin is rapidly degraded in neutral phosphate buffer, up to 90 percent within 30 minutes (Wang et al. 1997; Rabanel et al. 2015a).

More recently, we have demonstrated the role and importance of polymer matrix composition (LA to GA ratio). The lactic to glycolic ratio in PLGA has appeared to play a role not only on encapsulation efficiency and release profile, as expected from early works (Doggui et al. 2012), but also on NPs size (Djiokeng-Paka et al. 2016).

Using NPs made from PLGA 50:50 we showed that NPs encapsulation enhanced the neuroprotective activity of curcumin upon induced oxidative stress by modulating survival pathways such as NF-κB, Nrf2, and synaptic activity with Akt and Tau phosphorylation. Interestingly both curcumin loaded and blank PLGA NPs were able to decrease Akt phosphorylation. Moreover, NPs encapsulated curcumin upregulated the expression of some oxidative-stress-related genes affected during NDDs such as apolipoprotein E (ApoE), apolipoprotein J (ApoJ), thioredoxine (TRX), glutaredoxine (GLRX), and Repressor Element-1/Neuron-Restrictive Silencing Element (RE-1/NRSE) REST. Finally in this study, it appeared that PLGA 50:50 was superior to PLGA 65:35 in counteracting the increase of REST and GLX expressions (Figure 12.3).

Others studies have demonstrated the interest of antioxidant encapsulation in polymer NPs. Tsai et al. (2011) showed that curcumin encapsulated in PLGA NPs, prepared by emulsion/evaporation using PVA as a stabilizer, can be later found in its free form in rat brain hippocampus following NPs injection. It is noteworthy that the curcumin doses found in the brain parenchyma were very low, even if NPs encapsulation somewhat increase the curcumin doses, as organ biodistribution

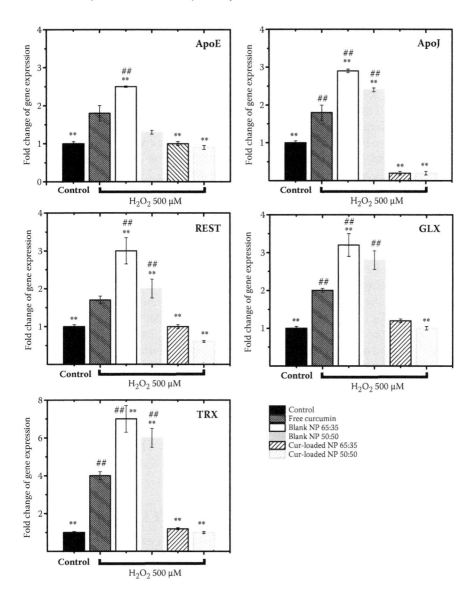

FIGURE 12.3 Effect of curcumin encapsulation in PLGA NPs with different LA/GA ratio on gene expression changes of several proteins implicated in oxidative stress response in neuronal cells. SK-N-SH cells were exposed to either free curcumin or curcumin loaded NPs (50:50, 65:35) in the presence of H_2O_2 (oxidative stress inductor). The results are presented as fold change with **, $p < 0.01$ in comparison with free curcumin in the presence of induced oxidative stress, while ##, $p < 0.01$ indicate statistical significant values with respect to control samples. (Adapted from Djiokeng-Paka G. et al., *Molecular Pharmaceutics*, 13(2), 391–403, 2016. With permission.)

data showed a curcumin accumulation mainly in liver, lung, and spleen (Tsai et al. 2011). Curcumin-loaded PLGA NPs were shown to increase curcumin neuronal cell uptake and differentiation *in vitro*. Moreover, *in vivo* these antioxidant-loaded NPs reverse learning and memory impairments in an Aβ-induced rat model of AD (Tiwari et al. 2014).

PLGA or PBCA NPs were also used to encapsulate the antioxidant enzyme superoxide dismutase (SOD). These NPs displayed a protective effect of the encapsulated enzyme *in vitro* and *in vivo*. SOD-loaded NPs limited the extent of apoptosis, enhanced protection by reducing the infarct volume in an ischemia-reperfusion rat models (Reddy and Labhasetwar 2009; Yun et al. 2013).

Besides synthetic polyesters and PACA, natural polymers have been also used for antioxidant encapsulation and brain delivery. For instance chitosan NPs were tested for gallic acid delivery and showed improved antioxidant and antidepressant activities in a mouse model (Nagpal et al. 2012). Gelatin NPs with layer-by-layer (LbL) polyelectrolytes coating were described for polyphenols delivery. High rates of encapsulation (20 to 70 percent w/w) were obtained as well as a certain *in vitro* controlled delivery (Shutava et al. 2009).

Although the first generation of PLGA NPs have several interesting features as vehicles for antioxidant molecules such as controlled release and protection from premature degradation, they suffer from several major limitations, starting with their instability in a saline medium without the help of steric stabilization, such as PVA. This is a major issue as NPs aggregation could lead to their modified biodistribution and thus active, premature elimination and rapid clearance. Another important issue is opsonization of NPs surface in biological medium; that is, binding of plasmatic proteins resulting in an increased of NPs size, macrophage uptake, premature elimination, and a limited time of circulation in the blood stream (Rabanel et al. 2012; Alexis et al. 2008). Moreover, PLGA or PLA NPs showed very low brain uptake (<1 percent) without surface modification (Li and Sabliov 2013).

12.4 SECOND GENERATION NANOPARTICLE SYSTEM

As early as the 90s, the addition of a hydrophilic polymeric coating (Figure 12.2) appeared as a solution to sterically stabilize NPs in saline media and prevent opsonization, that is, plasma protein adsorption on NP surfaces (Vonarbourg et al. 2006). PEG coating covalently anchored on NPs surface has become the gold standard as attempts to use other hydrophilic polymers did not provide properties suitable for biological applications (Vonarbourg et al. 2006). Surface PEG effect, is characterized by a significant reduction in mononuclear phagocyte system (MPS) uptake, resulting in an increase of the systemic circulation time and the distribution into organs.

Despite many advantages, PEG coating is not without flaws (Rabanel et al. 2014). The observed limitations of PEG coating effect in some studies (limited protein stealth effect, interference with endocytosis) may be due to under-characterized surface properties. The key question here is about the best PEG content, the optimal surface density or the optimal copolymer architecture to provide at the same time, stealth properties, colloidal stability, and optimal antioxidant encapsulation and release properties.

With the objective to determine the best polymer architecture, optimal PEG content, and surface PEG density, we encapsulated the antioxidant curcumin in polymeric NPs by nanoprecipitation using a library of PEGylated PLA polymers (Rabanel et al. 2015b; Rabanel et al. 2015a). The polymer library was composed of diblock made of PEG 2kD and PLA chains (PEG-PLA), and comb-like (PEG-g-PLA) copolymer with different PEG/PLA ratio. We have previously described a transition for NPs physicochemical properties (change in NPs size, PEG surface density and NPs morphology) around 15 percent PEG (w/w) polymer composition (Rabanel et al. 2015b). As PEG polymer content increased, we observed an increase in polyphenol curcumin encapsulation levels. This phenomenon was hypothesized to result from preferential interactions of curcumin with PLA, while increased PEG layer at the NPs surface retained curcumin inside the NPs. Diblock polymer architecture contributed to superior encapsulation levels than comb polymers for similar PEG content (w/w). Curcumin release properties were also influenced similarly as coefficients of diffusion were varying with architecture and PEG content. Even biological effects were found linked to polymer and NPs properties, since the decrease of intracellular ROS levels was correlated with PEG content and NPs morphology (Figure 12.4).

Overall, these studies indicate that polymer architecture (i.e., the position at which PEG chains are attached to the hydrophobic backbone) and PEG content of copolymer are controlling and modulating curcumin concentration and thus level of antioxidant activity. Diblock polymer and high PEG content comb polymers appeared to be the most efficient to reduce oxidative stress (Figure 12.4). In a short term exposition study like this work (1 hour), diblock and micelle-like NPs were found as effective as free curcumin in the condition of the experiments. However, NPs formulation may prove to be more efficient in longer exposition conditions (24 to 48 hours), thanks to their protective effect on curcumin and slow release properties (Rabanel et al. 2015a).

The benefit of NPs PEGylation has been assessed *in vivo* for brain biodistribution. Poly(alkyl cyanoacrylates)-Poly(ethylene glycol)(PACA-PEG) NPs were shown to penetrate mouse brain tissues in a larger extend than non-PEGylated NPs without perturbing BBB permeability. This was demonstrated by biodistribution studies following ^{14}C radiolabeling of NPs and by visualization of fluorescent NPs on histological brain sections (Calvo et al. 2001). The penetration of PEGylated NPs was enhanced in pathological conditions (allergic encephalomyelitis in rat) where the BBB permeability was compromised allowing NPs passive diffusion and macrophages infiltration (Calvo et al. 2002). Later it was determined that the surface PEG layer (or Polysorbate 80, a surfactant with PEG moieties used as a NP stabilizer in some studies) could recruit apolipoproteins E or B (ApoE or ApoB) *in vivo*. The increased brain uptake of PEGylated NPs appeared to be due, at least in part, to an increase in receptor-mediated transport involving apolipoproteins and the LDL receptors (LDL-r) (Kim et al. 2007).

PEG-PLA micelles encapsulating curcumin were also produced by flash nanoprecipitation and tested on an *in vitro* BBB. The NPs formulation led to much higher

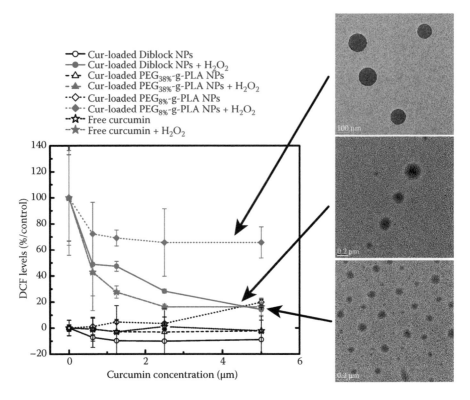

FIGURE 12.4 Encapsulated curcumin antioxidant efficacy as a function of polymer PEGylation level and NPs architecture. (Adapted from Rabanel, J. M. et al., *European Journal of Pharmaceutics and Biopharmaceutics*, 96, 409–420, 2015a. With permission.)

BBB permeability than free curcumin. Moreover, when orally given to Tg2576 mice, a transgenic model of Aβ deposition, NPs administration leads to increased brain bioavailability of curcumin, and improvement of mice memory (Cheng et al. 2013).

In the literature other PEGylated systems have been proposed for antioxidant encapsulation and release. Resveratrol (RES), a polyphenol notably found in wine, has been reported to protect several types of neuronal cells against Aβ peptide toxicity by scavenging ROS and inactivating Caspase-3 (Carrizzo et al. 2013). However, RES use is hampered by its short half-time in biological medium and low solubility in aqueous medium. Polycaprolactone-polyethyleneglycol (PCL-PEG) polymeric micelles have been tested for RES delivery. It was shown that a 12-hour pre-incubation of RES-loaded NPs protected PC12 cells from Aβ-induced damage in a dose dependent manner by attenuating intracellular oxidative stress and caspase-3 activity (Lu et al. 2009).

RES has also been reported as a potential antioxidant for the treatment of ischemia/reperfusion injury. A simple way to produce RES loaded NPs based on poly(N-vinylpyrrolidone)-*b*-poly(γ-caprolactone) polymer (PVP-*b*-PCL) was reported by Lu et al. In this study, PVP was used as the hydrophilic segment of the copolymer instead of PEG. The RES-loaded NPs were evaluated for the protective effect of RES on H_2O_2-induced oxidative stress and apoptosis in rat cortical cell coculture (containing neurons and astrocytes). RES-NPs demonstrated an enhanced neuroprotection compared to an equivalent dose of free RES (Lu et al. 2013).

In conclusion, regarding the use of hydrophilic polymer layer on NPs aimed to deliver antioxidants, several studies have pointed out interesting results particularly in regards to NPs colloidal stability, levels of encapsulation, interaction of PEG with some plasmatic proteins *in vivo* (ApoB, ApoE) which enable brain targeting and antioxidant efficacy for NDDs. So, the NPs PEGylation appears compatible with neuronal or vascular endothelial cell uptake and seems to contribute to enhance NPs and encapsulated antioxidants brain biodistribution. The mechanisms involved in NPs uptake *in vivo* are not clearly identified. The two main mechanisms could operate by transcytosis across the MECs or convection across BBB pores (Kreuter 2014). Long-circulating PEGylated NPs can accumulate at sites of leaky vasculature by the virtue of the enhanced permeation and retention (EPR) effect as demonstrated for tumor vessels (Fang et al. 2011). Brain tumor development, inflammation, and traumatic brain injuries as well as some treatments applied deliberately to increase brain uptake (ultrasound, osmotic shock, etc.) could cause these openings to the otherwise very tight BBB. However, although these openings are usually temporary, their adverse effects on brain homeostasis and their possible contributions to NPs or drug accumulation in the brain tissues are still controversial.

12.5 THIRD GENERATION OF NANOPARTICLE SYSTEM

A PEG layer confers more colloidal stability and longer residence time in blood circulation to NPs, as well as some passive targeting capabilities by the virtue of EPR effect at sites of leaky vasculature. Nevertheless, to achieve higher drug specificity and accumulation, the so-called "active targeting" has emerged as a novel strategy. Active targeting is based on the assumption that a specific ligand, installed on the NPs surface, having an affinity for a specific receptor in a particular tissue could lead to a specific accumulation of NPs or an increase of drug concentration at the targeted site (Figure 12.2). For this purpose, a plethora of strategies have been studied. The described attachments between the targeting moieties and the surface of the NPs are mainly covalent, although noncovalent interactions have been proposed too (Kreuter 2014). The challenge of active targeting for NDD is at two levels: (1) target the MECs of the BBB in order to enter and cross the endothelial barrier toward the brain parenchyma using cellular vesicular transport pathways and (2) target and enter the diseased neuronal cells over normal cells.

12.5.1 TARGETING NEURONAL CELLS

One major challenge in the field of nanotherapeutics is to increase the selective delivery of cargo to targeted cells avoiding unwanted side effects and decrease doses. The route of cell internalisation of polymeric NPs is another key component to consider in the elaboration of targeted devices as the intracellular fate of NPs may determine the encapsulated drug release and efficacy (Sahay et al. 2010).

Targeting neuronal cells (and BBB as discussed in the following section) has been proposed by different approaches and with different ligand-receptor couples. Amongst them, GSH, an endogenous thiolated tripeptide reputed for its powerful antioxidant properties against reactive oxygen and nitrogen species (ROS and NOS), has been proposed for its brain targeting capabilities (Gaillard et al. 2014; Rip et al. 2014).

Very recently, we effectively synthesized and characterised GSH-functionalized PLGA-PEG NPs (GSH-NPs) for the neuronal delivery of curcumin (GSH-NPs-Cur). GSHs were covalently bound to the distal end of PEG chains using thiol-maleimide click reaction. We found that GSH functionalization did not affect the drug loading efficiency (DLE), the size, the polydispersity index (PDI), the zeta potential, the release profile and the stability of the formulation (Djiokeng-Paka and Ramassamy 2017). While being nontoxic, the presence of GSH on the surface of the formulations exhibits a better neuroprotective property against acrolein, a by-product of lipid peroxidation found in the early stage of the disease hippocampus of AD patients. The neuronal internalisation of GSH-NPs-Cur was higher than with free curcumin. GSH-functionalization increases the uptake by neuronal cells and resulted in higher intracellular curcumin concentration as determined by fluorescence microscopy (Figure 12.5). Furthermore, we found that GSH-conjugation modifies the route of internalisation enabling them to escape the uptake through macropinocytosis and therefore avoiding the lysosomal degradation (Djiokeng-Paka and Ramassamy 2017).

Other targeting ligands, specific to neuronal cells, have been proposed (Table 12.1). Synthesized peptide has been used in several studies as brain targeting ligands. Tet-1, a 12-amino acid peptide (HLNILSTLWKYR), identified by Boulis and coworkers through phage-display (Liu et al. 2005), is known to have affinity to moto neurons and possesses retrograde delivery properties. Therefore, by coupling Tet-1 peptide to PLGA-NPs, Matthew et al. found that entrapped curcumin in Tet-1 conjugated PLGA NPs exhibited the ability to destroy Aβ aggregates, had antioxidative properties, and were safe for neuronal cells (Mathew et al. 2012). However, the upstream challenge is still to overcome the BBB.

12.5.2 Targeting the Blood–Brain Barrier

There is a lot of evidence that targeting receptors on the BBB could be an effective strategy for brain drug delivery as receptor-mediated endocytosis could lead to transcytosis and effective transport of NPs or their content in the brain parenchyma (Saraiva et al. 2016). This can further be explained by the fact that the uptake mechanisms could easily escape the lysosomal degradation (Masserini 2013).

It is now widely accepted and proved that conjugation of NPs surface by specific ligands able to recognize and interact with equivalent receptors on the brain endothelial cells of the BBB may be internalized through either the transporters or receptor-mediated endocytosis (Saraiva et al. 2016). The principal limitation with internalization through transporters is the size of NPs. Several attempts have been proposed with numerous types of ligands such as synthesized or endogens peptides, some antibodies and some endogenous proteins with well-characterized receptors such as transferrin, lactoferrin (Tf), insulin, and lipoprotein (Saraiva et al. 2016).

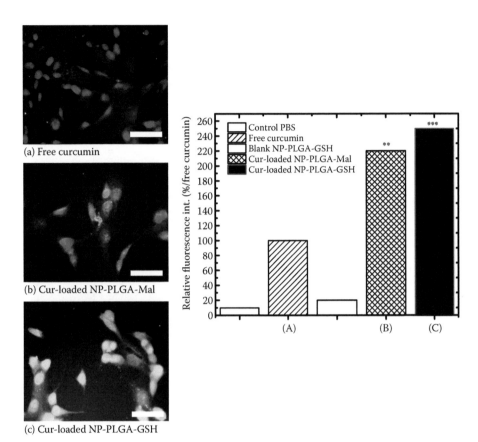

(a) Free curcumin

(b) Cur-loaded NP-PLGA-Mal

(c) Cur-loaded NP-PLGA-GSH

FIGURE 12.5   Effect of GSH modification of PLGA NPs on neuronal internalisation of cur-cumin: fluorescence microscopy imaging of curcumin uptake by SK-N-SH cells. (a) Control cells; (b) curcumin loaded NPs-PLGA-PEG-Mal; (c) curcumin loaded NPs-PLGA-PEG-*Mal*-GSH. The concentration of curcumin used in each condition was 1 μM. Fluorescence of curcumin is observed in green and cell nucleus DAPI in blue. The histogram represents quan-tification of the curcumin fluorescence with data representing mean ± SEM from at least three independent experiments; **p ≤ 0.01 and ***p ≤ 0.001. (Adapted from Djiokeng-Paka, G., and Ramassamy, C., *Molecular Pharmaceutics*, 14(1), 96–106, 2017. With permission.)

The expression of GSH transporters has also been reported on the BBB and there is an increasing interest in the use of GSH as ligand for the selective delivery of nanomedicines (Rip et al. 2014). Several *in vivo* studies found that the surface pres-ence of GSH on nanoformulations increases its cerebral bioavailability. Actually, a PEGylated formulation using GSH as a brain targeting ligand for the treatment of glioma, 2B3-101, is currently undergoing phase I/IIa trials (van der Meel et al. 2013). However, the exact mechanism of GSH on the BBB permeability is still unclear.

Several studies have reported the large distribution of GSH transporters on the BBB, namely EAC1 transporter (Aoyama et al. 2006). This is the principal reason why GSH is being investigated as a potential molecule to increase the cerebral tropism

TABLE 12.1
Some Examples of Ligands Used to Target the Neuronal Cells or the BBB

Ligands	Type of NPs	Encapsulated Active	Targeted Receptor/ Transporter	Limitations	Reference
		Neuronal Cells			
GSH	PLGA NPs	Curcumin	GSH transporter	Route of internalization	Djiokeng-Paka et al. 2016
Tet-1	PLGA NPs	Curcumin	Motor neuron receptor	Dose	Mathew et al. 2012
		Blood–Brain Barrier			
Transferrin	SLN	Quinine dihydrocloride	Tf-R	Iron	Gupta et al. 2007
Transferrin (OX26)	Polymerosomes	NC-1900	Tf-R	Iron	Pang et al. 2011
Lactoferrin (Lf)	PEG-PLGA NPs	Urocortin	Lf-R	Iron	Hu et al. 2011
ApoA-1	HSA	Loperamide	LDL-R	Ligand size	Zensi et al. 2010
ApoE, Apo B	HSA	HSA	LDL-R	Ligand size	Kreuter et al. 2007
ApoE3	Liposome	siRNA	LDL-R	Ligand size	Tamaru et al. 2014
ApoE3	PBCANPs	Curcumin	LDL-R	Ligand size	Mulik et al. 2010
Synthetic opioids peptides	PLGA NPs	None	ND		Costantino et al. 2005
GSH	Liposomes	Doxorubicin	GSH transporter	Route of internalization	Gaillard et al. 2014

of drugs. Very recently, Geldenhuys et al. (2015) synthesized doxorubicin PLGA-NPs coated with GSH in order to enhance brain tropism through GSH transporters on the BBB. Using a transwell system, they found a greater drug accumulation in the receiver compartment at 48 hours, with constant rate suggesting a time-dependent transport mechanism in comparison with free drug solution. Nowadays, several promising formulations using GSH as a targeting ligand are undergoing clinical evaluation (van der Meel et al. 2013). In proof-of-concept studies in rats, it was demonstrated that increasing amounts of GSH conjugated to PEGylated liposomes resulted in higher amounts of free drugs in the brain (Rip et al. 2014). A certain distribution of GSH transporters has been described on BBB namely EAC1 transporter (Aoyama et al. 2006). However, one study has revealed the potential involvement of GSH in the activation of FALS-linked mutant SOD1 during chronological aging. So GSH supplementation in terms of ligand-targeting may not be suitable for all NDD especially in ALS (Brasil et al. 2013).

LDL receptors (LDL-r) are a family of endocytosis receptors insuring supply of cholesterol toward different organs including brain. Some LDL-r are specifically overexpressed on endothelial cells forming the BBB (Dehouck et al. 1997a; Dehouck et al. 1997b; Lucarelli et al. 2002). Some works had shown that these receptors can be used for targeted administration of antioxidant to the CNS (Zensi et al. 2009; Mulik et al. 2010).

LDL-r possesses mainly two ligands: ApoB100 and ApoE. Following binding of ApoB100 (or ApoE) to the receptor, the cholesterol-containing lipid NPs are internalized by endocytosis. The afinity of ApoE is 10 to 100 fold higher for the LFDL-r than ApoB100 (Innerarity and Mahley 1978). Moreover, it is known that the absence of ApoE triggers oxidative damages in the CNS (Ramassamy et al. 2001).

Apolipoproteins have been grafted to liposomes to target cells expressing the LDL-r in order to deliver methotrexate or paclitaxel (Malcor et al. 2012) but also Mangostin (α-M) in biomimetic ApoE reconstituted high density lipoproteins (Song et al. 2016). In this last work, the authors showed *in vitro* uptake of the biomimetic antioxidant nanocarriers by brain endothelial cells and *in vivo* in mouse brain parenchyma (Song et al. 2016).

PEGylated polyhexadecylcyanoacrylate (PHDCA) NPs have been shown to translocate across BBB as mentioned in the previous section (Calvo et al. 2001). A more detailed analysis had shown later that ApoE from plasma adsorbed more onto PEG-PHDCA NPs surface than on PHDCA NPs surface. This adsorption, leading to a non-covalent functionalization, was directly linked to the enhanced brain transport (Kim et al. 2007). Several studies showed the advantage of nanoformulations with ApoE3 at the surface with, for instance, enhanced neuronal internalization of curcumin (Zensi et al. 2009, Mulik et al. 2010).

PEG-PLGA NPs modified with Lactoferrin (Lf), an iron binding protein and a ligand of the Lf-receptor found on the BBB was proposed for CNS delivery of peptide for the PD treatment (Hu et al. 2011). The authors showed an enhanced accumulation of NPs when modified by the Lf, *in vitro* (in a bEnd3 BBB mouse cell model) and *in vivo* in mouse brain parenchyma (Hu et al. 2011).

The use of protein (over 20kD) as targeting ligand, is costly, leads to complex NPs preparation and introduces some stability issues. Specific peptides (less than

30 amino acids) are more advantageous in term of cost and stability. Several studies make use of particular peptides for BBB or neuronal cell targeting. For instances, Li et al. screen a library of peptides with brain tropism generated by phage-display (Li et al. 2011). They identified a peptide (Pep TGN) allowing a significant increased accumulation of functionalized NPs *in vitro* in bEnd3 cells and *in vivo* in mouse brain as determined by fluorescence measurements (Li et al. 2011).

Besides receptor-mediated endocytosis, absorptive-mediated endocytosis (AME), an uptake process based on nonspecific charge-based interactions, has been used in some studies to increase NPs BBB translocation. AME can be triggered by polycationic molecules binding to the membrane or by the binding of extracellular lectins. For instance, delivery of Coenzyme Q10 was improved by trimethylated chitosan-conjugated PLGA (TMC/PLGA) NPs. Fluorescent microscopy showed a higher accumulation of TMC/PLGA NPs loaded with coumarin-6 in different structure of the brain, while no brain uptake of plain PLGA NPs was observed. Coenzyme Q10 loaded TMC/PLGA NPs improved memory impairment, restoring it to a normal level (Wang et al. 2010).

In conclusion, the "active" targeting of NPs for antioxidant delivery to neuronal cells and across the BBB has been described in numerous studies. Enhanced concentration of NPs have been detected in a few studies by microscopy in brain tissues (Calvo et al. 2001) or by tracking fluorescent probes encapsulated in NPs (Hu et al. 2011; Li et al. 2011). Therapeutic and behaviour studies supported an increased delivery of encapsulated antioxidants to the brain tissues (Wang et al. 2010; Yun et al. 2013; Cheng et al. 2013). However, many questions remained unsolved. The question regarding the effective dose of NPs or the effective dose of active compounds found in brain parenchyma stays in most studies unsolved. Also, the exact mechanism of the NPs encapsulation effect on brain biodistribution is unclear. It can be hypothesized that we have translocation of intact NPs across the BBB and release of active in the parenchyma. Some microscopic evidences have detected NPs in different part of the CNS (Calvo et al. 2002; Zensi et al. 2009; Calvo et al. 2001). Alternatively, we could have endocytosis of NPs at the BBB, intracellular destruction of the NPs and release of active in the brain parenchyma. Lastly, we could have a reservoir effect where the NPs do not necessarily cross the BBB. The beneficial effect here is the result of longer residence time, which protects the antioxidant from degradation and allows higher concentration around the organ or cellular target. NPs encapsulating antioxidant are therefore providing a blood compartment reservoir and a concentration gradient resulting in higher concentration in the brain (Tsai et al. 2011; Gaudin et al. 2015).

12.6   THE FOURTH GENERATION: STIMULI-RESPONSIVE NANOPARTICLES

After reaching the pathological site, nanocarriers should deliver their contents in an efficient manner to achieve a sufficient therapeutic response as only "free" antioxidants can exert their activity. One more reason that makes NPs attractive in medicinal chemistry is the possibility to insert specific structures with specific chemical, physical, and biological properties (Petkar et al. 2011). A new approach is currently being investigated and relies mostly on the intrinsic properties of the pathological sites which can differ from healthy tissues with lower interstitial pH, higher temperature or very low redox potential (Strong and West 2011; Quesada et al. 2013; Brülisauer et al. 2012). By using "smart stimulus sensitive polymers," researchers are expecting to finely tune and monitor the release of the encapsulated antioxidant compounds at a particular site.

An example of such a stimuli-responsive system are the redox-sensitive NPs. Indeed, NDDs are clearly characterized with the disturbance of the redox potential and therefore an oxidative stress situation prevails in affected tissues and cells (Ramassamy et al. 2000; Markesbery 1997). Based on the redox-sensing thiols, redox-responsive drug delivery NPs can be designed to specifically provide antioxidants in the injury sites of NDDs. So, the compartment displaying disturbance of the redox balance will destabilize the nanomaterial and the therapeutic drugs will be released. Very recently, Quesada and coworkers proposed PLGA NPs covered with a thin layer (6–10 nm) of a redox-responsive amorphous organo-silica shell with disulfides bridges inserted. Using electronic microscopy, they reveal a monodispersed population with average diameter between 35–165 nm, a size suitable for brain drug delivery. They reported a release profile close to Higuchi's square root model implying that the release was mainly through the diffusion process with minor contribution of degradation (Quesada et al. 2013). This silica sealed structure provides enough cargo stability before reaching the target cells due to the presence of intercalated disulfide molecular bridges. Also this device can be a very good approach to avoid the burst release observed with colloids. The limit with the redox-responsive approach is the need of free thiolated compounds in the blood in order to trigger the release of drugs through the destabilisation of disulfides bridges. In this study, the authors used dithiothreitol, a powerful antioxidant, to induce the redox-responsive release of pyrene, a model compound. Knowing the drastic decrease of glutathione and thiolated compounds reported in patients suffering from NDDs, the question to know whether it would be a release with this rigid system is unsolved.

It's worth noting that pH-responsive NPs have been suggested to deliver various antioxidants. Tang et al. (2015) proposed a pH-responsive carrier of tannic acid. Another pH responsive system was proposed for the delivery of silymarin with PLGA NPs embedded in an alginate microhydrogel (El-Sherbiny et al. 2011). Chitosan-g-poly (N-isopropylacrylamide) NPs can provide thermos-responsiveness as curcumin delivery become prominent above polymer lower critical solution temperature (LCST is the temperature at which the polymer change its solubility; Sanoj Rejinold et al. 2011a; Sanoj Rejinold et al. 2011b).

To conclude this section, it is important to stress that to be completely useful as vehicles for antioxidant delivery to the CNS, the stimuli-responsive NPs should integrate several characteristics: furtivity, selectivity, stability, and responsiveness. The incorporation of these features in the same NPs is a challenge in terms of fabrication and characterization. At this time, several proofs of concept have been put forward but the integration of multiple functions in a clinically relevant device is still an unreached goal.

12.7 CONCLUSION

Synoptically, antioxidant delivery to the brain parenchyma stays a challenge for a number of causes, starting with the chemical stability of the antioxidant molecules in biological media and their physico-chemistry resulting in a low brain availability. The challenges associated with the delivery of antioxidant-loaded NPs are to cross the BBB to the brain parenchyma with a sufficient dose to fully exercise antioxidant effects, to achieve timely release, and eventually to obtain selective neuronal cells uptake.

The toxicity of degradable polymer material is a question often overlooked. Few *in vivo* data are available regarding the fate and effect of polymer NPs on very sensitive brain tissues, including their effects on the integrity of the BBB and their neurotoxicity. On the other hand, it appears that the positive effect when encapsulating active molecules is, at this time, predominantly caused by the longer blood circulation of NPs. Brain exposition to NPs in this case will be limited, and therefore, a higher concern has to be put on the safety of clearance organs (liver, spleen, and kidney). More exhaustive *in vivo* results are needed, particularly for repeated dose administration, long term exposure, and tissue accumulation.

Once the NPs have reached the brain parenchyma, a last challenge is its diffusion within brain tissue in order to be able to interact with targeted cells. This step is not to be neglected, as diffusion of NPs in the interstitial tissue is quite limited by the extracellular matrix and apparently depends on surface properties (Nance et al. 2012; Mastorakos et al. 2015).

REFERENCES

Abbott, N. J., and Revest, P. A. 1991. Control of brain endothelial permeability. *Cerebrovascular and Brain Metabolism Reviews* 3(1):39–72.

Alexis, F., Pridgen, E., Molnar, L. K., and Farokhzad, O. C. 2008. Factors affecting the clearance and biodistribution of polymeric nanoparticles. *Molecular Pharmaceutics* 5(4):505–515.

Anderson, J. M., and Shive, M. S. 1997. Biodegradation and biocompatibility of PLA and PLGA microspheres. *Advanced Drug Delivery Reviews* 28(1):5–24.

Aoyama, K., Suh, S. W., Hamby, A. M., Liu, J., Chan, W. Y., Chen, Y., and Swanson, R. A. 2006. Neuronal glutathione deficiency and age-dependent neurodegeneration in the EAAC1 deficient mouse. *Nature Neuroscience* 9(1):119–126.

Arce-Varas, N., Abate, G., Prandelli, C., Martinez, C., Cuetos, F., Menendez, M., Marziano, M., Cabrera-Garcia, D., Fernandez-Sanchez, M. T., Novelli, A., Memo, M., and Uberti, D. 2016. Comparison of extracellular and intracellular blood compartments highlights redox alterations in Alzheimer's and Mild Cognitive Impairment patients. *Current Alzheimer Research* 14(1):112–122.

Athanasiou, K. A., Niederauer, G. G., and Agrawal, C. M. 1996. Sterilization, toxicity, biocompatibility and clinical applications of polylactic acid/polyglycolic acid copolymers. *Biomaterials* 17(2):93–102.

Banks, W. A., Kastin, A. J., and Barrera, C. M. 1991. Delivering peptides to the central nervous system: Dilemmas and strategies. *Pharmaceutical Research* 8(11):1345–1350.

Barnham, K. J., Masters, C. L., and Bush, A. I. 2004. Neurodegenerative diseases and oxidative stress. *Nature Reviews Drug Discovery* 3(3):205–214.

Begum, A, N., Jones, M. R., Lim, G. P., Morihara, T., Kim, P., Heath, D. D., Rock, C. L., Pruitt, M. A., Yang, F., Hudspeth, B., Hu, S., Faull, K. F., Teter, B., Cole, G. M., and Frautschy, S. A. 2008. Curcumin structure—Function, bioavailability, and efficacy in models of neuroinflammation and Alzheimer's disease. *Journal of Pharmacology and Experimental Therapeutics* 326(1):196–208.

Belkacemi, A., and Ramassamy, C. 2012. Time sequence of oxidative stress in the brain from transgenic mouse models of Alzheimer's disease related to the amyloid-beta cascade. *Free Radical Biology and Medicine* 52(3):593.

Belkacemi, A., Doggui, S., Dao, L., and Ramassamy, C. 2011. Challenges associated with curcumin therapy in Alzheimer disease. *Expert Reviews in Molecular Medicine* 13: e34.

Blesa, J., Trigo-Damas, I., Quiroga-Varela, A., and Jackson-Lewis, V. R. 2015. Oxidative stress and Parkinson's disease. *Frontiers in Neuroanatomy* 9(91):1–9.

Brasil, A. A., Belati, A., Mannarino, S. C., Panek, A. D., Eleutherio, E. C. A., and Pereira, M. D. 2013. The involvement of GSH in the activation of human Sod1 linked to FALS in chronologically aged yeast cells. *FEMS Yeast Research* 13(5):433–440.

Brülisauer, L., Kathriner, N., Prenrecaj, M., Gauthier, M. A., and Leroux, J.-C. 2012. Tracking the bioreduction of disulfide-containing cationic dendrimers. *Angewandte Chemie International Edition* 51(50):12454–12458.

Calvo, P., Gouritin, B., Chacun, H., Desmaële, D., D'Angelo, J., Noel, J.-P., Georgin, D., Fattal, E., Andreux, J. P., and Couvreur, P. 2001. Long-circulating PEGylated poly-cyanoacrylate nanoparticles as new drug carrier for brain delivery. *Pharmaceutical Research* 18(8):1157–1166.

Calvo, P., Gouritin, B., Villarroya, H., Eclancher, F., Giannavola, C., Klein, C., Andreux, J. P., and Couvreur, P. 2002. Quantification and localization of PEGylated polycyanoacrylate nanoparticles in brain and spinal cord during experimental allergic encephalomyelitis in the rat. *European Journal of Neuroscience* 15(8):1317–1326.

Carrizzo, A., Forte, M., Damato, A., Trimarco, V., Salzano, F., Bartolo, M., Maciag, A., Puca, A. A., and Vecchione, C. 2013. Antioxidant effects of resveratrol in cardiovascular, cerebral and metabolic diseases. *Food and Chemical Toxicology* 61:215–226.

Celia, C., Cosco, D., Paolino, D., and Fresta, M. 2011. Nanoparticulate devices for brain drug delivery. *Medicinal Research Reviews* 31(5):716–756.

Cheng, K. K., Yeung, C. F., Ho, S. W., Chow, S. F., Chow, A. H. L., and Baum, L. 2013. Highly stabilized curcumin nanoparticles tested in an in vitro blood–brain barrier model and in Alzheimer's disease Tg2576 mice. *The AAPS Journal* 15(2):324–336.

Costantino, L., Gandolfi, F., Tosi, G., Rivasi, F., Vandelli, M. A., and Forni, F. 2005. Peptide-derivatized biodegradable nanoparticles able to cross the blood–brain barrier. *Journal of Controlled Release* 108(1):84–96.

Cuajungco, M. P., Goldstein, L. E., Nunomura, A., Smith, M. A., Lim, J. T., Atwood, C. S., Huang, X., Farrag, Y. W., Perry, G., and Bush, A. I. 2000. Evidence that the beta-amyloid plaques of Alzheimer's disease represent the redox-silencing and entombment of abeta by zinc. *Journal of Biological Chemistry* 275(26):19439–19442.

Dehouck, B., Fenart, L., Dehouck, M.-P., Pierce, A., Torpier, G., and Cecchelli, R. 1997a. A new function for the LDL receptor: Transcytosis of LDL across the blood–brain barrier. *The Journal of Cell Biology* 138(4):877–889.

Dehouck, M. P., Vigne, P., Torpier, G., Breittmayer, J. P., Cecchelli, R., and Frelin, C. 1997b. Endothelin-1 as a mediator of endothelial cell-pericyte interactions in bovine brain capillaries. *Journal of Cerebral Blood Flow and Metabolism* 17(4):464–469.

Devore, E. E., Grodstein, F., van Rooij, F. J., Hofman, A., Stampfer, M. J., Witteman, J. C., and Breteler, M. M. 2010. Dietary antioxidants and long-term risk of dementia. *Archives of Neurology* 67(7):819–825.

Di Domenico, F., Pupo, G., Giraldo, E., Badia, M. C., Monllor, P., Lloret, A., Schinina, M. E., Giorgi, A., Cini, C., Tramutola, A., Butterfield, D. A., Vina, J., and Perluigi, M. 2016. Oxidative signature of cerebrospinal fluid from mild cognitive impairment and Alzheimer disease patients. *Free Radical Biology and Medicine* 91:1–9.

Djiokeng-Paka, G., Doggui, S., Zaghmi, A., Safar, R., Dao, L., Reisch, A., Klymchenko, A., Roullin, V. G., Joubert, O., and Ramassamy, C. 2016. Neuronal uptake and neuroprotective properties of curcumin-loaded nanoparticles on SK-N-SH cell line: Role of poly(lactide-co-glycolide) polymeric matrix composition. *Molecular Pharmaceutics* 13(2):391–403.

Djiokeng-Paka, G., and Ramassamy, C. 2017. Optimization of curcumin loaded-PEG-PLGA nanoparticles by GSH functionalization. Investigation of the internalization pathway in neuronal cells. *Molecular Pharmaceutics* 14(1):93–106.

Doggui, S., Sahni, J. K., Arseneault, M., Dao, L., and Ramassamy, C. 2012. Neuronal iptake and neuroprotective effect of curcumin-loaded PLGA nanoparticles on the human SK-N-SH cell line. *Journal of Alzheimers Disease* 30(2):377–392.

El-Sherbiny, I. M., Abdel-Mogib, M., Dawidar, A.-A. M., Elsayed, A., and Smyth, H. D. C. 2011. Biodegradable pH-responsive alginate-poly (lactic-co-glycolic acid) nano/micro hydrogel matrices for oral delivery of silymarin. *Carbohydrate Polymers* 83(3):1345–1354.

Fang, J., Nakamura, H., and Maeda, H. 2011. The EPR effect: Unique features of tumor blood vessels for drug delivery, factors involved, and limitations and augmentation of the effect. *Advanced Drug Delivery Reviews* 63(3):136–151.

Gaillard, P. J., Appeldoorn, C. C. M., Dorland, R., van Kregten, J., Manca, F., Vugts, D. J., Windhorst, B., van Dongen, G. A. M. S., de Vries, H. E., Maussang, D., and van Tellingen, O. 2014. Pharmacokinetics, brain delivery, and efficacy in brain tumor-bearing mice of glutathione pegylated liposomal doxorubicin (2B3-101). *PLoS ONE* 9(1):e82331.

Gaudin, A., Lepetre-Mouelhi, S., Mougin, J., Parrod, M., Pieters, G., Garcia-Argote, S., Loreau, O., Goncalves, J., Chacun, H., Courbebaisse, Y., Clayette, P., Desmaële, D., Rousseau, B., Andrieux, K., and Couvreur, P. 2015. Pharmacokinetics, biodistribution and metabolism of squalenoyl adenosine nanoparticles in mice using dual radiolabeling and radio-HPLC analysis. *Journal of Controlled Release* 212:50–58.

Geldenhuys, W., Wehrung, D., Groshev, A., Hirani, A., and Sutariya, V. 2015. Brain-targeted delivery of doxorubicin using glutathione-coated nanoparticles for brain cancers. *Pharmaceutical Development and Technology* 20(4):497–506.

Gilgun-Sherki, Y., Melamed, E., and Offen, D. 2004. The role of oxidative stress in the pathogenesis of multiple sclerosis: The need for effective antioxidant therapy. *Journal of Neurology* 251(3):261–268.

Gupta, Y., Jain, A., and Jain, S. K. 2007. Transferrin-conjugated solid lipid nanoparticles for enhanced delivery of quinine dihydrochloride to the brain. *Journal of Pharmacy and Pharmacology* 59(7):935–940.

Harrison, F. E. 2012. A critical review of vitamin C for the prevention of age-related cognitive decline and Alzheimer's disease. *Journal of Alzheimer's Disease* 29(4):711–726.

Hu, K., Shi, Y., Jiang, W., Han, J., Huang, S., and Jiang, X. 2011. Lactoferrin conjugated PEG-PLGA nanoparticles for brain delivery: Preparation, characterization and efficacy in Parkinson's disease. *International Journal of Pharmaceutics* 415(1–2):273.

Huber, J. D., Egleton, R. D., and Davis, T. P. 2001. Molecular physiology and pathophysiology of tight junctions in the blood-brain barrier. *Trends in Neuroscience* 24(12):719–725.

Innerarity, T. L., and Mahley, R. W. 1978. Enhanced binding by cultured human fibroblasts of apo-E-containing lipoproteins as compared with low density lipoproteins. *Biochemistry* 17(8):1440–1447.

Kamaly, N., Yameen, B., Wu, J., and Farokhzad, O. C. 2016. Degradable controlled-release polymers and polymeric nanoparticles: Mechanisms of controlling drug release. *Chemical Reviews* 116(4):2602–2663.

Kim, H., Park, B.-S., Lee, K.-G., Choi, C. Y., Jang, S. S., Kim, Y.-H., and Lee, S.-E. 2005. Effects of naturally occurring compounds on fibril formation and oxidative stress of β-Amyloid. *Journal of Agricultural and Food Chemistry* 53(22):8537–8541.

Kim, H. R., Andrieux, K., Gil, S., Taverna, M., Chacun, H., Desmaële, D., Taran, F., Georgin, D., and Couvreur, P. 2007. Translocation of poly(ethylene glycol-co-hexadecyl)cyanoacrylate nanoparticles into rat brain endothelial cells: Role of apolipoproteins in receptor-mediated endocytosis. *Biomacromolecules* 8(3):793–799.

Kniesel, U., and Wolburg, H. 2000. Tight junctions of the blood–brain barrier. *Cellular and Molecular Neurobiology* 20(1):57–76.

Kreuter, J. 2014. Drug delivery to the central nervous system by polymeric nanoparticles: What do we know? *Advanced Drug Delivery Reviews* 71:2–14.

Kreuter, J., Hekmatara, T., Dreis, S., Vogel, T., Gelperina, S., and Langer, K. 2007. Covalent attachment of apolipoprotein A-I and apolipoprotein B-100 to albumin nanoparticles enables drug transport into the brain. *Journal of Controlled Release* 118(1):54–58.

Li, J., Feng, L., Fan, L., Zha, Y., Guo, L., Zhang, Q., Chen, J., Pang, Z., Wang, Y., Jiang, X., Yang, V. C., and Wen, L. 2011. Targeting the brain with PEG–PLGA nanoparticles modified with phage-displayed peptides. *Biomaterials* 32(21):4943–4950.

Li, J., and Sabliov, C. 2013. PLA/PLGA nanoparticles for delivery of drugs across the blood–brain barrier. *Nanotechnology Reviews* 2(3):241–257.

Liu, J. K., Teng, Q., Garrity-Moses, M., Federici, T., Tanase, D., Imperiale, M. J., and Boulis, N. M. 2005. A novel peptide defined through phage display for therapeutic protein and vector neuronal targeting. *Neurobiology of Disease* 19(3):407–418.

Lu, X., Ji, C., Xu, H., Li, X., Ding, H., Ye, M., Zhu, Z., Ding, D., Jiang, X., Ding, X., and Guo, X. 2009. Resveratrol-loaded polymeric micelles protect cells from Aβ-induced oxidative stress. *International Journal of Pharmaceutics* 375(1–2):89–96.

Lu, X., Xu, H., Sun, B., Zhu, Z., Zheng, D., and Li, X. 2013. Enhanced neuroprotective effects of resveratrol delivered by nanoparticles on hydrogen peroxide-induced oxidative stress in rat cortical cell culture. *Molecular Pharmaceutics* 10(5):2045–2053.

Lucarelli, M., Borrelli, V., Fiori, A., Cucina, A., Granata, F., Potenza, R. L., Scarpa, S., Cavallaro, A., and Strom, R. 2002. The expression of native and oxidized LDL receptors in brain microvessels is specifically enhanced by astrocytes-derived soluble factor(s). *FEBS Letters* 522(1–3):19–23.

Makadia, H. K., and Siegel, S. J. 2011. Polylactic-co-glycolic acid (PLGA) as biodegradable controlled drug delivery carrier. *Polymers (Basel, Switz.)* 3(3):1377.

Malcor, J.-D., Payrot, N., David, M., Faucon, A., Abouzid, K., Jacquot, G., Floquet, N., Debarbieux, F., Rougon, G., Martinez, J., Khrestchatisky, M., Vlieghe, P., and Lisowski, V. 2012. Chemical optimization of new ligands of the low-density lipoprotein receptor as potential vectors for central nervous system targeting. *Journal of Medicinal Chemistry* 55(5):2227–2241.

Markesbery, W. R. 1997. Oxidative stress hypothesis in Alzheimer's disease. *Free Radical Biology and Medicine* 23(1):134–147.

Masserini, M. 2013. Nanoparticles for brain drug delivery. *ISRN Biochemistry* 2013:18.

Mastorakos, P., Zhang, C., Berry, S., Oh, Y., Lee, S., Eberhart, C. G., Woodworth, G. F., Suk, J. S., and Hanes, J. 2015. Highly PEGylated DNA nanoparticles provide uniform and widespread gene transfer in the brain. *Advanced Healthcare Materials* 4(7):1023–1033.

Mathew, A., Fukuda, T., Nagaoka, Y., Hasumura, T., Morimoto, H., Yoshida, Y., Maekawa, T., Venugopal, K., and Kumar, D S. 2012. Curcumin loaded-PLGA nanoparticles conjugated with Tet-1 peptide for potential use in Alzheimer's disease. *PLoS ONE* 7 (3):e32616.

Mulik, R. S., Monkkonen, J., Juvonen, R. O., Mahadik, K. R., and Paradkar, A. R. 2010. ApoE3 mediated poly(butyl) cyanoacrylate nanoparticles containing curcumin: Study of enhanced activity of curcumin against beta amyloid induced cytotoxicity using in vitro cell culture model. *Molecular Pharmaceutics* 7(3):815–825.

Nagpal, K., Singh, S. K., and Mishra, D. N. 2012. Nanoparticle mediated brain targeted delivery of gallic acid: In vivo behavioral and biochemical studies for improved antioxidant and antidepressant-like activity. *Drug Delivery* 19(8):378–391.

Nair, L. S., and Laurencin, C. T. 2007. Biodegradable polymers as biomaterials. *Progress in Polymer Science* 32(8–9):762–798.

Nance, E. A., Woodworth, G. F., Sailor, K. A., Shih, T.-Y., Xu, Q., Swaminathan, G., Xiang, D., Eberhart, C., and Hanes, J. 2012. A dense poly(ethylene glycol) coating improves penetration of large polymeric nanoparticles within brain tissue. *Science Translational Medicine* 4(149):149ra119–149ra119.

Pang, Z., Gao, H., Yu, Y., Chen, J., Guo, L., Ren, J., Wen, Z., Su, J., and Jiang, X. 2011. Brain delivery and cellular internalization mechanisms for transferrin conjugated biodegradable polymersomes. *International Journal of Pharmaceutics* 415(1–2):284–292.

Petkar, K. C., Chavhan, S. S., Agatonovik-Kustrin, S., and Sawant, K. 2011. Nanostructured materials in drug and gene delivery: A review of the state of the art. *Critical Reviews in Therapeutic Drug Carrier Systems* 28(2):101–164.

Quesada, M., Muniesa, C., and Botella, P. 2013. Hybrid PLGA-organosilica nanoparticles with redox-sensitive molecular gates. *Chemistry of Materials* 25(13):2597–2602.

Rabanel, J.-M., Aoun, V., Elkin, I., Mokhtar, M., and Hildgen, P. 2012. Drug-loaded nanocarriers: Passive targeting and crossing of biological barriers. *Current Medicinal Chemistry* 19(19):3070–3102.

Rabanel, J.-M., Faivre, J., Paka, G. D., Ramassamy, C., Hildgen, P., and Banquy, X. 2015a. Effect of polymer architecture on curcumin encapsulation and release from PEGylated polymer nanoparticles: Toward a drug delivery nano-platform to the CNS. *European Journal of Pharmaceutics and Biopharmaceutics* 96:409–420.

Rabanel, J.-M., Faivre, J., Tehrani, S. F., Lalloz, A., Hildgen, P., and Banquy, X. 2015b. Effect of the polymer architecture on the structural and biophysical properties of PEG-PLA nanoparticles. *ACS Applied Materials & Interfaces* 7(19):10374–10385.

Rabanel, J.-M., Hildgen, P., and Banquy, X. 2014. Assessment of PEG on polymeric particles surface, a key step in drug carrier translation. *Journal of Controlled Release* 185:71–87.

Ramassamy, C. 2006. Emerging role of polyphenolic compounds in the treatment of neurodegenerative diseases: A review of their intracellular targets. *European Journal of Pharmacology* 545(1):51–64.

Ramassamy, C., Averill, D., Beffert, U., Theroux, L., Lussier-Cacan, S., Cohn, J. S., Christen, Y., Schoofs, A., Davignon, J., and Poirier, J. 2000. Oxidative insults are associated with apolipoprotein E genotype in Alzheimer's disease brain. *Neurobiology of Disease* 7(1):23–37.

Ramassamy, C., Krzywkowski, P., Averill, D., Lussier-Cacan, S., Theroux, L., Christen, Y., Davignon, J., and Poirie, J. 2001. Impact of apoE deficiency on oxidative insults and antioxidant levels in the brain. *Molecular Brain Research* 86(1–2):76–83.

Ramchandani, M., and Robinson, D. 1998. In vitro and in vivo release of ciprofloxacin from PLGA 50:50 implants. *Journal of Controlled Release* 54(2):167–175.

Rapoport, S. I. 1996. Modulation of blood–brain barrier permeability. *Journal of Drug Targeting* 3(6):417–25.

Reddy, M. K., and Labhasetwar, V. 2009. Nanoparticle-mediated delivery of superoxide dismutase to the brain: An effective strategy to reduce ischemia-reperfusion injury. *The FASEB Journal* 23(5):1384–1395.

Ringman, J. M., Frautschy, S. A., Teng, E., Begum, A. N., Bardens, J., Beigi, M., Gylys, K. H., Badmaev, V., Heath, D. D., Apostolova, L. G., Porter, V., Vanek, Z., Marshall, G. A., Hellemann, G., Sugar, C., Masterman, D. L., Montine, T. J., Cummings, J. L., and Cole, G. M. 2012. Oral curcumin for Alzheimer's disease: Tolerability and efficacy in a 24-week randomized, double blind, placebo-controlled study. *Alzheimer's Research & Therapy* 4(5):43.

Rip, J., Chen, L., Hartman, R., van den Heuvel, A., Reijerkerk, A., van Kregten, J., van der Boom, B., Appeldoorn, C., de Boer, M., Maussang, D., C. M. de Lange, E., and Gaillard, P. J. 2014. Glutathione PEGylated liposomes: Pharmacokinetics and delivery of cargo across the blood–brain barrier in rats. *Journal of Drug Targeting* 22(5):460–467.

Sahay, G., Alakhova, D. Y., and Kabanov, A. V. 2010. Endocytosis of nanomedicines. *Journal of Controlled Release* 145(3):182–195.

Sanoj R. N., Muthunarayanan, M., Divyarani, V. V., Sreerekha, P. R., Chennazhi, K. P., Nair, S. V., Tamura, H., and Jayakumar, R. 2011a. Curcumin-loaded biocompatible thermoresponsive polymeric nanoparticles for cancer drug delivery. *Journal of Colloid and Interface Science* 360(1):39–51.

Sanoj R. N., Sreerekha, P. R., Chennazhi, K. P., Nair, S. V., and Jayakumar, R. 2011b. Biocompatible, biodegradable and thermo-sensitive chitosan-g-poly (N-isopropylacrylamide) nanocarrier for curcumin drug delivery. *International Journal of Biological Macromolecules* 49(2):161–172.

Saraiva, C., Praça, C., Ferreira, R., Santos, T., Ferreira, L., and Bernardino, L. 2016. Nanoparticle-mediated brain drug delivery: Overcoming blood–brain barrier to treat neurodegenerative diseases. *Journal of Controlled Release* 235:34–47.

Scheff, S. W., Ansari, M. A., and Mufson, E. J. 2016. Oxidative stress and hippocampal synaptic protein levels in elderly cognitively intact individuals with Alzheimer's disease pathology. *Neurobiology of Aging* 42:1–12.

Shutava, T. G., Balkundi, S. S., Vangala, P., Steffan, J. J., Bigelow, R. L., Cardelli, J. A., O'Neal, D. P., and Lvov, Y. M. 2009. Layer-by-layer-coated gelatin nanoparticles as a vehicle for delivery of natural polyphenols. *ACS Nano* 3(7):1877–1885.

Singh, M., Arseneault, M., Sanderson, T., Murthy, V., and Ramassamy, C. 2008. Challenges for research on polyphenols from foods in Alzheimer's disease: Bioavailability, metabolism, and cellular and molecular mechanisms. *Journal of Agricultural and Food Chemistry* 56(13):4855–4873.

Song, Q., Song, H., Xu, J., Huang, J., Hu, M., Gu, X., Chen, J., Zheng, G., Chen, H., and Gao, X. 2016. Biomimetic ApoE-reconstituted high density lipoprotein nanocarrier for blood–brain barrier penetration and amyloid beta-targeting drug delivery. *Molecular Pharmaceutics* 13(11):3976–3987.

Soppimath, K. S., Aminabhavi, T. M., Kulkarni, A. R., and Rudzinski, W. E. 2001. Biodegradable polymeric nanoparticles as drug delivery devices. *Journal of Controlled Release* 70(1–2):1–20.

Strong, L. E., and West, J. L. 2011. Thermally responsive polymer–nanoparticle composites for biomedical applications. *Wiley Interdisciplinary Reviews: Nanomedicine and Nanobiotechnology* 3(3):307–317.

Swomley, A. M., and Butterfield, D. A. 2015. Oxidative stress in Alzheimer disease and mild cognitive impairment: Evidence from human data provided by redox proteomics. *Archives of Toxicology* 89(10):669–1680.

Tamaru, M., Akita, H., Kajimoto, K., Sato, Y., Hatakeyama, H., and Harashima, H. 2014. An apolipoprotein E modified liposomal nanoparticle: Ligand dependent efficiency as a siRNA delivery carrier for mouse-derived brain endothelial cells. *International Journal of Pharmaceutics* 465(1–2):77–82.

Tang, C., Amin, D., Messersmith, P. B., Anthony, J. E., and Prud'homme, R. K. 2015. Polymer directed self-assembly of pH-responsive antioxidant nanoparticles. *Langmuir* 3(12):3612–3620.

Tiwari, S. K., Agarwal, S., Seth, B., Yadav, A., Nair, S., Bhatnagar, P., Karmakar, M., Kumari, M., Singh Chauhan, L. K., Patel, D. K., Srivastava, V., Singh, D., Gupta, S. K., Tripathi, A., Chaturvedi, R. K., and Gupta, K. C. 2014. Curcumin-loaded nanoparticles potently induce adult neurogenesis and reverse cognitive deficits in Alzheimer's disease model via canonical Wnt/β-Catenin pathway. *ACS Nano* 8(1):76–103.

Tsai, Y. M., Chien, C. F., Lin, L. C., and Tsai, T. H. 2011. Curcumin and its nano-formulation: The kinetics of tissue distribution and blood–brain barrier penetration. *International Journal of Pharmaceutics* 416(1):331.

Van der Meel, R., Vehmeijer, L. J. C., Kok, R. J., Storm, G., and van Gaal, E. V. B. 2013. Ligand-targeted particulate nanomedicines undergoing clinical evaluation: Current status. *Advanced Drug Delivery Reviews* 65(10):1284–1298.

Vina, J., Lloret, A., Giraldo, E., Badia, M. C., and Alonso, M. D. 2011. Antioxidant pathways in Alzheimer's disease: Possibilities of intervention. *Current Pharmaceutical Design* 17(35):3861–3864.

Vonarbourg, A., Passirani, C., Saulnier, P., and Benoit, J. P. 2006. Parameters influencing the stealthiness of colloidal drug delivery systems. *Biomaterials* 27(24):4356–4373.

Wang, Y. J., Pan, M. H., Cheng, A. L., Lin, L. I., Ho, Y. S., Hsieh, C. Y., and Lin, J. K. 1997. Stability of curcumin in buffer solutions and characterization of its degradation products. *Journal of Pharmaceutical and Biomedical Analysis* 15(12):1867–1876.

Wang, Z. H., Wang, Z. Y., Sun, C. S., Wang, C. Y., Jiang, T. Y., and Wang, S. L. 2010. Trimethylated chitosan-conjugated PLGA nanoparticles for the delivery of drugs to the brain. *Biomaterials* 31(5):908–915.

Yun, X., Maximov, V. D., Yu, J., Zhu, G., Vertegel, A. A., and Kindy, M. S. 2013. Nanoparticles for targeted delivery of antioxidant enzymes to the brain after cerebral ischemia and reperfusion injury. *Journal of Cerebral Blood Flow & Metabolism* 33(4):583–592.

Zensi, A., Begley, D., Pontikis, C., Legros, C., Mihoreanu, L., Büchel, C., and Kreuter, J. 2010. Human serum albumin nanoparticles modified with apolipoprotein A-I cross the blood-brain barrier and enter the rodent brain. *Journal of Drug Targeting* 18(10):842–848.

Zensi, A., Begley, D., Pontikis, C., Legros, C., Mihoreanu, L., Wagner, S., Buechel, C., von Briesen, H., and Kreuter, J. 2009. Albumin nanoparticles targeted with Apo E enter the CNS by transcytosis and are delivered to neurones. *Journal of Controlled Release* 137(1):78–86.

13 Application of Nanomaterials in Photodynamic Therapy

Olayemi J. Fakayode, Ncediwe Tsolekile,
Sandile P. Songca, and Oluwatobi Samuel Oluwafemi

CONTENTS

13.1 INTRODUCTION

Photodynamic therapy is a noninvasive method for the treatment of cancer malaise. It involves generation of reactive oxygen species which interact with the cancer cells to a transformational point of cell death by apoptosis or necrosis (Van Driel et al. 2016). The reactive oxygen species are generated via interaction of a nontoxic light (red or near-infrared) of a suitable wavelength with a photosensitizer and molecular oxygen. The interaction of light with photosensitizer often leads to photochemical generation of excited triplet state which interacts with molecular oxygen causing outbursts of reactive oxygen species via type I and type II reactions (Chiaviello et al. 2011). The type I reactive oxygen species, namely superoxide anion $\left(O_2^-\right)$, hydrogen peroxide (H_2O_2), and hydroxyl radical ($\cdot$OH) are generated through transfer of electron to molecular oxygen and abstraction of hydrogen from nearby biomolecules while the most prominent reactive oxygen species, singlet oxygen ($^1O_2$), is generated via direct transfer of photon energy to molecular oxygen (Chiaviello 2011; Ormond and Freeman 2013; Scheme 13.1).

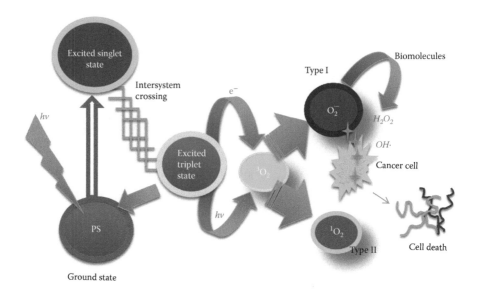

SCHEME 13.1 The mechanism of photodynamic therapy. PS = Photosensitizer; $^3O_2$ = molecular oxygen; $^1O_2$ = singlet oxygen; O_2^- = superoxide anion; $\cdot OH$= hydroxyl radical; H_2O_2 = hydrogen peroxide.

The apoptosis cell death pathway has been described as a naturally controlled energy-dependent programmed cell death (Allison and Moghissi 2013) associated with mitochondrion shut down. It involves release of cytochrome c from the mitochondrion leading to formation of apoptosome complex which triggers caspase's activation (Chiaviello et al. 2011) and subsequently a cascade of complex events that eventually cause induction of cell death (Elmore 2007).

The decrease in mitochondrion activities often leads to reduction in ATP production causing interruption of many cellular activities and subsequently disordered events which trigger natural regulatory cell deaths. For example, it has been shown that apoptosis is associated with decrease in the activities of the ATP-dependent ion (Na^+/K^+; Ca^{2+}) channel regulatory pumps leading to increase in the intracellular accumulation of these ions (Dogra et al. 2016). On the other hand, necrosis is a non-controlled cell death pathway that often occurs when the conditions that prompt apoptosis are extensive or extremely harsh (Elmore 2007); for example, a high light or photosensitizer dose, extreme heat, and intracellular accumulation of Ca^{2+} ions (Dogra et al. 2016). Also, necrosis has been reported to be associated with direct shut down of tumor vasculature (Van Driel et al. 2016).

The clinical procedure for photodynamic therapy involves time-controlled topical or intravenous administration of the photosensitizer (for superficial or deep-seated application respectively), followed by irradiation of the target site with light (Allison and Moghissi 2013) and monitoring of the reduction in tumor size with time. For topical administration, the irradiation can be immediate or a few minutes after administration, whereas intravenous routing requires some time for it to get to target site before irradiation, usually 24 hours or less depending on the nature of the photosensitizer and the site where the photodynamic therapeutic action is required. Furthermore, for intravenous administration, it is essential that the photosensitizer is nontoxic or exhibits insignificant toxicity in the absence of light (Ormond and Freeman 2013) as it travels through the body to the target site so as to avoid toxicity on normal cells.

13.2   PHOTOSENSITIZERS USED IN PHOTODYNAMIC THERAPY

13.2.1   PORPHYRIN MACROMOLECULES

Porphyrin and its derivatives such as hydroxyphenyl porphyrins and chlorins are by far the most commonly used photosensitizers in photodynamic therapy (PDT). The use of porphyrins in PDT has been in existence for many years. They are the first and oldest photosensitizers to be clinically accepted for human use. The first clinically accepted photosensitizer (PS) was photofrin which was a mixture of hematoporphyrin and derivatives (Schuitmaker et al. 1996). However, purity disintegrity, optical absorption limitation, non-directional toxicity, and prolonged photosensitivity are some of the challenges associated with this first generation PS. This has led to the development of second generation porphyrin derivatives capable of circumventing some of these challenges (Mccarthy et al. 2009). The second-generation porphyrin PS exhibit high purity, absorption of longer optical wavelength, and reduced period of photosensitivity (Schuitmaker et al. 1996). Examples of second generation porphyrin PS are meta-tetra(hydroxyphenyl)porphyrin, chlorins, and bacteriochlorins (Ormond and Freeman 2013). However, despite this huge breakthrough displayed by second-generation porphyrin PSs, non-directional light-associated toxicity still remains a challenge. This has prompted a move to develop third-generation porphyrin PS where porphyrins will be structured in such a way that they can be guided through the body to the target site without any form of interference. This is achieved by either receptor-mediated approach or magnetic targeting. The former involves joining of certain biomolecules such as carbohydrate (Mccarthy et al. 2009), antibody (Van Driel et al. 2016), peptide or protein (Hu et al. 2011) to the structure of a porphyrin in order to target the tumor site where the receptors of the attached biomolecules are overexpressed. By this, the porphyrin is safely delivered into tumor. On the other hand, magnetic targeting involves attachment of a biocompatible superparamagnetic nanomaterial to the structure of a porphyrin which aids the delivery of the porphyrin into a tumor via magnetic response to an external magnetic field (Li et al. 2013). The third generation porphyrin-PDT has more advantages than the second or first generation porphyrin-PDT. These include cost-effectiveness in terms of requirement of low-dose of PS, multifunctional characteristics via joining of different materials to porphyrin and directional specific toxicity to tumor cells.

13.2.2   NON-PORPHYRIN PHOTOSENSITIZERS

Besides porphyrin photosensitizers, there are many non-porphyrin photosensitizers such as methylene blue, hypericin, rose bengal (Ormond and Freeman 2013), and certain boronated dyes (Adarsh et al. 2010). These differ from porphyrin in structure but also have relatively unique photodynamic effects. However, the non-porphyrin photosensitizers do have one thing in common with the porphyrin PS. This is non-specific light-associated toxicity. As a result, they are currently being subjected to receptor-mediated approach and magnetic targeting strategy in order to improve their therapeutic efficiency (Zhao et al. 2014).

13.3 NANOMATERIALS IN PHOTODYNAMIC THERAPY

Nanomaterials are a specialized-class of functional materials with a dimensional size of less than or equal to 100 nm. They could be pristine or functionalized materials depending on their applications. Generally, for biomedical application, functionalized nanomaterials are used. This is due to many reasons, including the requirement to evade the body defense system (Weinstein et al. 2010), cellular penetration, water solubility (Penon et al. 2015), site localization, longer circulation half-life, and aqueous stability (Daou et al. 2009). The currently employed functionalized nanomaterials in photodynamic therapy will be briefly discussed under this section. These nanomaterials include the superparamagnetic iron oxide nanoparticles, gold nanoparticles, quantum dots, and lanthanide series nanoparticles. Their challenges and future perspective will also be discussed.

13.3.1 Superparamagnetic Iron Oxide Nanoparticles (SPIONs)

SPIONs are characterized with a core diameter usually less than 16 nm (Mürbe, Rechtenbach, and Töpfer 2008). However, functionalized SPIONs usually exhibit hydrodynamic diameters less than or equal to 300 nm (Corot et al. 2006). Biomedically, they may be classified in terms of their hydrodynamic sizes as orally administered SPIONs (300 nm; Corot et al. 2006), intravenously administered standard SPIONs (50–180 nm), ultrasmall (10–50 nm), and very small (<10 nm; Weinstein et al. 2010) and injectable SPIONs (10–180 nm; Cortajarena et al. 2014). They are excellent magnetic resonance imaging, magnetic hyperthermia, and drug delivery agents (Mouli et al. 2013).

SPIONs for biomedical applications are synthesized majorly via coprecipitation. This involves the generation of iron (II) and iron (III) oxide by heating a mixture of iron (II) and iron (III) salts (Tajabadi et al. 2013), partial reduction of iron (III) salts by a suitable reductants (Lu et al. 2010) or partial oxidation of iron (II) salts by a suitable oxidant (Shete et al. 2014) at a temperature usually below the boiling point of water in such a way that iron (II) and iron (III) ions exist at a stoichiometric ratio of 0.5 in the final oxide product. To avoid aggregation, SPIONs are usually covered with biocompatible polymers such as polyvinyl pyrrolidone (Arsalani et al. 2010), liposomes (Plassat et al. 2013), dextran (Saraswathy et al. 2014), polyethylene glycol (Silva et al. 2016), or carboxylic acid such as gluconic acid (Lu et al. 2010) or citric acid (Klein et al. 2012). The capping agent may be added during or after the synthesis.

In photodynamic therapy, due to their high surface to volume ratio, SPIONs have been successfully employed for the delivery of porphyrin (Li et al. 2013) and non-porphyrin (Zeng et al. 2013) photosensitizers into their tumor-target sites. They also have a platform where other targeting moieties such as enzymes, antibodies, carbohydrates, and peptides can be attached on their surface, making them a tool for the development of a multifunctional conjugate system (Zhao et al. 2014). Sometimes, SPIONs are covered with gold colloids (Wagstaff et al. 2012) or silica nanoparticles (Andrade et al. 2013) to passivate their surface and prevent leaching of their ions into the surrounding environment. This passivation may sometimes be required to prevent their toxicity *in vivo*.

Conjugation of SPIONs to PS in PDT may have some challenges. These may include aggregation (water-solubility issue), inefficient loading of targeting moiety or PS on SPIONs, and hydrodynamic size expansion. In order to resolve these challenges, a new synthesis and conjugation pathway may be explored. Also, encapsulation of SPIONs-PS conjugate into polymers such as polyethylene glycol may be fully maximized.

13.3.2 Gold Nanoparticles

Gold nanoparticles are specialized-plasmonic materials with variable size-dependent color characteristics. They have a long history in biomedical applications usually as drug delivery (Zhao et al. 2016) and photothermal agents (Huang and El-sayed 2011). They exhibit size-dependent tunable variant shapes such as spherical, rod, and cages (Huang and El-sayed 2011). However, for biomedical purposes, the spherical gold nanoparticles and gold nanorods are commonly employed. Moreover, gold nanorods are majorly used for photothermal application and thus will not be discussed in this chapter. The spherical gold nanoparticles are usually synthesized using sodium borohydride (Shervani and Yamamoto 2011), citrate (Verissimo et al. 2016), and carbohydrate (Pienpinijtham et al. 2011) reduction methods. However, for biomedical purposes, the citrate and carbohydrate reduction strategies are best employed due to their biocompatibility physiognomies. The citrate method involves reduction of gold precursor salt by citrate ion at boiling temperature of water (Zhao et al. 2016). In this approach, the citrate ion serves as both reducing and capping agent. On the other hand, the carbohydrate-reduction involves reduction of gold salt using reducing carbohydrates such as glucose or starch (Pienpinijtham et al. 2011), usually in an alkaline medium at a suitable temperature. Similar to the citrate approach, carbohydrate reductants also generate in situ capping agents making the approach cost-effective.

In PDT applications, spherical gold nanoparticles are usually used as passivating agent for SPIONs (Wagstaff et al. 2012) or carriers of PS (Penon et al. 2015; Meyers et al. 2015). However, aggregation of gold nanoparticles in physiological medium may be a challenge. Nonetheless, this may be prevented by optimizing the capping efficiency of the capping material on the surface of gold nanoparticles. Another challenge that may be encountered is the plasmonic effect of the spherical gold nanoparticles. Due to their plasmonic characteristics, they are capable of reducing the amount of light needed by the photosensitizers to achieve a complete therapeutic efficacy if they absorb light within the same wavelength range as the photosensitizers. Thus, it is essential to tune the surface plasmon resonance peak of the gold nanoparticles far away from the absorption wavelength peaks of the photosensitizers in order to avoid optical absorption interference which could lead to reduction in therapeutic function.

13.3.3 QUANTUM DOTS

Quantum dots are a specialized type of nanomaterials with unique quantum confinement effect characteristics (Drbohlavova et al. 2009). As a result, they exhibit exceptional optical properties (Sun et al. 2014). Quantum dots (QDs) have excellent broad light absorptions with unique narrow emissions (Zhang et al. 2014), strong photostability background (Dong et al. 2016), and large conjugable surfaces (Liang et al. 2009) for chemical attachment and tunable fluorescent properties (Oluwafemi et al. 2016; Liang et al. 2009). Thus, they are extensively employed in biological applications for biosensing (Wegner and Hildebrandt 2015), cell labeling (Chang et al. 2008), cellular imaging (Biju et al. 2010), and cancer diagnosis (Malik et al. 2013). Stereotypically, for biomedical purposes, QDs may be synthesized using a direct aqueous approach (Sun et al. 2014) via suitable reducing agent and hydrophillic capping agents or hot injection thermal decomposition of organometallic precursor (Mohan et al. 2014), followed by ligand exchange (Gao et al. 2014) via interaction with water-soluble materials which helps to solubilize them in aqueous solution.

In photodynamic therapy application, quantum dots can be employed as both diagnostic as well as therapeutic agents. Due to their unique fluorescence properties, they can be used to indicate the location of a tumor site within the body when applied alongside targeting moieties such as antibody or peptides (Lu et al. 2013). Therapeutically, QDs can be employed as fluorescence resonance energy transfer (FRET) agent to aid a nearby photosensitizer (PS) absorb light under two-photon irradiation (Fowley et al. 2012). This helps the PS to carry out its therapy efficacy at a wavelength where normally the photosensitizer does not absorb light. This helps an inherent visible light absorbing photosensitizer to function excellently well under near-infrared light irradiation without having to manipulate its structure. Nonetheless, the use of QDs in PDT may be prone to some few challenges. For example, toxicity of heavy metals such as cadmium usually employed as part of the core or shell edifice of QDs has been a long term concern. Thus, development of a new strategy which synergizes efforts to fabricate cadmium free QDs of comparable or better optical properties has become an inevitable task (Mandal et al. 2013). Also, poor loading efficiency of both cancer-targeting agents and photosensitizers on QDs is another difficulty. To this end, new tactics should be fabricated to increase the loading value of these materials on QDs.

13.3.4 LANTHANIDE SERIES NANOPARTICLES

Lanthanide series nanoparticles are specialized ultraviolet, visible or near infrared light emitting agents when irradiated with near infrared (up-conversion; Yang et al. 2015) or X-ray (down-conversion; Chen et al. 2015) light of appropriate wavelength. As a result, they are usually employed for up- or down-conversion optical applications under two-photon optical procedures. They are typically synthesized by doping lanthanide series salts in a suitable host compound (Yang et al. 2015) under microemulsion (Guo et al. 2007), reflux (Zeng et al. 2013) or thermal breakdown of a precursor salt (Wang et al. 2011) conditions, usually in the presence of a suitable organic stabilizing agents (Guo et al. 2007). However, for biomedical applications,

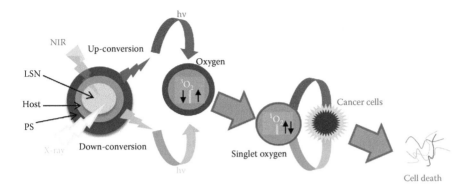

SCHEME 13.2 Up- and down- conversion "Type II-PDT" by lanthanide series nanomaterials. LSN = Lanthanide series nanomaterial; PS = photosensitizer; $^3O_2$ = molecular oxygen; $^1O_2$ = singlet oxygen.

biocompatible carbohydrate materials (Tian et al. 2013) or polymers (Zeng et al. 2013) may be employed via ligand exchange to avoid toxicity and ensure aqueous stability. The make-up of lanthanide series nanomaterials exhibits a core-shell assembly consisting of an inner lanthanide series nanoparticle embedded in host matrix core and the outer functionalized shell used for passivation of the core surface for reduction of toxicity and augmenting hydrophilicity (Scheme 13.2).

Application of lanthanide series nanomaterials in PDT probably arises as a result of ongoing exertions in circumventing the inability of some photosensitizers to treat deep-seated tumors due to their drawback in absorbing near infrared light (Yang et al. 2015). In up-conversion PDT, near infrared absorbing lanthanide series nanoparticles are excited by near infrared light of appropriate wavelength leading to an emission of visible light that is absorbable by a photosensitizer (PS). By this approach, the PS does not need to absorb within the therapeutic biological window before it can be used to treat deep-seated tumors. In contrast, the down-conversion PDT strategy involves excitation of the lanthanide series nanoparticles by a light of shorter wavelength (e.g., X-ray) than the wavelength absorbed by an inherent PS leading to an emission capable of exciting the PS (Chen et al. 2015). The use of X-ray light for PDT has been prone to debate. However, it has been argued that since X-ray is currently being employed for deep-seated body part imaging, it should be suitable for deep-seated PDT treatment (Tang et al. 2015). However, the nervousness about the safety of lanthanide series nanoparticles and toxicity associated with prolong exposure to X-ray light may limit the future acceptability of this PDT approach. Moreover, visible—visible light emitting down conversion and near-infrared—visible light emitting up-conversion PDTs will be points of attractions for improvement in many years to come.

13.4 CONCLUSION AND FUTURE PERSPECTIVES

The introduction of nanomaterials in photodynamic therapy has enabled a broad spectrum of enhancement of the treatment modality in the areas of tumor-targeting and therapeutic specificity, optical absorption improvement, treatment of deep-seated tumors, and local tumor sightings. Superparamagnetic iron oxide nanoparticles (SPIONs) are exceptional for the magnetic targeting while quantum dots (QDs), spherical gold nanoparticles, and lanthanide series nanoparticles (LS-NPs) have unique surface platforms to effect receptor-mediated tumor targeting approach. Both QDs and LS-NPs are effective agents for two-photon PDT, which is relatively more cost-effective than the conventional PDT. As the search for better involvement of nanomaterials in PDT continues, improvement of the existing nanomaterials in terms of reduction in toxicity and fabrication of new nanomaterials of better efficacies will govern many reports in many years to come.

ACKNOWLEDGMENTS

The authors thank National Research Foundation (NRF), South Africa, under the Nanotechnology Flagship Programme (grant no: 97983) for the financial support.

REFERENCES

Adarsh, N., Avirah, R. R., and Ramaiah, D. 2010. Tuning photosensitized singlet oxygen generation efficiency of novel Aza-BODIPY dyes. *Organic Letters* 12(24):5720–5723.

Allison, R. R., and Moghissi, K. 2013. Photodynamic therapy (PDT): PDT mechanisms. *Clin Endosc* 46:24–29.

Andrade, A. L., Fabris, J. D., Pereira, M. C., Domingues, R. Z., and Ardisson, J. D. 2013. Preparation of composite with silica-coated nanoparticles of iron oxide spinels for applications based on magnetically induced hyperthermia. *Hyperfine Interactions* 218(1–3):71–82.

Arsalani, N., Fattahi, H., and Nazarpoor, M. 2010. Synthesis and characterization of PVP-functionalized superparamagnetic Fe_3O_4 nanoparticles as an MRI. *eXPRESS Polymer Letters* 4(6):329–338.

Biju, V., Mundayoor, S., Omkumar, R. V., Anas, A., and Ishikawa, M. 2010. Bioconjugated quantum dots for cancer research: Present status, prospects, and remaining issues. *Biotechnology Advances* 28(2):199–213.

Chang, Y.-P., Pinaud, F., Antelman, J., and Weiss, S. 2008. Tracking bio-molecules in live cells using quantum dots. *Journal of Biophotonics* 1(4):287–298.

Chen, H., Wang, G. D., Chuang, Y. J., Zhen, Z., Chen, X., Biddinger, P., Hao, Z. et al. 2015. Nanoscintillator-mediated x-ray inducible photodynamic therapy for in vivo cancer treatment. *Nano Letters* 15(4):2249–2256.

Chiaviello, A., Postiglione, I., and Palumbo, G. 2011. Targets and mechanisms of photodynamic therapy in lung cancer cells: A brief overview. *Cancers* 3(1):1014–1141.

Corot, C., Robert, P., Idée, J. M., and Port, M. 2006. Recent advances in iron oxide nanocrystal technology for medical imaging. *Advanced Drug Delivery Reviews* 58(14):1471–1504.

Cortajarena, A. L., Ortega, D., Ocampo, S. M., Gonzalez-García, A., Couleaud, P., Miranda, R., Belda-Iniesta, C., and Ayuso-Sacido, A. 2014. Engineering iron oxide nanoparticles for clinical settings. *Nanobiomedicine* 1(2):1–20.

Daou, T. J., Bertin, A., Felder-Flesch, D., Daou, T. J., Pourroy, G., Greneche, J. M., Bertin, A., Felder-Flesch, D., and Begin-Colin, S. 2009. Water soluble dendronized iron oxide nanoparticles. *Dalton Transactions* 4442–4449.

Dogra, Y., Ferguson, D. C. J., Dodd, N. J. F., Smerdon, G. R., Curnow, A., and Winyard, P. G. 2016. The hydroxypyridinone iron chelator CP94 increases methyl-aminolevulinate-based photodynamic cell killing by increasing the generation of reactive oxygen species. *Redox Biology* 9:90–99.

Dong, H., Tang, S., Hao, Y., Yu, H., Dai, W., Zhao, G., Cao, Y., Lu, H., Zhang, X., and Ju, H. 2016. Fluorescent MoS2 quantum dots: Ultrasonic preparation, up-conversion and down-conversion bioimaging, and photodynamic therapy. *ACS Applied Materials and Interfaces* 8(5):3107–3114.

Drbohlavova, J., Adam, V., Kizek, R., and Hubalek, J. 2009. Quantum dots—Characterization, preparation and usage in biological systems. *International Journal of Molecular Science* 10:656–673.

Driel, P. B. A. A. V., Boonstra, M. C., Slooter, M. D., Heukers, R., Stammes, M. A., Snoeks, T. J. A., De Bruijn, H. S. et al. 2016. EGFR targeted nanobody-photosensitizer conjugates for photodynamic therapy in a pre-clinical model of head and neck cancer. *Journal of Controlled Release* 229:93–105.

Elmore, S. 2007. Apoptosis: A review of programmed cell death. *Toxicology Pathology* 35:495–516.

Fowley, C., Nomikou, N., McHale, A. P., McCarron, P. A., McCaughan, B., and Callan, J. F. 2012. Water soluble quantum dots as hydrophilic carriers and two-photon excited energy donors in photodynamic therapy. *Journal of Materials Chemistry* 22:6456–6462.

Gao, B., Shen, C., Yang, Y., and Yuan, S. 2014. Green synthesized CdSe quantum dots capped by 3-mercaptopropionic acid sensitized solar cells, in International Congress on Energy Efficiency and Energy Related Materials (ENEFM2013), eds. A. Y. Oral et al. *Springer Proceedings in Physics* 155:9–18.

Guo, Y., Kumar, M., and Zhang, P. 2007. Nanoparticle-based photosensitizers under CW infrared excitation. *Chemistry of Materials* 19(25):6071–6172.

Hu, Z., Rao, B., and Chen, S. 2011. Selective and effective killing of angiogenic vascular endothelial cells and cancer cells by targeting tissue factor using a factor VII-targeted photodynamic therapy for breast cancer. *Breast Cancer Research Treat* 126:589–600.

Huang, X., and El-sayed, M. A. 2011. Plasmonic photo-thermal therapy (PPTT). *Alexandria Journal of Medicine* 47(1):1–9.

Klein, S., Sommer, A., Distel, L. V. R., Neuhuber, W., and Kryschi, C. 2012. Superparamagnetic iron oxide nanoparticles as radiosensitizer via enhanced reactive oxygen species formation. *Biochemical and Biophysical Research Communications* 425(2):393–397.

Li, Z., Wang, C., Cheng, L., Gong, H., Yin, S., Gong, Q., Li, Y., and Liu, Z. 2013. PEG-functionalized iron oxide nanoclusters loaded with chlorin e6 for targeted, NIR light induced, photodynamic therapy. *Biomaterials* 34(36):9160–9170.

Liang, G.-X., Gu, M.-M., Zhang, J.-R., and Zhu, J.-J. 2009. Preparation and bioapplication of high-quality, water-soluble, biocompatible, and near-infrared-emitting CdSeTe alloyed quantum dots. *Nanotechnology* 20:415103.

Lu, W., Shen, Y., Xie, A., and Zhang, W. 2010. Green synthesis and characterization of super-paramagnetic Fe_3O_4 nanoparticles. *Journal of Magnetism and Magnetic Materials* 322(13):1828–1833.

Lu, Y., Zhong, Y., Wang, J., Su, Y., Peng, F., Zhou, Y., Jiang, X., and He, Y. 2013. Aqueous synthesized near-infrared-emitting quantum dots for RGD-based in vivo active tumour targeting. *Nanotechnology* 24:135101–135110.

Malik, P., Gulia, S., and Kakkar, R. 2013. Quantum dots for diagnosis of cancers. *Advanced Materials Letters* 4(11):811–822.

Mandal, G., Darragh, M., Wang, Y. A., and Heyes, C. D. 2013. Cadmium-free quantum dots as time-gated bioimaging in highly-autofluorescent human breast cancer cells. *Chemical Communications* 49(6):624–626.

Mccarthy, J. R., Bhaumik, J., Merbouh, N., and Weissleder, R. 2009. High-yielding syntheses of hydrophilic conjugatable chlorins and bacteriochlorins. *Organic and Biomolecular Chemistry* 7:3430–3436.

Meyers, J. D., Cheng, Y., Broome, A.-M., Agnes, R. S., Schluchter, M. D., Margevicius, S., Wang, X., Kenney, M. E., Burda, C., and Basilion, J. P. 2015. Peptide-targeted gold nanoparticles for photodynamic therapy of brain cancer. *Particle and Particle Systems Characterization* 32(4):448–457.

Mohan, S., Oluwafemi, O. S., Songca, S. P., Osibote, O. A., George, S. C., Kalarikkal, N., and Thomas, S. 2014. Facile synthesis of transparent and fluorescent epoxy–CdSe–CdS–ZnS Core–multi shell polymer nanocomposites. *New Journal of Chemistry* 38(1):155–162.

Mouli, S. K., Tyler, P., McDevitt, J. L., Eifler, A. C., Guo, Y., Nicolai, J., Lewandowski, R. J. et al. 2013. Image-guided local delivery strategies enhance therapeutic nanoparticle uptake in solid tumors. *ACS Nano* 7(9):7724–7733.

Mürbe, J., Rechtenbach, A., and Töpfer, J. 2008. Synthesis and physical characterization of magnetite nanoparticles for biomedical applications. *Materials Chemistry and Physics* 110(2–3):426–433.

Oluwafemi, O. S., Mohan, S., Olubomehin, O., Osibote, O. A., and Songca, S. P. 2016. Size tunable synthesis of HDA and TOPO capped ZnSe nanoparticles via a facile aqueous/thermolysis hybrid solution route. *Journal of Materials Science: Materials in Electronics* 27(4):3880–3887.

Ormond, A. B., and Freeman, H. S. 2013. Dye sensitizers for photodynamic therapy. *Materials* 6:817–840.

Penon, O., Patiço, T., Barrios, L., Noguøs, C., Amabilino, D. B., Wurst, K., and Perez-Garcia, L. 2015. A new porphyrin for the preparation of functionalized water-soluble gold nanoparticles with low intrinsic toxicity. *Chemistry Open* 4:127–136.

Pienpinijtham, P., Han, X. X., Ekgasit, S., and Ozaki, Y. 2011. Highly sensitive and selective determination of iodide and thiocyanate concentrations using surface-enhanced Raman scattering of starch-reduced gold nanoparticles. *Analytical Chemistry* 83:3655–3662.

Plassat, V., Renoir, J.-M., Autret, G., Marsaud, V., Ménager, C., Clément, O., and Lesieur, S. 2013. Systemic magnetic targeting of pure-antiestrogen-loaded superparamagnetic nanovesicles for effective therapy of hormone-dependent breast cancers. *Journal of Bioanalysis & Biomedicine* 05(02):28–35.

Saraswathy, A., Nazeer, S. S., Nimi, N., Arumugam, S., Shenoy, S. J., and Jayasree, R. S. 2014. Synthesis and characterization of dextran stabilized superparamagnetic iron oxide nanoparticles for in vivo MR imaging of liver fibrosis. *Carbohydrate Polymers* 101:760–768.

Schuitmaker, J. J., Baas, P., van Leengoed, H. L., van der Meulen, F. W., Star, W. M., and van Zandwijk, N. 1996. Photodynamic therapy: A promising new modality for the treatment of cancer. *Journal of Photochemistry and Photobiology. B, Biology* 34(1):3–12.

Shervani, Z., and Yamamoto, Y. 2011. Carbohydrate-directed synthesis of silver and gold nanoparticles: Effect of the structure of carbohydrates and reducing agents on the size and morphology of the composites. *Carbohydrate Research* 346(5):651–658.

Shete, P. B., Patil, R. M., Thorat, N. D., Prasad, A., Ningthoujam, R.S., Ghosh, S.J., and Pawar, S.H. 2014. Magnetic chitosan nanocomposite for hyperthermia therapy application: Preparation, characterization and in vitro experiments. *Applied Surface Science* 288:149–157.

Silva, A. H., Lima, E., Vasquez Mansilla, M., Zysler, R. D., Troiani, H., Mojica Pisciotti, M. L., Locatelli, C. et al. 2016. Superparamagnetic iron-oxide nanoparticles mPEG350- and mPEG2000-coated: Cell uptake and biocompatibility evaluation. *Nanomedicine: Nanotechnology, Biology, and Medicine* 12(4):909–919.

Sun, X., Dai, R., Chen, J., Zhou, W., Wang, T., Kost, A. R., Tsung, C.-K. F., and An, Z. 2014. Enhanced thermal stability of oleic-acid-capped PbS quantum dot optical fiber amplifier. *Optics Express* 22(1):519–524.

Tajabadi, M., Khosroshahi, M. E., and Bonakdar, S. 2013. An efficient method of SPION synthesis coated with third generation PAMAM dendrimer. *Colloids and Surfaces A: Physicochemical and Engineering Aspects* 431:18–26.

Tang, Y., Hu, J., Elmenoufy, A. H., and Yang, X. 2015. Highly efficient FRET system capable of deep photodynamic therapy established on x-ray excited mesoporous LaF3:Tb scintillating nanoparticles. *ACS Applied Materials and Interfaces* 7(22):12261–12269.

Tian, G., Ren, W., Yan, L., Jian, S., Gu, Z., Zhou, L., Jin, S., Yin, W., Li, S., and Zhao, Y. 2013. Red-emitting upconverting nanoparticles for photodynamic therapy in cancer cells under near-infrared excitation. *Small (Weinheim an Der Bergstrasse, Germany)* 9(11):1928–1938.

Verissimo, T. V., Santos, N. T., Silva, J. R., Azevedo, R. B., Gomes, A. J., and Lunardi, C. N. 2016. In vitro cytotoxicity and phototoxicity of surface-modi Fi Ed gold nanoparticles associated with neutral red as a potential drug delivery system in phototherapy. *Materials Science & Engineering C* 65:199–204.

Wagstaff, A. J., Brown, S. D., Holden, M. R., Craig, G. E., Plumb, J. A., Brown, R. E., Schreiter, N., Chrzanowski, W., and Wheate, N. J. 2012. Cisplatin drug delivery using gold-coated iron oxide nanoparticles for enhanced tumour targeting with external magnetic fields. *Inorganica Chimica Acta* 393:328–333.

Wang, C., Tao, H., Cheng, L., and Liu, Z. 2011. Near-infrared light induced in vivo photodynamic therapy of cancer based on upconversion nanoparticles. *Biomaterials* 32(26): 6145–6154.

Wegner, K. D., and Hildebrandt, N. 2015. Quantum dots: Bright and versatile in vitro and in vivo fluorescence imaging biosensors. *Chemical Society Reviews* 44(14):4792–4834.

Weinstein, J. S., Varallyay, C. G., Dosa, E., Gahramanov, S., Hamilton, B., Rooney, W. D., Muldoon, L. L., and Neuwelt, E. A. 2010. Superparamagnetic iron oxide nanoparticles: Diagnostic magnetic resonance imaging and potential therapeutic applications in neurooncology and central nervous system inflammatory pathologies, a review. *Journal of Cerebral Blood Flow and Metabolism: Official Journal of the International Society of Cerebral Blood Flow and Metabolism* 30(1):15–35.

Yang, G., Yang, D., Yang, P., Lv, R., Li, C., Zhong, C., He, F., Gai, S., and Lin, J. 2015. A single 808 nm near-infrared light-mediated multiple imaging and photodynamic therapy based on titania coupled upconversion nanoparticles. *Chemistry of Materials* 27(23):7957–7968.

Zeng, L., Xiang, L., Ren, W., Zheng, J., Li, T., Chen, B., Zhang, J., Mao, C., Li, A., and Wu, A. 2013. Multifunctional photosensitizer-conjugated core-shell $Fe_3O_4@NaYF_4:Yb/Er$ nanocomplexes and their applications in T2-weighted magnetic resonance/upconversion luminescence imaging and photodynamic therapy of cancer cells. *RSC Advances* 3(33): 13915–13925.

Zhang, L., Zhang, Y., Kershaw, S. V., Zhao, Y., Wang, Y., Jiang, Y., Zhang, T. et al. 2014. Colloidal PbSe quantum dot-solution-filled liquid-core optical fiber for 1.55 μM telecommunication wavelengths. *Nanotechnology* 25:105704–105711.

Zhao, L., Kim, T.-H., Kim, H.-W., Ahn, J.-C., and Yeon, S. 2016. Enhanced cellular uptake and phototoxicity of verteporem Fi N-conjugated gold nanoparticles as theranostic nanocarriers for targeted photodynamic therapy and imaging of cancers. *Materials Science & Engineering C* 67:611–622.

Zhao, X., Chen, Z., Zhao, H., Zhang, D., Tao, L., and Lan, M. 2014. Multifunctional magnetic nanoparticles for simultaneous cancer near-infrared imaging and targeting photodynamic therapy. *RSC Advances* 4:62153–62159.

14 Nanomedicine
A Complex Interplay between Patients, Science, and Society

Jean-Claude André, Jonathan Simon,
and Bertrand Henri Rihn

CONTENTS

Nanotechnology applied to medicine or nanomedicine is a field that has been growing rapidly over recent years as can be seen in Figure 14.1. A search of the library resources of the University of Lorraine identified more than 50,000 articles classified as "nanomedicine," with a constant rise in the number of publications in this area since the beginning of the twenty-first century. The articles featured in the present volume provide a much-needed synthesis and a helpful analysis of this emerging field, which has yet to assume its definitive form.

Nevertheless, a closely related area, the NBIC (Nano Biology, Information technology, and Cognitive sciences) convergence has already elicited warnings over questions of ethics and responsibility. Researchers in ethics and risk have alerted the public, focusing on projected developments that they believe might be put on the market in the near future (André 2016). There are two lessons to be drawn from these alerts. First, that nanotechnology is an area that arouses suspicion and fear among the public, and second, that it is difficult, if not impossible, to predict future directions of research and development with precision. Like other areas of scientific research, the nanosciences have proved resistant to planned projects.

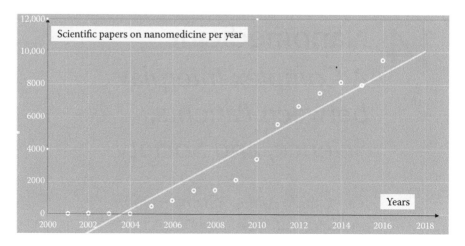

FIGURE 14.1   Number of publications in nanomedicine against time.

14.1   FROM NANOTECHNOLOGY TO PERSONALIZED MEDICINE

The recent term *personalized medicine* covers a wide program that, over the last fifteen years or so, has mobilized actors throughout the medical sector around the common goal of improving the diagnosis and treatment of patients (whether sick or, in the case of preventative treatment, healthy) using new technologies oriented towards molecular analysis such as genome sequencing, high-volume screening of biomolecules, or computer modeling. This program initially crystallized around the human genome project in the 1990s, based on the medical potential of drawing up an exhaustive map of individual nucleotide polymorphisms and correlating these genetic variations with the probable response to specific treatments. At the same time, this genetic information was used to develop early detection of disease and to improve the accuracy of prognosis in the context of multifactorial disease (Guchet and André 2017).

Nanotechnology has since contributed to a range of associated domains classified under the heading of personalized medicine, including high-volume sequencing, new diagnostic techniques involving the analysis of biomolecules, and targeted therapies and techniques for drug-delivery, as is illustrated by the chapters collected in the present volume. Indeed, convergence between personalized medicine and nanomedicine (NM) has become one of the explicit political objectives of health and technology policy, as we can see in the vision paper published by the European Technology Platform on Nanomedicine in 2005, where they present three priority domains—diagnostics, drug delivery, and regenerative medicine—under the global heading of personalized medicine (European Technology Platform on Nano-Medicine 2005). In this context, NM is seen as a transversal research field that promises to revolutionize healthcare (Noury and Lafontaine 2014), with some seeing it as the means to arrive at making human enhancement a reality (Roco and Bainbridge 2002).

The therapeutic payoffs predicted at the beginning of this movement have not, however, yet been realized in terms of clinical applications. While the applications in pharmacogenetics—for example, the correlation between genes and response to specific anticancer drugs—have undeniably progressed, the domains of predictive biomarkers or other early diagnostic techniques remain limited when compared with the ambitious promises that were made at the outset. What has become clear over this period is the inadequacy of an approach based exclusively on the genome. A more global perspective is called for, combining different levels of the life process, for example, integrating information on the epigenome, transcriptome, proteome, or interactome. Today, researchers are turning more and more to systemic or integrative approaches to these problems.

Furthermore, the development of personalized medicine has rapidly run up against difficulties that stem precisely from the ambiguity of this concept (Guchet 2016). Does personalized medicine simply mean identifying and characterizing molecular targets for diagnosis and treatment, or does it mean placing the patient at the center of the healthcare system? In order to avoid any misunderstanding, some have suggested replacing the term personalized medicine with individual medicine or precision medicine to cover the approaches based on genetic profiling, thereby reducing the risk of confusion with the various forms of the patient-centered medicine movement.

These developments around personalized medicine have their parallels in NM, which also finds itself confronted with scientific and technological problems as well as economic and ethical ones. From the scientific point of view, as with genetic profiling, NM will have to take the complexity of the living organism into account as well as dealing with problems of pharmacokinetics and evaluating the specificity and long-term efficacy of targeted therapies (pharmacodynamics). Economic problems already include high production costs in general as well as the elevated costs of diagnostic tools and targeted treatment. On the side of ethics, one can ask whether NM is a form of human-centered medicine, with the patient taken into account as a human being rather than being considered just another element in a techno–scientific system. Thus, despite its enormous potential, NM still faces significant obstacles on its way to any significant clinical applications in human subjects.

14.1.1 THE SCIENCE OF NANOMEDICINE

Approaching human health from the perspective of complexity signals a break with a long tradition in medical science, and requires acknowledging the exceptional and problematic nature of living organisms. Two features of this approach via complexity are an increased level of incertitude and a greater reliance on heuristic strategies when dealing with "complex" problems concerning the health of a single individual (and not a population). This means paying more attention to qualitative and even the emotive aspects of the situation, as well as relying on a heuristic orientation rather than limiting considerations to quantifiable parameters. Working on the nanoscale potentially allows the researcher to penetrate to the very material core of any physical situation, opening up unlimited therapeutic horizons through the possibility of specific combinations between atoms, molecules, neurons, and genes. Nevertheless, the vertiginous narratives associated with the NBIC convergence need to be treated with caution, and rendering explicit the implicit assumptions that lie behind them has

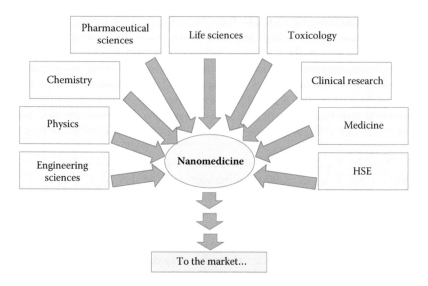

FIGURE 14.2 The interdisciplinary nature of nanomedicine. HSE: Hygiene, Safety, Environment.

become an important task. These assumptions include a particular vision of power that is both concentrated in few hands and based on secrecy, as well as a certain posture with respect to the natural world as a domain to be reconstructed, which is in turn based on a vision of nature itself as imperfect. Leaders in this area tend to have a rather narrow vision of what counts as appropriate knowledge (usually reduced to engineering), and a limited vision of the human subject (considered as cybernetic and connected), preconceptions with significant ethical and even political consequences. Last but not least, the NBIC convergence implies a transformation of the conceptual categories of human, animal, and artifact (Guchet and André 2017; André 2017).

If we consider the disciplinary configuration of NM as represented in Figure 14.2, we can see that it is a frontier-object lying at the intersection of a large number of disciplines, providing a focus for an interdisciplinary collaboration aimed at achieving certain concrete goals. Many supporters of NM hope to impose mathematical rigor in the field, confident in the belief that precise experimentation can establish a new conceptual doctrine at the interface of technology, science, and medicine (LEEM 2014). Achieving this goal clearly will not be easy, particularly in light of the interdisciplinary nature of the field. In order to reinforce cooperation across disciplines, the different partners need to agree on a common language that they can then use to explore promising leads, but without any guarantee of particular concrete results. In any case, researchers will have to manage the slippage between the projected goals and the projects that will effectively be put into place.

14.1.2 FROM THE PATIENT'S PERSPECTIVE

As the chapters of this book make clear, and despite the difficulties related to its interdisciplinary nature, NM is making real scientific progress, particularly in terms of proof of concept. It is now no longer possible to reduce the whole NM system to its constitutive elements, and researchers are increasingly adopting more global (albeit reductive) approaches. Such engineering-inspired analyses suffer from the shortcomings of a paradigm in which the engineer seeks to identify the determinant parameters as the gateway to an effective solution. The predictions of a system's utility are based on an underlying model of "technological solutions" that underpins the push to constantly develop new technologies that will, as they have in the past, resolve the consumers' problems and effectively respond to their needs. Thus, from this perspective, the faults of any technological system can only be resolved by an innovative technological solution.

From the perspective of their individual disciplines and with their inherent conservatism, researchers tend to be cautious about such global views. Their objections are based on their specialist knowledge, including the use of specific instruments, particular evaluation methods, among other considerations. This kind of tension poses the questions of the financing of interdisciplinary projects and the integration of appropriate research teams, with individual researchers always under pressure to remain within their discipline for reasons of peer-recognition and credibility in the eyes of the wider community. This issue of disciplinary identity is also reflected in the problems of evaluation, in particular publication, with peer-review always favoring disciplinary specialization (Vianin 2016). In general, work on theoretical or conceptual problems in interdisciplinary fields receives little credit, either in terms of financing projects or in terms of advancing one's career.

The introduction of New Public Management policies into the world of science means that money for research is now largely procured through competition for limited funding (Bruno 2008) a context in which interdisciplinary projects are usually at a disadvantage. Research around interdisciplinary questions and convergence requires more time for reflection and construction, not to mention additional research staff, trends that fit poorly with the current austerity of national and European funding agencies. The favored mechanisms of competition for funding can also result in negative outcomes, favoring research in areas that guarantee more deliverables in a shorter time frame and in general work in the most fashionable domains, as well as possibly inciting less rigorous publishing practices.

After having determined appropriate conditions for the evaluation and treatment of patients (theranostics), the introduction of nanotechnologies into the healthcare field calls for a significant degree of implication on the part of the human sciences. The issue of individual health cannot be treated without taking into account the much wider question of the desirability of these technologies, which is an ethical rather than a technical problem. Opening the reflection to cover real-world concerns also raises issues in the Hygiene Safety Environment domain (protection of healthcare staff, citizens, and the environment), as well as demanding cost–benefit and "quality-by-design" studies to guarantee the quality of the NM pharmaceutical products that eventually come to market. It is essential therefore to encourage initiatives to mediate between research and application, despite the difficulty and unglamorous nature of this work. As with other drugs, NM products will require preclinical and clinical trials as well as the development of new industrial production processes, time-consuming steps that will lead to long unproductive periods before the realization of any clinical applications. One can ask whether investors will be prepared to accept the risks and extended time frame associated with all these steps.

14.2 CONVERGENCE

The phrase *convergent technologies* suggests the integration of a variety of independently developed components and concepts into a single technological system. There are numerous examples of how the cross-fertilization of convergent technologies leads to innovation (e.g., the multiple uses of the Global Positioning System). In the case of NBIC, the interdisciplinary convergence would be between microelectronics, bioinformatics, nanotechnologies, and cognitive science. The technology is being pushed toward the frontiers of scientific knowledge, even while it remains quite speculative, by powerful commercial and political interests. The essential idea of convergence is to extract diverse elements from different disciplinary fields to bring them together in industrial applications, thereby forcing a juncture between scientific, economic, and social actors in the interests of technological innovation.

According to Roco and Bainbridge, the reflections of the National Nanotechnology Initiative (2001, 2002, 2013) aim to establish an ethical vision of the methods deployed to integrate knowledge in favour of groups or individuals, and are particularly concerned with human relations—humans and systems—and the environment. The solution envisaged by these authors is a holistic (integrated or interdisciplinary) approach. In the present state of affairs, researchers have already realized passive and active nanostructures as well as some molecular nanosystems, which, while admittedly complex and impressive achievements, do not represent very high levels of systemic integration. Nevertheless, commentators have already identified possible blockages that need to be dealt with in order to facilitate further innovation and integration, pointing out, for example, the need for a common language shared by researchers across different disciplines (Jeonga and Lee 2015). Appropriate forms of organization capable of coping with a new "holistic" approach cannot, Roco and Bainbridge (2013) argue, be expected to be put in place before 2020.

14.3 NBIC, INTERDISCIPLINARITY, AND CONVERGENCE

As a general rule, and despite the attendant problems of communication and cooperation, interdisciplinary collaborations are expected to bring benefits proportional to the distance that separates the disciplines concerned, and this is what has been observed for the collaborations that have already taken place across different components of NBIC (Llerena and Meyer-Krahmer 2003). These authors conclude that R&D projects will only be undertaken if the expected benefit is superior to the estimated costs, explaining in part the rarity of such projects. Other researchers have shown how the interdisciplinary aspects of research in the nanohubs has been hindered by the scientific knowledge specific to each discipline, as well as by discipline-specific apparatus and practices (Porter and Youtie 2009; Battard 2012). Thus, cross-fertilization usually only takes place between disciplines on a pairwise basis (Jeonga and Lee 2015), far from the ideal of the NBIC convergence, although this has not hampered the development of the field (Jeong et al. 2015).

TABLE 14.1
Contribution of the Different Areas N, B, I, C to Ongoing Scientific and Technological Projects

NBIC—Areas	N	B	I	C	Other Domains
Neuronal enhancement			+	+	
Nanomedicine					
• Diagnostics	+	+			Instrumentation
• Therapy	+	+			Medicine
• Tissue engineering		+			Engineering
• Nano motors/nano-robots	+				Robotics
Man–machine communication; artificial intelligence			+	+	Human sciences
Language recognition			+	+	Human sciences
Nano-sensors	+		+		Medicine, automata, Internet of Things
Nanoelectronics	+				Electronics
Microfluidics	+				Process engineering, fluid mechanics
Protection of privacy	+ ?		+		Big Data

Several reports have analysed the products or systems derived from NBIC concepts. Table 14.1 has been drawn up using several such publications (e.g., Beckert et al. 2007; Lymberis 2010; Van Est et al. 2014) and allows us to see the weak interpenetration between the different disciplines. The reality is that the NBIC convergence is today far from realizing either the ambitious predictions that have been made for it or the fears associated with this convergence, as, for the time being at least, there are almost no projects in which all four areas interact simultaneously.

Curbatov and Louyot-Gallicher (2016) wrote that "The interactions between these different disciplinary forms of scientific knowledge are not, however, legion [...]." Indeed, the NBIC convergence serves what we call *performativity*, a tool needed to mobilize resources and minds, to mobilize, to formulate objectives, to define research priorities, to alert the public and politicians, and so on. The number of publications in the human and social sciences on the subject of "convergence" is much higher than the number of publications dealing with any concrete achievements in convergence across NBIC. Van Est and Stemerding (2014) have proposed an explanation of this phenomenon, suggesting that a NBIC convergence means that biology becomes technology, rendering everything quantitative, and thereby introducing ethical and political problems into society.

14.4 NM CONVERGENCE

As we have just explained, the NBIC convergence has not yet led to any projects actually being put into place across all four domains, although this has not prevented a considerable number of publications by philosophers and sociologists on the subject, underlining the difficulty of mounting collaborations between researchers from four distinct disciplines, each with their own paradigms, and different temporalities for their research. NM is, therefore, still at the beginning of its interdisciplinary development, and it is doubtless thanks to a greater degree of integration that it will succeed in delivering more socially significant applications (cf. Figure 14.2).

The fact that NBIC has yet to achieve full maturity leaves plenty of room for philosophers and other social scientists, as well as researchers in the so-called "exact" sciences to contribute to shaping the field, although it will be hard to avoid hierarchies being put into place. Such hierarchies will undoubtedly be both in terms of disciplines and in terms of targets. We can already note that much of the research investment, as is the case for other domains of healthcare, is being directed towards oncology. Nevertheless, the overall goal of NM is the massive application of biomedical science and technology to help the sick and also their healthy peers. While no one is opposed to this overall goal, many ask whether it obscures more questionable objectives. Will the development of NM usher in an era of even more impersonalised medicine, a domain governed by nanoelectronic sensors, diagnostic programs, statistical algorithms, wiring humans into the ever-growing Internet of Things (IoT)? There seems to be a real risk that the patient will fade out of the picture altogether, lost behind the driving force of the industrial interests that are at stake through such things as new apparatus and software or new models for insurance. Finally, what place will the health authorities occupy in tomorrow's NM (André 2017a)?

14.5 CONCLUSION

It is rare to witness a new scientific and technological field like NM being put into place, but the excitement of the commentators is also necessarily mitigated by fears about the consequences of the unchecked development of technological applications in the field. The present collected volume seeks to give an overview of current directions of research in this rapidly growing field, thereby not only providing important elements for understanding these current areas of interest but also providing a basis for thinking about how best to manage and integrate this new domain from the wider perspective of the state and society. It is tempting to let one's imagination run wild and project a futuristic world repaired or destroyed by freely replicating "nanobots," but it is just as easy to be cynical and dismissive and to observe that not much has been realized in terms of any concrete applications across the NBIC convergence. We encourage the reader to adopt an intermediary approach, trying to understand the current trends in NM as well as distinguishing between fact and fiction in the NBIC convergence. We need also to recognize that while the NBIC convergence is only at its beginning, its inevitable growth will transform significant aspects of our lives. Thus, while it seems unrealistic to control or predict the development in this field in any detail, it remains important to insist on making realistic demands concerning its deployment in society. This global reflection can have a positive effect in advancing this convergence by consciously working to overcome both institutional and professional resistance to the application of interdisciplinary work. This same reflection can also allow us to predict ethical or social problems linked to the rollout of NM technologies in the future, giving the possibility to make democratic decisions concerning these applications rather than just letting the industries involved dictate their development and use. The successful introduction of NM will ultimately depend on a wider engagement with the issues on the part of the patients and the public in general, requiring a level of information and reflection on these issues that is far from being in place today. We hope that the present volume will contribute positively to this engagement with NM.

REFERENCES

André, J. C. 2016. Santé connectée. *Environ Risque Santé* 15:380–385.

André, J.C. 2017. *Convergence NBIC : Risques et conditions de possibilité au regard d'autres risques silencieux. Environ Risques Santé* 16:178–1091.

Battard, N. 2012. Convergence and multi-disciplinarity in nanotechnology: Laboratories as technological hubs. *Technovation* 32:234–244.

Beckert, B., Blümel, C., and Friedewald, M. 2007. Visions and realities in converging technologies. Innovation. *Eur J Soc Sci* 20:375–394.

Bruno, I. 2008. *A Vos Marques, Prêts... Cherchez ! La Stratégie Européenne de Lisbonne, Vers un Marché de la Recherche.* Paris: Éditions du Croquant, Coll. Savoir/Agir, ISBN:9782914968379.

Curbatov, O., and Louyot-Gallicher, M. 2016. Convergence NBIC et knowledge marketing: Champs expérimentaux d'applications; exemple du domaine biomédical. Venice: International Marketing Trends Conference.

European Technology Platform on NanoMedicine. 2005. Nanotechnology for Health. Luxembourg: Office for Official Publications of the European Communities.

Guchet, X. 2016. *La Médecine personnalisée. Un essai philosophique.* Paris: Les Belles Lettres Edition, ISBN:9782251430379.

Guchet, X., and André, J. C. 2017, in press. Nano-médecine translationnelle (French). Observatory for Micro & NanoTechnologies.

Jeong, S., Kim, J. C., and Choi, J. Y. 2015. Technology convergence: What developmental stage are we in? *Scientometrics* 104:841–871.

Jeonga, S., and Lee, S. 2015. What drives technology convergence? Exploring the influence of technological and resource allocation contexts. *J Eng Technol Manage* 36:78–96.

Lymberis, A. 2010. Micro-nano-biosystems: An overview of European research. *Minimally Invasive Ther* 19:136–143.

LEEM. 2014. Applications des nanotechnologies à la médecine. Accessed from http://www.leem.org/applications-des-nanotechnologies-medecine.

Llerena, P., and Meyer-Krahmer, F. 2003. Interdisciplinary research and the organization of the university: General challenges and a case study, in *Science and Innovation: Rethinking the Rationales for Funding and Governance*, eds. A. Geuna, J. A. Salter, and W. Steinmueller, pp. 69–88. Cheltenham, UK: Edward Elgar Ed. ISBN:9781843761099.

Noury, M., and Lafontaine, C. 2014. De la nano-médecine à la nano-santé: Vers un nouveau paradigme biomédical. *Soc-Anthropol* 29:13–35. Accessed from https://socio-anthropologie.revues.org/1635.

Porter, A. L., and Youtie, J. 2009. How interdisciplinary is nanotechnology? *J Nanopart Res*, 11:1023–1041.

Roco, M. C., and Bainbridge, W. S. 2013. The new world of discovery, invention, and innovation: Convergence of knowledge, technology, and society. *J Nanopart Res* 15:1946. doi: 10.1007/s11051-013-1946-1.

Roco, M. C., and Bainbridge W. S. 2002. Converging technologies for improving human performance: Integrating from the nanoscale. *J Nanopart Res* 4:281–295.

Roco, M. C., and Bainbridge, W. S. (Eds). 2001. Societal implications of nanoscience and nanotechnology. Dordrecht: Springer Ed. Accessed from http://www.wtec.org/loyola /nano/NSET.Societal.Implications.

Van Est, R., Stemerding, D., Rerimassie, V., Schuijff, M., Timmer, J., and Brom, F. 2014. De BIO à la convergence NBIC; de la pratique médicale à la vie quotidienne. Report for the Council of Europe prepared by the Bioethics committee of the Rathenau Institute. Institut Rathenau, La Haye, Pays-Bas.

Vianin, A. 2016. Quand l'interdisciplinarité naît de la croisée des regards. L'Interdisciplinaire. Accessed from http://www.ihqeds.ulaval.ca/fileadmin/fichiers/fichiersIHQEDS/Public ations/LintErDiSciplinaire/IHQEDS_Journal_No10_lres.pdf.

Index

A

AAS, *see* Atomic absorption spectroscopy (AAS)
Abelect®, 54
Abraxane®, 54
Absorption, distribution, metabolism, and
        excretion (ADME) data, 107
AD, *see* Alzheimer's disease (AD)
AFM, *see* Atomic force microscopy (AFM)
Airborne substances, in vitro exposure systems to
        assess toxicity of, 209–222
    advantages of in vitro testing using cells from
        the respiratory tract, 210
    automated exposure system, 213–215
    background, 209
    deposition enhancement by electrical field,
        216–217
    dose monitoring, 215–216
    examples, 219
    manual exposure systems, 212–213
    sampling ports for particle analyzers, 217–218
    submerged exposure conditions versus ALI
        exposure, 210–212
Air–liquid interface (ALI) exposure, 210–212,
        218
Alzheimer's disease (AD), 68, 277
AmBisome®, 54
Anticancer drugs, 9, 54, 315
Antioxidants, delivery of, *see* Brain, delivery of
        antioxidants in
Apolipoprotein E (ApoE), 282
Apolipoprotein J (ApoJ), 282
Asialoglycoprotein receptor (ASGP-R), 259–260
Atomic absorption spectroscopy (AAS), 26
Atomic force microscopy (AFM), 25, 39, 102
AuNPs, *see* Gold (Au) nanoparticles
AuroShell® particles, 60
Autoimmune diseases, 70–71
Autophagy, NPs and, 136–143
    autophagy activation by NPs, 136–138
    autophagy blockade by NPs, 138–139
    lysosome membrane permeabilization, 139
    mechanisms of autophagy and lysosomal
        dysfunction induced by
Axitinib, 67

B

Bafilomycin A1, 139
Bimodal nanoparticles, 82–83
Biological characterization, 105–107

Blood–brain barrier (BBB), 54, 177; *see also*
        Brain, delivery of antioxidants in
Brain, delivery of antioxidants in, 277–300
    blood–brain barrier, properties of, 279
    first generation nanoparticle system, 281–284
    fourth generation (stimuli-responsive
        nanoparticles), 292–293
    general aspects of nanoparticles, 280
    polymer and nanoparticle preparation, 281
    second generation nanoparticle system,
        284–287
    targeting the blood–brain barrier, 288–292
    targeting neuronal cells, 287–288
    third generation nanoparticle system,
        287–292

C

CAGR, *see* Compound annual growth rate (CAGR)
Cancer
    cell uptake, intracellular trafficking and,
        247–261
    nanoparticle use in, 67–68
    therapeutics, see Transbarrier trafficking of
        nanoparticles
Carbon nanotubes (CNTs), 64
Cardiovascular diseases (CVD), 73–74
Characterization of nanoparticles, *see* Dispersion
        and characterization of nanoparticles
Clariscan®, 61
Clinical and preclinical use (nanomedicine),
        53–96
    active and passive targeting, 67
    autoimmune diseases, 70–71
    bi- and multimodal nanoparticles, 82–83
    biodegradable polymeric particles, 57
    cancer, nanoparticle use in, 67–68
    carbon nanocarriers, 63–64
    cardiovascular diseases, 73–74
    dendrimers, 64–66
    emulsification–diffusion, 57
    emulsion–solvent extraction, 57
    global nanomedicine market, 55
    inorganic nanoparticles, 58–62
    lipid-based nanoparticles, 55
    magnetic hyperthermia, 61
    magnetic nanoparticles, 79–80
    metabolic disorders, 71–73
    metal and metal oxides nanoparticles, 58–62
    micro- and nanoparticulate delivery systems,
        55–66

323